Vaccination Programmes

Vaccination programmes are of vital importance to public health and are present in virtually every country in the world. By promoting an understanding of the diverse effects of vaccination programmes, this textbook discusses how epidemiologic methods can be used to study, in real life, their impacts, benefits and risks.

Written by expert practitioners in an accessible and concise style, this book is interspersed with practical examples that allow readers to acquire understanding through real-life data and problems. Part I provides an overview of basic concepts in vaccinology, immunology, vaccination programmes, infectious disease transmission dynamics, the various impacts of vaccination programmes and their societal context. Part II covers the main field tools used for the epidemiological evaluation of vaccination programmes: monitoring coverage and attitudes towards vaccination, surveillance of vaccine-preventable diseases and pathogens, seroepidemiological studies, methods to assess impact and outbreak investigation. Part III is dedicated to vaccine effectiveness and its assessment. Part IV includes an overview of the potential risks of vaccination and how to study these. Lastly, Part V deals with methods for an integrated assessment of benefits and risks of vaccination programmes. Suitable for professionals working in public health, epidemiology, biology and those working in health economics and vaccine development, *Vaccination Programmes* also serves as a textbook for postgraduate students in public health, epidemiology and infectious diseases.

The book is aimed at all those involved in the many aspects of vaccination programmes, including public health professionals and epidemiologists. Its primary target audiences are master and doctoral students in infectious disease epidemiology and public health, post-doctoral participants of field epidemiology training programmes and public health professionals working in the post-implementation epidemiological evaluation of vaccines and vaccination programmes.

Susan Hahné is a senior epidemiologist in the National Immunisation Programme Department at the Centre for Epidemiology and Surveillance of Infectious Diseases of the National Institute for Public Health and the Environment (RIVM) in the Netherlands.

Kaatje Bollaerts is the head of data science at P95 Belgium, a scientific service-providing company focused on pharmacovigilance and epidemiology related to vaccines and infectious diseases.

Paddy Farrington is an emeritus professor of statistics at the Open University (OU), UK. Prior to joining the OU in 1998, he was a statistician at the Immunisation Division of the Communicable Disease Surveillance Centre in the UK for 11 years.

Vaccination Programmes

Epidemiology, Monitoring, Evaluation

Susan Hahné, Kaatje Bollaerts and Paddy Farrington

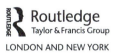

LONDON AND NEW YORK

First published 2022
by Routledge
2 Park Square, Milton Park, Abingdon, Oxon OX14 4RN

and by Routledge
605 Third Avenue, New York, NY 10158

Routledge is an imprint of the Taylor & Francis Group, an informa business

© 2022 Susan Hahné, Kaatje Bollaerts and Paddy Farrington

The right of Susan Hahné, Kaatje Bollaerts and Paddy Farrington to be identified as authors of this work has been asserted by them in accordance with sections 77 and 78 of the Copyright, Designs and Patents Act 1988.

The Open Access version of this book, available at www.taylorfrancis.com, has been made available under a Creative Commons Attribution-NonCommercial-NoDerivatives (CC-BY-NC-ND) 4.0 International license. Funded by CEPI and P95.

Trademark notice: Product or corporate names may be trademarks or registered trademarks, and are used only for identification and explanation without intent to infringe.

British Library Cataloguing-in-Publication Data
Names: Hahné, Susan, author. | Farrington, Paddy, author. | Bollaerts, Kaatje, author.
Title: Vaccination programmes : epidemiology, monitoring, evaluation/ Susan Hahné, Paddy Farrington, Kaatje Bollaerts.
Description: Milton Park, Abingdon, Oxon; New York, NY: Routledge, 2021. | Includes bibliographical references and index. |
Identifiers: LCCN 2021008974 (print) | LCCN 2021008975 (ebook) | ISBN 9781138054844 (hardback) | ISBN 9781138054851 (paperback) | ISBN 9781315166414 (ebook)
Subjects: LCSH: Vaccination. | Vaccines. | Epidemiology. | Monitoring. | Evaluation.
Classification: LCC RA638 .H34 2021 (print) | LCC RA638 (ebook) | DDC 614.4/7–dc23
LC record available at https://lccn.loc.gov/2021008974
LC ebook record available at https://lccn.loc.gov/2021008975

ISBN: 978-1-138-05484-4 (hbk)
ISBN: 978-1-138-05485-1 (pbk)
ISBN: 978-1-315-16641-4 (ebk)

DOI: 10.4324/9781315166414

Typeset in Times New Roman
by Newgen Publishing UK

Contents

List of acronyms and abbreviations	vii
List of boxes	xi
Preface	xxi
Acknowledgements	xxiii
Introduction	1

PART I: Background — 3

1	Vaccines	5
2	How vaccines work: immune responses and vaccine failure	18
3	Vaccination programmes: aims and strategies	34
4	Dynamics of vaccine-preventable infectious diseases	55
5	Impact of mass vaccination programmes	75
6	Vaccination: a societal perspective	97

PART II: Field tools for monitoring vaccination programmes — 113

7 Monitoring vaccine coverage and attitudes towards vaccination — 115

8 Surveillance of vaccine-preventable diseases and pathogens — 131

9 Serological surveillance — 154

10 Assessing and monitoring impact — 172

11 Outbreak investigation of vaccine-preventable diseases — 195

PART III: Vaccine effectiveness — 221

12 Vaccine effectiveness — 223

13 Estimating vaccine effectiveness: general methodological principles — 245

14 Estimating vaccine effectiveness: cohort and household contact studies — 264

15 Estimating vaccine effectiveness: case-control and screening studies — 289

16 Waning vaccine effectiveness and modes of vaccine action — 309

PART IV: Risks associated with vaccination programmes — 337

17 Vaccine safety: an introduction — 339

18 Surveillance of adverse events following immunisation — 347

19 Estimating vaccination risks: general methodological principles — 364

20 Epidemiological study designs for evaluating vaccine safety — 383

PART V: Benefit–risk assessment of vaccination programmes — 405

21 Benefit–risk assessment of vaccination programmes — 407

Index — 437

Acronyms and abbreviations

AEFI	Adverse event following immunisation
AF	Attributable fraction
AFP	Acute flaccid paralysis
AIN	anal intraepithelial neoplasia
AR	Attributable risk
aVDPV	Ambiguous vaccine-derived poliovirus
AWD	Acute watery diarrhoea
BCG	Bacille Calmette-Guérin
BRAT	Benefit risk action team
BRR	Benefit risk ratio
BSE	Bovine spongiform encephalopathy
CDC	Centers for Disease Control and Prevention
CI	Confidence interval
CIN	Cervical intraepithelial neoplasm
CIR	Cumulative incidence ratio
CLL	Complementary log-log link
CNS	Central nervous system
COPD	Chronic obstructive pulmonary disorder
COVID-19	Coronavirus disease 2019
CPRD	Clinical Practice Research Datalink
CRS	Congenital rubella syndrome
cVDPV	Circulating vaccine-derived poliovirus
DALY	Disability-adjusted life year
DHS	Demographic health survey
DIVA	Differentiating infected from vaccinated animals
DTaP	Diphtheria, tetanus, acellular pertussis

EC	European Commission
ECDC	European Centre for Disease Prevention and Control
EDS	Excessive daytime sleepiness
EIA	Enzyme-linked immunosorbent assay
ELISA	Enzyme-linked immunosorbent assay
EMA	European Medicines Agency
EPI	Expanded Programme on Immunization
EU	European Union
FAIR	Findable, accessible, interoperable and reusable
FDA	Food and Drug Administration
FNI	First Nation and Inuit
GACVS	Global Advisory Committee on Vaccine Safety
GAVI	Global alliance for vaccination and immunisation
GBD	Global burden of disease
GBS	Guillain-Barré syndrome
GMP	Good manufacturing practice
GMT	Geometric mean titre
GP	General practitioner
GPEI	Global polio eradication initiative
GPS	Global positioning system
HAV	Hepatitis A virus
HBsAg	Hepatitis B surface antigen
HBV	Hepatitis B virus
Hib	*Haemophilus influenzae* type b
HIV	Human immunodeficiency virus
HMO	Health maintenance organisation
HPV	Human papillomavirus
HR	Hazard ratio
ICD	International classification of diseases
IgA/D/E/G/M	Immunoglobulin A/D/E/G/M
ILI	Influenza-like illness
IMPACT	Immunization monitoring programme, active
IPD	Invasive pneumococcal disease
IR	Incidence rate
IRR	Incidence rate ratio
IS	Intussusception
ITP	Idiopathic thrombocytopenic purpura
iVDPV	Immunodeficiency-associated vaccine derived poliovirus
JRF	Joint reporting form
LMIC	Low- and middle-income country
LQAS	Lot quality assurance sampling
MAH	Marketing authorisation holder
MCC	Meningococcal serogroup C conjugate
MenC	Meningococcal serogroup C
MHC	Major histocompatibility complex

MICS	Multiple indicator cluster survey
MIV	Monovalent inactivated vaccine
MMR	Measles, mumps, rubella
MMRV	Measles, mumps, rubella, varicella
MR	Measles and rubella
MS	Multiple sclerosis
MSM	Men who have sex with men
NHB	Net health benefit
NID	National immunisation day
NITAG	National immunisation technical advisory group
NNH	Number needed to harm
NNV	Number needed to vaccinate
NRA	National regulatory authority
NUTS	Nomenclature of territorial units for statistics
OR	Odds ratio
PAHO	Pan American Health Organization
PBMC	Peripheral blood mononuclear cell
PCR	Polymerase chain reaction
PCVn	n-valent pneumococcal conjugate vaccine
PFU	Plaque forming unit
POCT	Point of care test
PPV	Positive predictive value
PrOACT-URL	Problems, objectives, alternatives, consequences, trade-offs, uncertainty, risk attitudes, and linked decisions
PRR	Proportional reporting ratio
PT	Programme impact on transmission
QALY	Quality-adjusted life year
RBR	Risk benefit ratio
RCA	Rapid cycle analysis
RDD	Regression discontinuity design
RI	Relative incidence
RIVM	Netherlands Institute for Public Health and the Environment
RNA	Ribonucleic acid
RR	Relative risk
RSV	Respiratory syncytial virus
RT-PCR	Reverse transcriptase polymerase chain reaction
RVGE	Rotavirus gastroenteritis
SAGE	Strategic advisory group of experts
SAR	Secondary attack rate
SARS-CoV-2	Severe acute respiratory syndrome coronavirus 2
SBA	Serum bactericidal antibody
SCCS	Self-controlled case series
SCRI	Self-controlled risk interval
SIA	Supplementary immunisation activity
SIDS	Sudden infant death syndrome

SIR	Susceptible infected recovered
SmPC	Summary of product characteristics
SMS	Short message service
SNID	Subnational immunisation day
Tdap	Tetanus, diphtheria, acellular pertussis
TIV	Trivalent influenza vaccine
UI	Uncertainty interval
UN	United Nations
UNICEF	United Nations Children's Fund
US(A)	United States (of America)
USAID	United States Agency for International Aid
VAED	Vaccine-associated enhanced disease
VAERS	Vaccine Adverse Event Reporting System
VAPP	Vaccine-associated paralytic polio
VDPV	Vaccine-derived poliovirus
VE	Vaccine effectiveness
VI	Vaccine effectiveness against infectiousness
VLP	Virus-like particle
VP	Vaccine effectiveness against progression
VP	Virus protein
VPDI	Vaccine-preventable disease incidence
VSD	Vaccine Safety Datalink
VZV	Varicella zoster virus
WHA	World Health Assembly
WHO	World Health Organization
WPV	Wild poliovirus
WPV1/2/3	Wild poliovirus type 1/2/3
WUENIC	WHO/UNICEF estimate of national immunisation coverage
YLD	Years lived with disability
YLL	Years of life lost

Boxes

1.1	Variolation, immunisation, vaccination and inoculation	6
1.2	The four types of antigenic components used in currently licensed vaccines	8
1.3	The four types of vaccine platforms used in currently licensed vaccines	9
1.4	Vaccine potency	10
1.5	The vaccine 'cold chain'	11
1.6	High-titre measles vaccines	12
1.7	Vaccine administration routes with examples	13
1.8	Vaccine trials: phase I, II, III and IV	14
1.9	The development and licensure of Ebola vaccines	15
1.10	Vaccine licensing authorities: examples	16
2.1	The main components of the immune system	19
2.2	Cross-reactivity	20
2.3	B cell responses to vaccination: T-dependent and T-independent antigens	21
2.4	Maternal antibodies	22
2.5	Maturation of antibodies: affinity, avidity maturation and isotype switching	23
2.6	Antigen recognition in T cell responses	24
2.7	Long-lasting protection induced by vaccination	26
2.8	Priming and boosting	27
2.9	Antibody tests: antibody-binding, avidity and functional assays	29
2.10	Differentiating vaccine-induced immunity from immunity induced by natural infection	30
2.11	Vaccine failure types	31
2.12	Laboratory testing to differentiate between primary and secondary vaccine failure	31
3.1	Variolation and vaccination programmes for military purposes	35
3.2	The smallpox eradication programme	36

3.3	The programme to eradicate poliomyelitis	37
3.4	Eradication, elimination or containment: definitions	39
3.5	Factors favouring the possibility of elimination and eradication	39
3.6	WHO Regional Office for Europe definitions for the elimination of measles (WHO, 2014)	40
3.7	Indications for selective vaccination programmes	41
3.8	Maternal vaccination	42
3.9	Role of national or subnational immunisation days in the eradication of poliomyelitis	43
3.10	Eliminating measles from the Americas: 'catch-up, keep-up, follow-up'	44
3.11	Ring vaccination	45
3.12	Reducing the number of doses in pneumococcal and HPV vaccination schedules	47
3.13	The WHO Strategic Advisory Group of Experts and the Vaccine Position Papers	48
3.14	The Global Alliance for Vaccination and Immunisation	49
3.15	Monitoring and evaluation of vaccination programmes: key areas and tools	49
3.16	Ceasing the RotaShield rotavirus vaccination programme in the United States	51
4.1	Routes of transmission of infectious diseases	56
4.2	Indirect effect of vaccination	57
4.3	Factors affecting the magnitude of the indirect effect of vaccination	58
4.4	Epidemic cycles for directly transmitted immunising infections	59
4.5	Outbreak of measles in healthcare workers	60
4.6	Ranges of values of R_0 for selected infections	62
4.7	The basic reproduction number and critical immunisation threshold	63
4.8	Proportion susceptible in a homogeneously mixing population	66
4.9	R_0 and critical immunisation threshold for hepatitis A in Bulgaria	67
4.10	Effect of heterogeneity of contacts on R_0	68
4.11	Contact surveys for close-contact infections	69
4.12	The SIR and other compartmental models	71
4.13	Impact of childhood vaccination on influenza in the elderly	72
5.1	Pertussis vaccination in England and Wales	76
5.2	Rubella vaccination in China	76
5.3	Protection of unvaccinated children against cholera by herd immunity	78
5.4	Herd immunity masking vaccine failure of Hib vaccine	78
5.5	Herd immunity and human papillomavirus vaccination	79

5.6	Ranges of values of R_0, vaccine effectiveness and the critical immunisation and vaccination threshold for selected infections	80
5.7	A post-honeymoon outbreak of measles in Muyinga, Burundi	82
5.8	Mumps vaccination in England and Wales	83
5.9	Chickenpox vaccination and shingles	85
5.10	Adult pertussis in the Netherlands	85
5.11	Impact of mass vaccination on the average age at infection in the United States	87
5.12	Persistence of CRS cases in Greece following mass rubella vaccination	87
5.13	Impact of vaccination on the dynamics of measles and whooping cough in Senegal	88
5.14	Pertussis in the Netherlands	90
5.15	Pneumococcal vaccination and serotype replacement	90
5.16	Contrasting socio-economic impacts of rotavirus vaccination	91
5.17	Hospital admissions due to rotavirus gastroenteritis in Bangladesh	92
5.18	Reduction in gonorrhoea hospitalisation following introduction of meningococcal B vaccination in New Zealand	93
5.19	The impact of live-attenuated influenza vaccine in reducing amoxicillin prescribing for children	93
6.1	Extension of compulsory vaccination in France in 2018	98
6.2	Opposition to smallpox vaccination in the United Kingdom in the 19th century	98
6.3	Whole-cell pertussis vaccine and brain damage	100
6.4	MMR vaccine and autism	101
6.5	The northern Nigerian polio vaccine boycott	102
6.6	Thiomersal and autism	103
6.7	Vaccine hesitancy and the life cycle of vaccination programmes	105
6.8	Measles vaccination worldwide: one step forward, two steps back?	106
6.9	Global levels of confidence in vaccines	106
6.10	Vaccine hesitancy in Europe	107
6.11	Is the MMR vaccine safe?	108
6.12	Setting out risks and benefits	109
7.1	Reporting vaccine coverage estimates	116
7.2	Monitoring vaccine coverage: register-based, survey and administrative methods	117
7.3	Demographic health surveys and multiple-indicator cluster surveys	118
7.4	Vaccine coverage estimates in Greece	119
7.5	The 'EPI coverage survey' and subsequent WHO guidance for vaccine coverage surveys	121

7.6	A population-based vaccine register in Norway	122
7.7	Monitoring vaccine coverage through health insurance claims data in Germany	123
7.8	WHO/UNICEF vaccine coverage estimates	125
7.9	Repeated surveys of parental attitudes towards vaccination in England, 2001–2015	126
7.10	Analyses of internet reports to assess public concerns about vaccines	127
7.11	Monitoring of vaccination-related social media messages in the Netherlands	128
8.1	Measures of validity of a case definition: sensitivity, specificity and positive predictive value	133
8.2	Clinical case definitions for measles: positive predictive value depends on the level of measles control achieved	134
8.3	Use of multiple data sources for the surveillance of rotavirus in the Netherlands	136
8.4	EuroMOMO: monitoring excess deaths due to respiratory diseases in Europe	137
8.5	Influenza sentinel surveillance in Australia	139
8.6	'GrippeNet', an example of citizen science-based surveillance in France	140
8.7	Descriptive analyses of the incidence of invasive *Haemophilus influenzae* type b infection in the United Kingdom	142
8.8	Surveillance to assess the impact of pneumococcal vaccination in Kenya	145
8.9	Surveillance for acute flaccid paralysis	148
8.10	The contribution of molecular surveillance to the elimination of poliomyelitis from India	149
8.11	Wild poliovirus type 2 infection in a laboratory worker after a spill, the Netherlands, 2017	150
9.1	Hepatitis A seroprevalence in Madagascar	155
9.2	Rubella immunity among women and the burden of congenital rubella syndrome in Cambodia	156
9.3	Monitoring immunity to polio in Kano state, Nigeria	158
9.4	Meningococcal serogroup C conjugate vaccination in the United Kingdom	159
9.5	The UK measles and rubella vaccination campaign	160
9.6	Human papillomavirus vaccine coverage in the United Kingdom	162
9.7	Mechanistic and non-mechanistic correlates of protection	163
9.8	Serological surveys based on residual sera and random sampling	165
9.9	Standardisation of hepatitis A assay results	166
9.10	Obtaining seroprevalence and GMTs	168

9.11	Analysis of varicella zoster virus seroprevalence data with mixture models	169
10.1	Individual effects and population impact of mass vaccination programmes	173
10.2	Impact of cholera vaccination in South Sudan	176
10.3	Impact of vaccinating school-age children against influenza in England	177
10.4	Impact of *Haemophilus influenzae* type b vaccination in the Gambia	178
10.5	Impact of human papillomavirus vaccination on anogenital warts in Québec	180
10.6	Obtaining evidence of indirect effects of vaccination	182
10.7	Impact of vaccination on diphtheria and poliomyelitis in the Netherlands	183
10.8	Impact of rotavirus vaccination in Kenya	185
10.9	Impact of herpes zoster vaccination in the United Kingdom	186
10.10	The RDD for estimating impact at cut-off	187
10.11	Early impact of HPV vaccination in Ontario, Canada	188
10.12	Measles surveillance post-elimination in the United States in the 1990s	190
10.13	WHO measles elimination status in the United Kingdom	192
11.1	A large measles outbreak in Pakistan	197
11.2	Diphtheria outbreaks in newly independent states of the former Soviet Union in the 1990s	198
11.3	A rubella outbreak due to failure to vaccinate	199
11.4	A poliomyelitis outbreak in Nigeria caused by a boycott of the vaccine	200
11.5	A measles outbreak in Polynesia due to cold chain problems	201
11.6	A mumps outbreak among vaccinated students in Norway, 2015 to 2016	202
11.7	Post-honeymoon outbreaks	203
11.8	A measles outbreak in northern Pakistan	205
11.9	The 10 steps of an outbreak investigation	206
11.10	Delays in laboratory diagnosis of cholera hampering outbreak control	207
11.11	Examples of case definitions used in vaccine-preventable disease outbreak investigations	208
11.12	Outbreak of meningococcal serogroup C disease in MSM	209
11.13	Descriptive epidemiology of a meningococcal disease outbreak investigation	211
11.14	An outbreak investigation assessing risk factors for failure to vaccinate	212
11.15	Relevant study questions during the meningococcal W outbreak investigation among Hajj pilgrims	214

11.16	A polio outbreak investigation assessing risk factors for dying	215
11.17	Public health campaign during mumps outbreak in Canada	217
12.1	Calculating vaccine effectiveness	225
12.2	Confidence intervals for *VE*	225
12.3	Influenza vaccine effectiveness in the community and in households	226
12.4	The potential impact of programmatic errors	227
12.5	The stepped-wedge design: hepatitis B vaccination in the Gambia	228
12.6	The Guinea Ebola ring vaccination trial	229
12.7	Efficacy and effectiveness of rotavirus vaccines vary by population studied	230
12.8	Effectiveness of Hib conjugate vaccination against colonisation	231
12.9	Effectiveness of influenza vaccines against hospitalisation in Canada	232
12.10	Effectiveness of pneumococcal polysaccharide vaccines against bacteraemia	233
12.11	The effectiveness of pertussis vaccination against progression to severe disease	234
12.12	Influenza vaccine effectiveness against influenza-like illness in pilgrims to the Hajj	236
12.13	Using the cholera vaccine as a probe in Bangladesh	236
12.14	Conjugate vaccines and nasopharyngeal carriage of bacterial infections	237
12.15	Effectiveness against infectiousness: mumps vaccine in the Netherlands	238
12.16	Impact of mumps vaccination on household transmission in the Netherlands	240
12.17	Is elimination of mumps achievable?	241
13.1	Pertussis vaccine effectiveness: the influence of case definitions	246
13.2	Measles vaccine effectiveness under routine conditions in Tanzania	248
13.3	Pertussis vaccine effectiveness and notifications in Wales	249
13.4	Sensitivity, specificity, PPV and bias in vaccine effectiveness	250
13.5	Case definition and ascertainment for the Tanzanian measles vaccine study	252
13.6	Measles vaccine effectiveness in Pakistan	253
13.7	Confounding bias in vaccine effectiveness studies	254
13.8	Effectiveness of rotavirus vaccination in the United Kingdom	255
13.9	Does vaccination against seasonal influenza reduce all-cause mortality?	256
13.10	Effectiveness and bias-indicator study of oral cholera vaccination in rural Haiti	257
13.11	Risks and rates	259

13.12	Risk-based and rate-based vaccine effectiveness	261
14.1	Effectiveness of post-exposure measles vaccination in Catalonia	265
14.2	Rubella vaccine effectiveness in Guangzhou, China	267
14.3	Effectiveness of adolescent booster acellular pertussis vaccination in Maine	268
14.4	Mumps vaccine effectiveness against orchitis in the Netherlands	269
14.5	Rate-based measles vaccine effectiveness in Catalonia outbreak	271
14.6	Rate-based and risk-based vaccine effectiveness estimates for pertussis vaccine	272
14.7	Effectiveness of group B meningococcal vaccine in New Zealand	274
14.8	Effectiveness of herpes zoster vaccination in elderly people in the United Kingdom	275
14.9	Effectiveness of vaccination in pregnancy to prevent infant pertussis	278
14.10	Household study of measles vaccine effectiveness in Bavaria	280
14.11	Effectiveness against infectiousness of pertussis vaccine in Senegal	281
14.12	Joint estimation of mumps vaccine effectiveness measures in the Netherlands	283
14.13	Joint estimation of pertussis vaccine effectiveness measures in Senegal	283
14.14	Varicella vaccination in California: the effects of interaction	285
15.1	Influenza vaccine effectiveness in Malaysian pilgrims attending the Hajj	291
15.2	Pneumococcal vaccine effectiveness in high-risk patients	293
15.3	Control selection for vaccine studies in outbreaks in Vietnam and Tanzania	294
15.4	Vaccine effectiveness of a cholera vaccine during a cholera outbreak in Guinea	295
15.5	Effectiveness of cholera vaccination during an outbreak in South Sudan	296
15.6	Effectiveness of inactivated quadrivalent influenza vaccine in Japan	298
15.7	Effectiveness of a 13-valent pneumococcal conjugate vaccine in Germany	299
15.8	Effectiveness of the 7-valent pneumococcal vaccine in England and Wales	300
15.9	Measles vaccine effectiveness in South Africa	302
15.10	Surveillance of influenza vaccine effectiveness in France	303
15.11	Effectiveness of Hib vaccine in England and Wales	305
16.1	Calculating age-specific vaccine effectiveness	310

16.2	Details of calculations of cases in Box 16.1	312
16.3	Waning of mumps vaccine effectiveness in England and Wales	312
16.4	Duration of BCG protection in England	313
16.5	Risk-based vaccine effectiveness when the rate-based VE is constant	315
16.6	Rate-based vaccine effectiveness when the risk-based VE is constant	316
16.7	Partial protection, all-or-nothing protection and other modes of vaccine action	319
16.8	Long-term effectiveness of varicella vaccine	320
16.9	Some mathematical formulas	322
16.10	Protective antibody threshold for measles	323
16.11	Serological correlate of protection for *Bordetella pertussis*	323
16.12	Estimating $VE(t)$ with high incidence: partial protection mode of vaccine action	325
16.13	Estimating $VE(t)$ with high incidence: all-or-nothing mode of vaccine action	326
16.14	How to handle prior infections: mathematical rationale	328
16.15	Rubella vaccine effectiveness and time since vaccination in Guangzhou, China	329
16.16	Whole-cell pertussis vaccine age-specific effectiveness in England and Wales	330
16.17	Sensitivity analysis for the whole-cell pertussis vaccine data	331
16.18	Assessing VE long after vaccination when prior infections are common	333
17.1	AEFIs: cause-specific classification	340
17.2	Frequencies of some severe vaccine product-related reactions	341
17.3	Side effects of live-attenuated polio vaccines: vaccine-associated paralytic poliomyelitis and vaccine-derived polioviruses	342
17.4	Vaccine-associated enhanced disease	343
17.5	The Cutter incident	344
17.6	WHO and global vaccine safety	345
18.1	Rotavirus vaccine and intussusception in the United States	348
18.2	Evidence of vaccine safety when no adverse events are observed	349
18.3	Passive AEFI surveillance in the United States: the VAERS system	349
18.4	Pandemic influenza vaccination and narcolepsy in children and adolescents	350
18.5	Aseptic meningitis after MMR vaccines in the United Kingdom	351
18.6	Increases in vaccine-associated narcolepsy diagnoses after media reports	351
18.7	Active surveillance for AEFIs: the Canadian IMPACT system	353

18.8	Vaccine safety monitoring through data linkage in the United States: the Vaccine Safety Datalink project	353
18.9	Active AEFI surveillance in Ethiopia, Guatemala, Taiwan and Vietnam	354
18.10	Rapid cycle analysis in the VSD: febrile convulsions after MMRV vaccine	355
18.11	Real-time surveillance of influenza vaccine safety in Australia by SMS and email	356
18.12	Disseminated BCG in First Nation and Inuit people in Canada	356
18.13	An MMR tragedy and a measles disaster in Samoa	357
18.14	WHO approach to causality assessment for individual AEFI	357
18.15	Bell's palsy and monovalent inactivated pandemic influenza vaccine in the United States	359
18.16	Bell's palsy and parenteral inactivated seasonal influenza vaccines	360
19.1	Risk periods for MMR and DTP safety studies in England	365
19.2	Risk periods for MMR vaccine and autism studies	366
19.3	Intussusception and rotavirus vaccination with the RotaShield vaccine	368
19.4	Relative and attributable risks of febrile convulsions after MMR vaccine in England	369
19.5	Relative and attributable risks of febrile convulsions after MMR vaccine in the United States	370
19.6	RotaShield vaccine and intussusception: dose effect	371
19.7	Hib booster vaccination, MMR and febrile convulsions	372
19.8	MMR vaccine and autism	373
19.9	Febrile convulsions and DTP vaccine	374
19.10	Intussusception and oral polio vaccine in Cuba	375
19.11	DTP vaccination, the healthy vaccinee effect and sudden infant death syndrome	376
19.12	Asthma exacerbations after influenza vaccination	377
19.13	Influenza vaccine, influenza-like illness and Guillain-Barré syndrome	378
19.14	Influenza vaccination, asthma and chronic obstructive pulmonary disorder in the General Practice Research Database	380
20.1	Febrile convulsions after DTaP vaccine in the United States	384
20.2	Autism and MMR vaccine in Denmark	385
20.3	Hepatitis B vaccination in children and risk of relapse of inflammatory demyelination	387
20.4	Oral polio vaccine and intussusception in the United Kingdom	388
20.5	HBV vaccination and MS in the United States	389
20.6	Narcolepsy and pandemic influenza vaccination in England	391

20.7	Bell's palsy and vaccinations in US children	392
20.8	ITP and MMR vaccines	393
20.9	MMR vaccine and autism	395
20.10	Adverse events following varicella vaccine in Taiwan	395
20.11	Influenza vaccination and Bell's palsy	397
20.12	Influenza vaccination and Guillain-Barré syndrome in France	398
20.13	Rotavirus vaccination and intussusception in sub-Saharan Africa	399
20.14	Vaccinations and the risk of relapse in MS in Europe	401
21.1	Rotavirus vaccination and intussusception	408
21.2	Hepatitis B vaccination in France and Italy	409
21.3	HPV vaccine controversy in Japan	410
21.4	PrOACT-URL framework	411
21.5	PrOACT-URL framework applied to HPV vaccination in boys	413
21.6	A value tree applied to HPV vaccination in boys	415
21.7	Benefit–risk table applied to HPV vaccination in boys	415
21.8	Benefit–risk of suspending routine childhood immunisation during the COVID-19 pandemic in Africa	418
21.9	Benefit–risk ratio of rotavirus vaccination in Latin America	419
21.10	*NNV* and *NNH* for a specific influenza vaccine	421
21.11	Benefit–risk difference of rotavirus vaccination in Japan	422
21.12	Benefits and risks of removing the age restrictions for rotavirus vaccination	423
21.13	Benefit–risk ratio of rotavirus vaccination in France	424
21.14	Calculating QALYs	427
21.15	Quantifying benefits and risks of HPV vaccination based on QALYs, Japan	427
21.16	Net health benefit of meningococcal vaccination based on QALYs	428
21.17	Calculating DALYs	430
21.18	Years lived with disability for adverse events following immunisation	431
21.19	DALYs for measles and rubella vaccination	432

Preface

Our intention in writing this book is to bring together the many different perspectives on the epidemiological evaluation of vaccination programmes, describe the methods used and illustrate them with practical examples drawn from the literature. We hope this will contribute to high-quality decision-making on vaccination programmes and help ensure that such programmes can optimally protect populations from death and suffering from vaccine-preventable diseases.

The book is aimed at all those involved in the many aspects of vaccination programmes, including public health professionals and epidemiologists. Its primary target audiences are master and doctoral students in infectious disease epidemiology and public health, post-doctoral participants of field epidemiology training programmes and public health professionals working in the post-implementation epidemiological evaluation of vaccines and vaccination programmes. Other target audiences include professionals and students in clinical medicine, public health policy, health economics, medicine regulatory practice and the pharmaceutical industry.

Some background knowledge of biology, epidemiology, statistics and infectious diseases will aid the understanding of this book, but we have tried to keep it accessible also for readers starting out in these areas. The style of the book is non-technical, and the use of mathematical formulas is kept to a minimum. We do take the reader to the frontier where the subject gets more seriously technical but, while giving an indication of what lies beyond that frontier, we do not venture over it.

The background and theory covered in this book are relevant to vaccines and vaccination programmes in all countries of the world. By including examples from high-, middle- and low-income countries, we have sought to make the learning points relevant to readers in these different settings.

The topics covered in this book and its outline broadly match those of the EPIET training course on the epidemiology of vaccine-preventable diseases on which one of the authors has taught over the past 15 years. The idea to write this book came about when the three authors met during the ADVANCE project, a European collaboration that aimed to facilitate decision-making on vaccination programmes by developing methods for assessing their benefits and risks, separately and in an integrated manner. The book has since grown to encompass other aspects of vaccination programmes, in resource-poor as well as resource-rich settings. Much of the book was finalised in 2020, the first year of the SARS-CoV-2 pandemic, which has brought to the fore the importance of mass vaccination in protecting public health.

Acknowledgements

We owe a huge debt of gratitude to the people we have met and have had the pleasure to work with over the years, for sharing their knowledge and experience, collaborating with us and providing stimulation and inspiration. This book is really the result of these encounters and interactions, and we particularly wish to thank Paul Fine, Elizabeth Miller, Alain Moren and Mary Ramsay.

We are further indebted to those we have worked with in ADVANCE, during EPIET training courses, and on all of our other vaccine epidemiology projects.

We thank Jossy van den Boogaard, Cécile van Els, Laura Nic Lochlainn, Elizabeth Miller and Alain Moren for reviewing earlier versions of (some) chapters in this book and providing helpful comments.

Furthermore, we would like to thank our employers (RIVM and P95 Belgium) for their support and granting us time.

Finally, we are very grateful to our parents, partners, children, family and friends, in particular Beckie, Bent, Betsy, Bram, Cathie, Dylan, Lore, Maginty, Marjo, Niel and Saar, for their kind support and patience throughout this project.

Introduction

Next to providing clean water, vaccination is the most effective intervention to prevent death and suffering from infectious diseases. The COVID-19 crisis starting in late 2019 painfully demonstrates the challenges of controlling a pandemic without vaccines.

The enormously beneficial potential of vaccination to improve public health and reduce health inequalities can best be realised by delivering vaccines as part of a planned vaccination programme. The public health triumph of smallpox eradication demonstrates what can be achieved by such a concerted effort. Programmatic vaccination implies that the aims of the programme have been specified, vaccine strategies and policies to achieve these aims have been determined and that an ongoing evaluation of the programme is undertaken throughout its lifetime. Once a vaccination programme has been introduced, continued assessment of its performance in terms of benefits and risks is required to provide evidence to maintain, modify or strengthen the programme.

Effects of vaccines are extensively studied in pre-clinical and clinical trials prior to their use in vaccination programmes. Nevertheless, post-implementation evidence is essential to guide programmes since their effects, impact, benefits and risks may differ from what can be anticipated based on results of these trials. For example, the impact of a vaccination programme may be limited by low vaccine coverage, rare adverse reactions may become apparent that trials were incapable of detecting owing to sample-size limitations, effectiveness in field conditions may be lower than in trials, changing pathogen populations may reduce the impact of the programme and unanticipated herd-immunity effects may make the programme more effective than expected.

The aim of this book is to guide readers through the methods commonly used for evaluating vaccines and vaccination programmes once they are implemented. Methods that are mainly relevant to the pre-implementation evaluation of vaccines and vaccination programmes, such as clinical trials and economic evaluation, are largely excluded from this book.

The primary purpose in the evaluation of a vaccination programme is to assess whether the programme is meeting its aims. A further purpose is to identify any factors that may limit its beneficial impact. Ongoing evaluation will also seek evidence of safety and effectiveness of vaccination, assess its risks and identify any additional beneficial

DOI: 10.4324/9781315166414-1
This Chapter has been made available under a CC-BY-NC-ND license.

or detrimental impacts of the programme as a whole. Such evidence will determine whether the programme needs to be modified in any way, and will underpin an integrated assessment of benefits and risks. This book covers the main methods relevant to all of these activities.

Vaccination programmes achieve their aims by altering the epidemiology of vaccine-preventable diseases. Epidemiology is therefore the main tool for studying the interactions between vaccination programmes and human populations: the epidemiology of vaccination programmes is about investigating, in real conditions of life, the impacts, benefits and risks of such programmes.

We have chosen to restrict the content of this book to the methodological subject area of epidemiology. Other disciplines, such as immunology, vaccinology, microbiology, health services research, psychology, anthropology and economic evaluation are all very relevant to the evaluation of vaccination programmes, and are occasionally touched upon where needed, but fall outside the scope of the book. When covering statistical and epidemiological methods, we have focused on specifying the methods most relevant for the evaluation of vaccination programmes, rather than providing a complete description, which may be found elsewhere.

The book is organised in five parts. We start in Part I by providing an overview of basic concepts in vaccinology, immunology, vaccination programmes, infectious disease transmission dynamics, the various impacts of vaccination programmes and their societal context. Part II covers the main field tools used for the epidemiological evaluation of vaccination programmes: monitoring coverage and attitudes towards vaccination, surveillance of vaccine-preventable diseases and pathogens, seroepidemiological studies, methods to assess impact and outbreak investigation. Part III is dedicated to vaccine effectiveness, and its assessment. Part IV includes an overview of the potential risks of vaccination and how to study these. Lastly, Part V deals with methods for an integrated assessment of benefits and risks of vaccination programmes.

Interspersed through the text are two types of boxes: those in which further details about a specific concept or method are provided (light-grey boxes) and those in which concepts and methods are illustrated or elaborated in real-life examples (light-blue boxes).

We hope you enjoy this journey through the varied landscapes of vaccine epidemiology as much as we have benefited from exploring them.

Part I

Background

Chapter 1

Vaccines

A key characteristic of infectious agents is that they may induce immunity, which means that upon a second exposure a person is, to a certain degree, protected. This feature is unique to infectious diseases: it does not occur with any other hazard such as chemicals or radiation. Centuries ago, observant individuals recognising the potential of immunity tried to find ways to induce it while avoiding having to go through the disease. This led to the development of vaccines and the practice of vaccination.

Key characteristics of vaccines (safety, immunogenicity and efficacy) are assessed in clinical trials prior to their implementation in vaccination programmes. Use of the vaccine in real-life programmes over time, however, may make some properties become apparent that may not have been observed before, such as waning of vaccine-induced immunity or very rare adverse reactions. Since these may require adaptation of the vaccination programme, assessing vaccine-induced immunity, effectiveness and safety remains essential during the lifetime of a vaccination programme, together with continued monitoring of vaccine coverage and impact.

We start this chapter by providing background information on vaccines: how they were invented and developed, the types of vaccines currently available and their components. We then define key properties of vaccines (potency, stability, immunogenicity and safety). While potency and stability are intrinsic properties of a vaccine, immunogenicity and safety also depend on the interaction of the vaccine with its recipient. Vaccine efficacy and vaccine effectiveness are determined not only by characteristics of the vaccine and its recipient, but also by the infectious agent and the epidemiological context of vaccination. Since the assessment of vaccine effectiveness is an important methodological subject in the epidemiological evaluation of vaccination programmes, several chapters of this book (Chapters 12–16) are dedicated to it.

We continue the chapter by providing an overview of the different routes of administration of currently licensed vaccines. Lastly, we present a brief overview of the steps before a vaccine is implemented in a vaccination programme and where vaccines are manufactured. Further details on the topics included in this chapter may be found in *Plotkin's Vaccines* (Plotkin, Orenstein, Offit, & Edwards, 2018).

DOI: 10.4324/9781315166414-2
This Chapter has been made available under a CC-BY-NC-ND license.

1.1 A brief history of vaccines

The first verified documentation about attempts to induce immunity to an infectious disease describes a 16th-century practice in India to introduce material from smallpox pustules into the skin of another person. It has been suggested that an even older, similar tradition, invented by a Taoist or Buddhist monk or nun, was practised in China around the year 1000, but this has not been well documented (Boylston, 2012). The virus causing smallpox is called variola virus, and the practice of immunising someone with materials from a smallpox patient is hence called 'variolation'. It was effective to protect against smallpox, but not surprisingly also carried a substantial (around 2%) risk of causing lethal smallpox in the variolated subject. When safer vaccines to prevent smallpox became available, variolation became obsolete.

The observation that people, often dairymaids, who had been infected with cowpox (caused by vaccinia virus) became immune to smallpox, led to the first practice of 'vaccination' in England in 1774 by Benjamin Jesty, a farmer. He administered materials from a herd with cowpox to his wife and two children (himself already having experienced cowpox), who subsequently remained free from smallpox. Edward Jenner developed the same hypothesis about the protective effects of cowpox infection against smallpox some years later, experimentally tested it and published the findings in 1789, reaching a large medical audience. In subsequent years, methods were developed to turn material from cows infected with cowpox into smallpox vaccines.

Following on from this, vaccines against many other infectious diseases were developed. Initially these were aimed at protecting animals (cholera and anthrax vaccines). The first human vaccine after the smallpox vaccine was against rabies, used from 1885 onwards but initially only as post-exposure vaccination. Several human vaccines based on killed bacteria or bacterial toxins were developed in subsequent years. The possibility of growing viruses in cell cultures, discovered in the 1950s, allowed the development of several new viral vaccines.

Throughout history, the terms 'immunisation' and 'vaccination' have changed their meaning according to practices at the time (see Box 1.1). Nowadays they are often used as synonyms. In this book, however, we do distinguish vaccination from immunisation, as vaccination does not always lead to immunity, and immunity can be induced by other means than vaccination.

Box 1.1 Variolation, immunisation, vaccination and inoculation

Variolation refers to the practice of administering materials from a patient with smallpox (caused by variola virus) to a healthy person aiming to induce immunity. This practice was abandoned when smallpox vaccination became available, which was much safer.

Immunisation refers to the induction of immunity against an infectious disease in someone by administering antibodies or a vaccine. Inducing immunity by administering antibodies is called 'passive immunisation'. This does not lead to long-term protection since the antibodies are gradually broken down by the host and there is no acquisition of immune memory. Inducing acquired immunity by vaccination is called 'active immunisation'. Here the immune response is the result of someone's own immune system being activated. This has the potential to induce long-term protection (see Chapter 2).

Immunisation always refers to prevention and does not apply to the administration of antibodies for therapeutic purposes. It does apply to the use of vaccines or antibodies as pre- and post-exposure methods of preventing infection.

Vaccination (or 'inoculation') refers to the act of administering a vaccine to someone (which may or may not lead to immunity in that person). Vaccination initially referred specifically to administering cowpox vaccine (based on the vaccinia virus), but the meaning of this term was later extended to all vaccines. The term 'inoculation' has become obsolete.

1.2 Vaccine antigens, platforms and excipients

Immunity to an infectious disease results from an exposed person's immune system specifically responding to antigens of its causal infectious agent while it is being stimulated by other parts of the pathogen. Antigens are recognised by the adaptive part of the immune system, while the stimuli are recognised by the innate part of the immune system (see Chapter 2). For vaccines to have the same effect, they therefore must include one or more antigens derived from the targeted infectious agent as well as stimulatory components, so that the immune system knows that the antigen is something foreign to respond to. In addition to antigens, vaccines may include adjuvants to stimulate and modulate the immune response and other components. In addition to the components of a vaccine (which are listed in the summary of product characteristics (SmPC)), its design is crucial for its effects and safety. In what follows we provide a brief overview of the main vaccine components and vaccine designs.

1.2.1 Vaccine antigens

The antigenic component of a vaccine is derived from the targeted pathogen. This can be the entire pathogen (containing many antigens), some of its components (those mainly used are proteins, polysaccharides or glycoproteins) or a toxin it produces. When an entire pathogen is used, it is killed or attenuated to make sure it can no longer cause disease. In the case of smallpox vaccine, a mild and related virus (cowpox virus) is used in a modified form. When a toxin is used, it similarly needs to be inactivated so as not to make the vaccine recipient ill. An inactivated toxin is called a toxoid. Examples of vaccines using these different types of antigens are listed in Box 1.2.

Box 1.2 The four types of antigenic components used in currently licensed vaccines

1. *Live-attenuated organisms*: these are mainly used in vaccines against viral infections. Examples include smallpox, measles, mumps, rubella, yellow fever and oral polio vaccines. Vaccines containing live-attenuated bacteria include BCG vaccine (Bacille Calmette-Guérin, a vaccine against tuberculosis), a cholera vaccine ('Vaxchora™') and a typhoid vaccine ('Ty21a vaccine').
2. *Killed organisms*: these are included in, for example, inactivated polio, rabies, hepatitis A and whole-cell pertussis vaccines.
3. *Subunits of organisms (polysaccharides, proteins or glycoproteins)*: examples of these are meningococcal, pneumococcal and *Haemophilus influenzae* type b vaccines (including polysaccharide antigens or polysaccharides conjugated to proteins (see below)); and acellular pertussis, hepatitis B and meningococcal B vaccines (including protein antigens). Viral proteins that are (naturally or synthetically) assembled into a virus-like structure are called 'virus-like particles' (VLPs). This is used in, for example, human papillomavirus (HPV) vaccines.
4. *Toxins secreted by organisms*: inactivated toxins are called toxoids. The only two examples of toxoids used in vaccines are diphtheria and tetanus toxoid.

Vaccines containing live-attenuated organisms are usually very immunogenic, meaning they are good at inducing an immune response. They therefore require relatively few doses for protection (two or even only one in the case of rubella vaccine) and do not need adjuvants to enhance the immune response. The duration of protection of this type of vaccine is usually long compared to the vaccines including other types of antigens.

Vaccine antigens based on polysaccharide subunits of organisms (type 3 in Box 1.2) have generally the weakest immunogenic potential. They therefore usually contain adjuvants (see Section 1.2.3), and the polysaccharides may be chemically coupled ('conjugated') to another substance to increase its immunogenicity (see Box 2.3 in Chapter 2). Examples of conjugates are tetanus toxoid, CRM197 (a non-toxigenic natural variant of diphtheria toxin) and protein D (obtained from non-typeable *Haemophilus influenzae*). Of note, conjugate vaccines induce immunity against both the antigen and the protein.

1.2.2 Vaccine platforms

In addition to the composition of their antigenic content, vaccines can also be classified according to the way they are designed, that is, which platform is used to make sure the antigen reaches the recipient's immune system. An overview of vaccine platforms of currently licensed vaccines protecting against infectious diseases is provided in Box 1.3. The particular platform used has implications for the way the immune response is stimulated, the immunogenicity and also safety of the vaccine.

Box 1.3 The four types of vaccine platforms used in currently licensed vaccines

1. *Live-attenuated pathogens*: this type of vaccine contains very small amounts of attenuated viruses or bacteria, which replicate in the recipient leading to an immune response. Vaccine-virus-associated effects only occur after an 'incubation period' during which replication takes place. Contraindications and side effects of live-attenuated vaccines are reviewed in Chapter 2. The live-attenuated organisms may be transmitted from the vaccinee to other people. This has been documented for the mumps vaccine virus and oral polio vaccine (OPV) strains. In the case of OPV, this has beneficial effects as it may lead to immunising contacts of OPV recipients.
2. *Killed (components of) pathogens or toxins*: in this type of vaccine, antigen classes 2, 3 or 4 as listed in Box 1.2 may be used. To enhance and modulate the immune response, adjuvants need to be included.
3. *Viral vector vaccines*: here a harmless virus is genetically engineered to contain genes coding for an antigen of the targeted pathogen. The virus, called the vector, replicates in the recipient whereby the antigen is produced. An example of this is Ervebo, protecting against Ebola virus disease, in which the vector virus is a weakened recombinant vesicular stomatitis virus, which in itself has little or no effect on humans.
4. *mRNA (messenger ribonucleic acid) vaccines*: this platform uses genetic material of the targeted infection coding for one of its antigens. Once inside the recipient's immune cells, these cells start to produce the pathogen's antigen, leading to an immune response. Vaccines of this type have been licensed to protect against COVID-19 (coronavirus disease-2019).

1.2.3 Adjuvants

Adjuvants are substances included in vaccines to strengthen and/or modulate the immune response following vaccination, by engaging with the innate immune system. They work by enhancing antigen presentation and/or by providing co-stimulation and maturation signals to the responding cells from the adaptive immune system. Adjuvants are not needed in live-attenuated vaccines, as explained above. The most widely used adjuvants are aluminium salts such as aluminium phosphate or aluminium hydroxide.

1.2.4 Other vaccine excipients

In addition to antigens and adjuvants, vaccines may also contain preservatives, antibiotics, stabilisers and components resulting from the vaccine manufacturing process. Preservatives and antibiotics can be added to vaccines to prevent them becoming contaminated by bacteria or fungi. Most currently used vaccines are, however, free from preservatives. These exclude vaccines available in multi-dose vials, where preservatives continue to be used. Trace amounts of preservatives and antibiotics may be present in vaccines as a result of their use in the manufacturing process. In this situation the vaccine can still be qualified as 'free from preservatives'. In the past, widely used preservatives were phenol and thiomersal.

Stabilisers are added to vaccines to bulk up the small amounts of antigens included in them and to protect against temperature changes during transportation and storage. Examples include proteins (such as gelatine), sugars (such as sucrose) and amino acids (such as glycine).

Components in vaccines that are left over in trace amounts by the manufacturing process are called residuals. These include, for example, residual cell-culture materials (such as egg protein) and compounds to inactivate toxins or kill viruses included in the vaccine (e.g., formaldehyde). Due to the way vaccines are manufactured (using biological products from animals and humans), micro-organisms from these hosts may inadvertently be included in the vaccine. An example is porcine circovirus found in rotavirus vaccines.

1.3 Vaccine potency, stability, immunogenicity and safety

In this section, we define the terms describing key attributes of vaccines. 'Potency' of a vaccine refers to the amount of immunogenic agents (and, in the case of live-attenuated vaccines, their viability) included in a dose (see Box 1.4).

Box 1.4 Vaccine potency

Vaccine potency is defined as the amount of antigen included in a vaccine dose. The unit used to indicate the amount of antigen depends on the type of antigen and which assay is used to assess potency. Potency assessments are quite variable, and reference reagents are therefore used for standardisation. Below we give some examples of potency units.

The potency of live-attenuated vaccines is called their 'titre', which is expressed in $TCID_{50}$ ('tissue culture infective dose 50', indicating the dilution of a virus suspension that will infect 50% of cell cultures), $CCID_{50}$ ('cell culture infective dose 50') or PFUs ('plaque forming units'), whereby a plaque is a circular zone of infected cells in a monolayer cell culture representative of one infective virus particle.

The potency of killed/subunit vaccines against bacteria is usually expressed in IU ('international units' of potency as determined in animal tests) or weight (μg) of the antigen included in a single dose.

The potency of inactivated polio vaccine is expressed in DU (appropriate 'D-antigen units') of a single dose.

The potency of BCG vaccine is expressed as the number of live particles in a single dose.

Vaccines lose their potency over time, and this process is hastened by inadequate storage. Temperature and light are key determinants of this: vaccines may lose their potency when they become too hot or too cold (see Box 1.5), or if they are exposed to light for too long. The sensitivity to extreme temperatures and light varies between vaccines. The stability of a vaccine is defined as its ability to sustain its potency under different conditions of storage. Chapter 11 provides an example where inadequate storage was the likely cause of a measles outbreak.

Box 1.5 The vaccine 'cold chain'

A vaccine's potency can diminish when it is kept at inappropriate (too high or too low) temperatures. The term 'cold chain' refers to all points of storage and transport between them, from manufacture to use of the vaccine, where the appropriate temperature range (as indicated in the SmPC, usually at +2 to +8 °C) must be maintained. The storage requirements for the first licensed mRNA vaccines against COVID-19 (coronavirus disease 2019) are exceptional (ranging from –20 to –80 °C). Vaccine vial monitors containing heat-sensitive material can be used on vaccine vials to indicate excessive cumulative heat exposure. Of note, an important cause for some vaccines to lose their potency in the field is when they freeze at the back of refrigerators, a problem that is not detected by vaccine vial monitors (Figure 1.1).

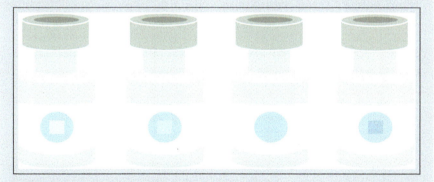

Figure 1.1 Vaccine vials with vaccine vial monitors.
Note: The monitor on the two left vials indicates that they have not been exposed to excessive heat. The indicator on the right two bottles indicates excessive heat exposure with likely loss of potency of the vaccine.

The ability of a vaccine to induce an immune response is called its immunogenicity. Determinants of immunogenicity are reviewed in Chapter 2.

Safety of a vaccine refers to its intrinsic potential to cause, trigger or worsen adverse events. Reactogenicity of a vaccine refers to its potential to cause a subset of adverse events that occur soon after vaccination and that are physical manifestations of the inflammatory response to vaccination. This can include injection site local reactions such as pain, redness or swelling, or systemic reactions such as fever, myalgia or headache. Tolerability of a vaccine is the opposite of its reactogenicity. The topic of adverse events following immunisation (AEFI) is further described in Chapters 2 and 17–20.

Potency, immunogenicity and safety are all determined by the vaccine's antigenic, adjuvant and other content and the way the vaccine was stored. In contrast to potency, immunogenicity and safety are also determined by characteristics of the vaccine's recipient and the way the vaccine was administered.

Most currently licensed vaccines have been developed by trial and error rather than by evidence-based design, since the way the immune system works was, at their time of development, to a large extent unknown. Potency is one factor that has been adjusted downwards to limit the amount of antigen needed, or upwards to increase immunogenicity. An example where this went wrong is the development of high-titre measles vaccines (Box 1.6). Their effect to increase mortality in girls only became apparent after their use in vaccination programmes, emphasising the importance of continued monitoring of benefits and risks throughout the lifetime of vaccination programmes.

Box 1.6 High-titre measles vaccines

The immunogenicity of measles vaccines increases, up to a certain age, with age at administration. This is thought to be due to maturation of the infant's immune system and the decrease of maternal antibodies in the infant over time.

Since young infants are an important risk group for measles, attempts were made to overcome this reduced immunogenicity by increasing the potency of measles vaccines. During the 1980s, several trials of high-titre measles vaccines reported good results in children as young as 4 months of age.

This led the World Health Organization (WHO) in 1989 to recommend high-titre measles vaccines ($>10^{4.7}$ PFU) be used for children of 6 months of age in areas of high measles incidence, in refugee camps and for HIV-infected children. This recommendation was withdrawn in 1992, after reports from several countries demonstrated increases in female mortality after the receipt of high-titre measles vaccines. To date, there is no consensus on the causes of this increased mortality among girls (Aaby, Jensen, Simondon, & Whittle, 2003).

1.4 Routes of administration of vaccines

Currently licensed vaccines can be administered by injection, ingestion or inhalation (see Box 1.7). The recommended route of administration is usually determined in pre-licensure studies (see Section 1.5) considering immunogenicity and safety. Oral and intranasal vaccines are also called 'mucosal vaccines', since they enter the body via a mucosal membrane. For some diseases, different vaccines with contrasting routes of administration are licensed (e.g., poliomyelitis and influenza).

> **Box 1.7 Vaccine administration routes with examples**
>
> *Injection (parenteral)*
>
> *Intramuscular (in a muscle)*: diphtheria, tetanus, acellular pertussis, *Haemophilus influenzae* type b, hepatitis B, inactivated polio and meningococcal conjugate vaccines.
>
> *Subcutaneous (under the skin)*: measles, mumps, rubella, varicella and herpes zoster vaccines.
>
> *Intradermal (in the skin)*: BCG vaccine, smallpox vaccine.
>
> *Oral (in the mouth)*: rotavirus vaccines, oral polio vaccines, some cholera and typhoid vaccines.
>
> *Intranasal (in the nose)*: live-attenuated influenza vaccine.

Adjuvant-containing vaccines are usually injected in the muscle to avoid local side effects in the skin, while the less reactogenic live viral vaccines can be administered subcutaneously, which has the advantage of a lower risk of local neurovascular injury. Mucosal vaccines (administered orally or intranasally) have several important advantages: their administration is needle-free and painless, avoiding the risk of transmission of blood-borne viruses. They can also be relatively good at inducing mucosal immunity (see Chapter 2). Unfortunately, most vaccines still need to be injected. Microneedles are an upcoming and promising, but not yet licensed, method of administration of vaccines.

1.5 Vaccine trials and licensure of vaccines

The life of a new vaccine starts by setting out a rationale for its use (Figure 1.2). When pre-clinical research with an experimental product has led to promising results, clinical trials with a batch prepared under good manufacturing practice and released for use in humans are needed to provide evidence for licensure. These trials can be distinguished into four types ('phases'), differing in design and the main end points studied (see Figure 1.2 and Box 1.8).

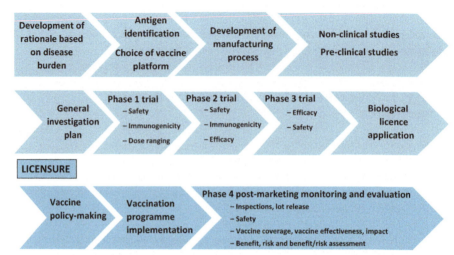

Figure 1.2 **Steps in the development and licensure of new vaccines.**
Source: Adapted from Plotkin et al. (2018, chap. 79).

Box 1.8 Vaccine trials: phase I, II, III and IV

Vaccine trials are conducted prior to licensure of a new vaccine for routine use, to obtain evidence on its safety, immunogenicity and efficacy. They share very many characteristics with clinical trials of other pharmaceutical products and are regulated by the same national and international authorities (see Box 1.10). Phase I trials are the first trials in humans and are typically small experiments undertaken in healthy adult volunteers to assess safety as the primary end point. Phase II trials are undertaken in the target population (e.g., children) but are small scale (up to a few hundred participants), focusing on safety and measuring the immune response to different doses and perhaps different candidate vaccines. Phase III trials are full-scale efficacy and safety trials and typically involve tens of thousands of participants. Post-licensure studies are sometimes called phase IV trials – but they are not experimental trials in the same sense as phase I, II and III trials.

Phase II and phase III trials are usually double-blind, randomised controlled studies. The control arm of the trial may receive a placebo or a vaccine in current use. If the comparison group receives a vaccine that protects against the same infection as the study vaccine, the trial may be a superiority or non-inferiority study, designed to demonstrate that the new vaccine is superior or not inferior to the vaccine currently in use, respectively. The latter is relevant when the study vaccine has additional benefits such as fewer adverse events or lower costs. In vaccine trials, participants are selected using clearly defined entry and exclusion criteria. At all trial phases, participants are monitored intensively according to strict, predetermined protocols to meet the exacting standards of regulatory authorities. Further information about the design and conduct of vaccine trials may be found in (Halloran, Longini, & Struchiner, 2010) and (Farrington & Miller, 2003). Adaptive trial designs, potentially combining several phases into a single study, are gaining popularity.

The process from development of the vaccine to its use in vaccination programmes usually takes over 10 years. However, in the case of, for example, Ebola and COVID-19 vaccines this process was much accelerated (see Box 1.9).

Box 1.9 The development and licensure of Ebola vaccines

The devastating Ebola virus outbreak in several West-African countries in 2014–2015 brought together multiple stakeholders involved in vaccine development, licensure and funding to make Ebola vaccines available for outbreak control in an unprecedented short period of time. Whereas in the 38 years since the discovery of Ebola virus there had only been four completed phase I trials, during the 2014–2015 outbreak phase III trials of new vaccines were initiated only months after these vaccines were first administered to humans (Venkatraman, Silman, Folegatti, & Hill, 2018).

From a vaccination programme point of view, the moment of licensure (also called 'marketing authorisation') is the key milestone in the development of a new vaccine, since from that moment on it can be marketed and used in national vaccination programmes. Companies, firms or non-profit organisations can be called marketing authorisation holders, which means they are allowed to market a specific medicinal product.

Licensure of vaccines is generally done by national, regional or global regulatory authorities (see Box 1.10), who review all available evidence on the product's safety, quality and efficacy to assess if this is acceptable. WHO carries out a specific type of licensure of vaccines, called 'pre-qualification'. This is a similar process of assuring the quality of new vaccines, after which these can be procured by United Nations (UN) agencies (such as the UN Children's Fund (UNICEF)) without the need for approval by other regulatory authorities. This process was developed to facilitate access to vaccines for national vaccination programmes in countries without an adequately functioning national regulatory authority.

> **Box 1.10 Vaccine licensing authorities: examples**
>
> - *National regulatory authorities (NRAs)*: such as the Food and Drug Administration (FDA) in the United States, the China Food and Drug Administration (CFDA), the Medicines Evaluation Board (MEB) in the Netherlands, the Tanzania Food and Drugs Authority (TFDA) and the National Administration of Drugs, Food and Medical Technologies (ANMAT) in Argentina.
> - *Regional medicine regulatory authority (Europe)*: the European Medicines Agency (EMA) evaluates market authorisation applications, and subsequently sends the resulting scientific opinion to the European Commission (EC). The EC may then issue a market authorisation.
> - *Global regulatory authority*: WHO, who can issue a 'pre-qualification'.

1.6 Vaccine manufacturing

The manufacturing of vaccines started by individual researchers in the early 19th century, some of whom did so for commercial purposes. The first vaccine companies were set up in the early 20th century, at a time when national public health institutes also started producing vaccines.

Vaccine manufacture usually requires more capital and investments than the production of other pharmaceutical products due to increasingly stringent regulatory directives. This has limited the involvement of public health institutes and smaller companies in vaccine manufacturing over time. Currently four large companies (GlaxoSmithKline (GSK), Merck, Pfizer and Sanofi) hold nearly the entire world market share of vaccines. From a public health point of view, this trend is unfavourable since these large companies are unlikely to cater for niche markets needing vaccines. Furthermore, vaccine prices are increased by reduced competition. This landscape is changing rapidly due to mergers and the arrival of new companies. Vaccine manufacturers in low- and middle-income countries, such as India, China, Brazil and Indonesia, are emerging.

Summary

- Vaccines were invented by trying to replicate disease-induced immunity while avoiding the disease.
- Variolation, in which material from smallpox pustules was introduced into the skin of another person to induce smallpox immunity, can be considered the first form of vaccination.
- Currently used vaccines include (genetic material coding for) antigens and other components. Antigens induce the immune system to generate a specific response. Antigens used in vaccines are derived from (components of) the targeted (or a closely related) pathogen.

- In addition to their content, the design of vaccines also determines their effects and safety. Currently licensed vaccine platforms are based on live-attenuated micro-organisms, killed (components of) micro-organisms, viral vectors and mRNA.
- Key attributes of vaccines include potency, immunogenicity and safety. All of these are determined by the content of the vaccine, their design and the way it was stored. Immunogenicity and safety are also determined by characteristics of the vaccine's recipient and the way the vaccine was administered.
- Currently licensed vaccines can be administered by injection (in the muscle, skin or under the skin), by ingestion or by inhalation. The latter two routes of administration of vaccines are referred to as mucosal vaccination.
- Vaccines can only be used in vaccination programmes after they have been licensed by a (national, regional or global) regulatory authority.
- Nowadays, vaccines are mostly manufactured by pharmaceutical companies, also called marketing authorisation holders.

References

Aaby, P., Jensen, H., Simondon, F., & Whittle, H. (2003). High-titer measles vaccination before 9 months of age and increased female mortality: Do we have an explanation? *Seminars in Pediatric Infectious Diseases*, *14*(3), 220–232. Retrieved from www.ncbi.nlm.nih.gov/pubmed/12913835.

Boylston, A. (2012). The origins of inoculation. *Journal of the Royal Society of Medicine*, *105*(7), 309–313. doi:10.1258/jrsm.2012.12k044.

Farrington, P., & Miller, E. (2003). Clinical trials. In A. P. Robinson, M. P. Cranage, & M. J. Hudson (Eds.), *Methods in molecular medicine: Vaccine protocols* (pp. 335–351). Totowa, NJ: Humana Press.

Halloran, M. E., Longini, I. M., & Struchiner, C. J. (2010). *Design and analysis of vaccine studies*. New York: Springer.

Plotkin, S. A., Orenstein, W. A., Offit, P. A., & Edwards, K. M. (Eds.) (2018). *Plotkin's vaccines* (7th ed.). Philadelphia, PA: Elsevier.

Venkatraman, N., Silman, D., Folegatti, P. M., & Hill, A. V. S. (2018). Vaccines against Ebola virus. *Vaccine*, *36*(36), 5454–5459. doi:10.1016/j.vaccine.2017.07.054.

Chapter 2

How vaccines work
Immune responses and vaccine failure

Vaccines work by inducing immunity, which is the body's ability to protect itself against infectious diseases. This protection arises through diverse processes taking place in the body's immune system. The immune response can prevent or clear an infection, which also results in the absence of infectiousness. The immune response may also only modify an infection by preventing or reducing the severity of disease manifestations. In this case, immunity may not prevent infectiousness.

For vaccine-preventable diseases where natural infection provides life-long immunity (such as smallpox, measles and rubella), vaccines aim to stimulate the immune system in a similar way as natural infection does. These vaccines are generally very effective and provide life-long immunity. For infections that do not induce long-term immunity (such as malaria and respiratory syncytial virus infection), vaccines have to induce immune mechanisms other than those involved in natural infection to be effective.

We start this chapter by providing a brief overview of the body's immune system and the main effector mechanisms activated by vaccination. We then describe how the presence of vaccine-induced immunity can be assessed. We end this chapter by describing types of vaccine failure and the importance of distinguishing these when monitoring vaccination programmes. Detailed information on the immunology of vaccine responses is available in *Plotkin's Vaccines* (Plotkin, Orenstein, Offit, & Edwards, 2018) and in the World Health Organization (WHO) series 'The Immunological Basis for Immunization' (WHO, 2020).

2.1 The immune system

The body's immune system is comprised of structures, free-ranging cells and molecules working together to protect against infectious diseases (see Box 2.1). The immune system can also cause diseases when it attacks the body's own cells in autoimmunity or when it overreacts causing allergies.

DOI: 10.4324/9781315166414-3
This Chapter has been made available under a CC-BY-NC-ND license.

Box 2.1 The main components of the immune system

- *Structures (organs, tissues and vessels)*: such as the thymus, bone marrow, mucosal tissues, lymph nodes and lymphatic vessels.
- *Free-ranging cells*: such as phagocytes, antigen presenting cells and lymphocytes (e.g., B cells and T cells).
- *Molecules*: such as antimicrobial proteins, complement-associated molecules, cytokines (e.g., interferons), antibodies and cytotoxic molecules.

Infection and vaccination induce immunity by stimulating the immune system to produce certain molecules and cells that limit the replication of pathogens or inactivate their toxins. Mounting an immune response to non-self substances can be lifesaving. To avoid the risk of self-attack, immune responses are carefully regulated.

Not all exposures to foreign substances lead to an immune response. First, there needs to be an effective exposure, meaning the body's natural barriers such as the skin have been breached. Second, the structures included in the substance need to be capable of inducing an immune response.

Immune responses can be divided into non-specific and specific processes, mediated by the innate and adaptive parts of the immune system, respectively. Innate immunity is present from birth and is fast, taking minutes to hours to respond after detecting classes of molecules representing an alarming situation. These can be 'pathogen-associated molecular patterns' (PAMPs), indicating the presence of a pathogen, or 'danger-associated molecular patterns' (DAMPs), indicating tissue damage. Until recently, the innate immune system was regarded as not having memory. Nowadays we know that it can be trained to a certain extent by encounters with particular pathogens or vaccines to maintain a higher level of alertness: this is called trained innate immunity. This phenomenon underlies non-specific effects (NSE) of vaccination, an area of much scientific debate.

Adaptive immunity is acquired, responses taking days to weeks to develop, generally recognising molecules unique for one organism (or a group of closely related organisms), known as 'antigens'. Adaptive immune responses acquired throughout life are maintained in the form of immune memory. This immune memory gives the adaptive immune system a head start in case an antigen is re-encountered upon infection. This secondary adaptive immune response will be very fast and highly vigorous, which is the principal mechanism behind vaccine-induced immune protection.

Adaptive immunity is the result of humoral and cellular immune responses, both of which are described in what follows. The assessment of immunity by laboratory testing is mostly done by assessing the humoral immune response in serum, since this is relatively straightforward to standardise. This has contributed to the misconception that the serological response is the main effector mechanism for immunity. The importance of mucosal and cell-mediated immunity is often overlooked just because they are more problematic to measure. The advantage of assessing the humoral response, however, is that for many vaccines it correlates with the inducement of immunity in general. Chapter 9 provides more information on correlates for protection.

Both the innate and adaptive immune response include the production and activation of certain molecules and cells. The key molecules involved in the innate response are antimicrobial proteins, complement-associated molecules and interferons, while main cell types are phagocytes and cells capable of antigen presentation. The main molecules of the adaptive immune response are antibodies and cytokines, the main cell types being lymphocytes (a type of white blood cell). There are three key types of lymphocytes involved in inducing and sustaining immunity: B cells, T helper cells and cytotoxic T cells. These are the major cell types among the peripheral blood mononuclear cell (PBMC) fraction of blood.

Innate and adaptive immunological processes are usually activated in parallel but there is important crosstalk: the magnitude and quality of the innate immune response strongly influence the magnitude and effectiveness of the adaptive immune response. The rest of this chapter is dedicated to adaptive immune responses, as vaccine-induced immunity is mainly derived through those.

2.2 The humoral immune response: antibodies

Most current vaccines provide protection by stimulating the immune system to produce specific antibodies. This is called the humoral immune response. Antibodies are proteins of the immunoglobulin (Ig) family that can help to clear pathogens and can inactivate toxins. They can do this only to pathogens that are present outside the body's cells (extracellular pathogens). This explains why vaccines against intracellular pathogens such as tuberculosis and HIV will not work if based only on antibody production. Intracellular pathogens require cell-mediated immunity as well (see Section 2.3).

Antibodies are Y-shaped molecules produced by plasma cells, which are B lymphocytes (B cells) that have differentiated to become effector cells. With their tail, antibodies interact with receptors on innate immune phagocytes. With their head, the antibody molecule can specifically bind to an antigen: the relation between the antibody and the antigen can be thought of as that between a lock and a key, although cross-reactivity does occur (see Box 2.2).

Box 2.2 Cross-reactivity

The specific immune system is characterised by activation in response to specific antigens. In addition to this, the specific immune response induced by certain vaccines can also provide protection against other non-targeted, but related, antigens or, in some cases, unrelated pathogens. 'Cross-reactivity' refers to reactivity of vaccine-induced antibodies or cell-mediated immunity against non-targeted subtypes of the targeted pathogen or an unrelated pathogen. Cross-reactivity may lead to cross-protection.

An example of cross-reactivity is of specific antibodies mounted against serotype 6B of the pneumococcus, which are also somewhat reactive against serotype 6A, or of smallpox vaccine that is based on vaccinia (cowpox) virus but also induces protection against smallpox and monkeypox. Whereas many examples of cross-reactivity are advantageous, there are also negative implications. Cross-reactivity of vaccine-induced immunity against 'self' antigens in the human body can cause damage. Furthermore, when occurring in diagnostic tests, cross-reactivity of antibodies can give false-positive results.

To recognise an antigen, each B cell expresses a unique receptor on its surface. B cell receptors are in fact antibody molecules still attached to the cell. The immune system creates billions of different B cell clones, each with a unique receptor and antigen specificity. Upon exposure to an antigen, B cells specifically recognising the antigen get stimulated and start a B cell response. This response includes differentiation of B cells into so-called plasma cells that produce and secrete high levels of specific antibodies. The B cell response can be either dependent or independent from help by T cells. Antigens that are able to induce both B and T cell responses are generally better at inducing long-lasting immunity than those eliciting only B cell responses (see Box 2.3).

Box 2.3 B cell responses to vaccination: T-dependent and T-independent antigens

The B cell response, leading to the production of antibodies, can be T-dependent or T-independent. The type of antigen and type of B cell determines which of these is activated. Only T-dependent B cell responses involve maturation of antibodies (see Box 2.5), form long-lasting antibody production and produce B cell memory. The key differences between these responses are outlined in Table 2.1.

Table 2.1 Main differences between T-independent and T-dependent B cell responses

T-independent B cell response	T-dependent B cell response
Mainly elicited by polysaccharide antigens	Mainly elicited by protein antigens, toxoids, inactivated or attenuated live viral vaccines, but also by polysaccharide antigens when conjugated to a protein
Rapid response (days), short-lived	Slow response (weeks), long-lived
Limited class switch, no affinity maturation of antibodies (see Box 2.5)	Class switch, affinity maturation of antibodies (see Box 2.5)
Low-affinity antibodies produced by short-lived plasma cells	High-affinity antibodies produced by long-lived plasma cells
No induction of immune B cell memory	Induction of immune B cell memory
Relatively ineffective in children <2 years of age	Relatively effective at all ages

An important benefit of vaccines that induce T-dependent B cell responses is that they are effective in young infants, a crucial requirement when aiming to prevent infections that occur in early childhood. Antigens that induce a T-independent response can be transformed into T-dependent antigens by coupling (conjugating) them to a carrier protein, a technique used in conjugate vaccines. Strikingly, some of these conjugate vaccines lead to a better immune response than natural infection, explaining, for example, why cases of meningococcal C disease benefit from meningococcal C vaccination upon their recovery.

Five isotypes of antibodies (IgD, IgM, IgG, IgA and IgE) have been identified, differing by the structure of their tail. Nearly all currently licensed vaccines work via the production of IgG, which is present in serum and plasma, saliva and on mucosal surfaces. Exceptions to this include BCG (Bacille Calmette-Guérin vaccine against tuberculosis (TB)) and varicella zoster vaccine, which work by inducing cell-mediated immunity. Vaccines may also induce IgA antibodies, which control viral shedding on mucosal surfaces (see Section 2.4) and are also present in a woman's colostrum and milk. The other three antibody classes (IgM, IgD and IgE) do not form a major part of the sustained immune response following vaccination.

For some diseases, administration of antibodies derived from human serum can also provide immunity. This is called passive immunisation (see Chapter 1). During pregnancy, some types of antibodies can cross the placenta, and, once in the foetus or infant, are called maternal antibodies (see Box 2.4).

Box 2.4 Maternal antibodies

During pregnancy, active transfer of antibodies in the pregnant woman's blood through the placenta protects the newborn and young infant against infections in early life. The largest amounts of antibodies are transferred during the third trimester.

After birth, maternal antibodies decay in the infant; the period they are present mainly depends on the antibody concentration in the mother's serum. The latter can be increased by vaccination in pregnancy (called 'maternal vaccination', see Chapter 3). The presence of maternal antibodies may inhibit the immune response to vaccines in infants, an effect that varies by vaccine.

If the antibody concentration in the mother's serum is higher when induced by natural infection rather than by vaccination, infants of vaccinated mothers become susceptible sooner after birth than infants of mothers who have had natural infection. Measles is an example of a disease where this was shown to be relevant (Waaijenborg et al., 2013). This may require modifying the vaccine schedule, by lowering the recommended age for the first vaccine dose.

The production of antibodies by the immune system 'matures' over time since the exposure to an antigen, even in the absence of repeated exposure. This means that antibodies become better at binding antigens, which is expressed by characteristics called 'affinity' and 'avidity' (see Box 2.5). This maturation provides a key explanation as to why immunity following exposure to antigens (in pathogens or vaccines) is so effective: upon a second encounter, B cells have matured and hence produce antibodies of relatively high affinity that are very functional. Signals to B cells by a certain type of T cell are essential for this maturation to happen (see Box 2.3).

Box 2.5 Maturation of antibodies: affinity, avidity maturation and isotype switching

During T-dependent B cell responses (Box 2.3), daughter cells of proliferating B cells can acquire specific functions, such as becoming antibody-secreting plasma cells or memory B cells. In a T-dependent response, B cells can also alter the gene segments encoding their antibody molecules: for the head part of the antibody molecule this process is called somatic hypermutation, while for the tail part it is called isotype switching. This improves the binding capacity of the antibody and its functionality, respectively.

The head part, or so-called antigen binding fragment (Fab), is capable of binding with each of its mirror ends to an antigen by making a connection with an epitope (which is the part of an antigen that the immune system can recognise). The strength of this binding per epitope is called the antibody's affinity. The total strength of the bond between an antibody molecule and an antigen is called the antibody's avidity. Avidity may be larger than the sum of affinities when a favourable repeated structural arrangement of epitopes is present or when antibodies form multimers, such as the pentameric IgM isotype. Affinity and avidity are important markers for how well the antibody is able to clear the antigen. In practice, affinity is difficult to measure whereas for avidity certain assays exist (see Box 2.9).

With its tail part, or so-called constant fragment (Fc), the antibody communicates with cells of the innate immune system that have receptors for these Fc tails. An increasing number of antibody-mediated immune mechanisms are being recognised, including virus neutralisation, antibody-dependent cellular cytotoxicity, antibody-dependent cellular phagocytosis, opsonophagocytosis and serum bactericidal activity (Lu, Suscovich, Fortune, & Alter, 2018). This research field is called systems serology.

Higher-affinity antibodies can be produced as time since exposure to antigens increases, an effect called 'affinity maturation'. As this maturation takes time, a certain minimum interval between the first and subsequent vaccine doses (see Box 2.8) is required for an optimal response. In general, the affinity and avidity of antibodies is an indicator of the quality of the immune response, meaning how well the pathogen can be destroyed and how long the immunity may last.

2.3 Cell-mediated immunity

In addition to stimulating B cells to differentiate into antibody producing plasma cells or become memory B cells, vaccines also work through T cells, leading to what is called cell-mediated (or cellular) immunity. Certain types of T cells can directly kill pathogen-infected cells ('cytotoxic T cells', also called 'CD8$^+$ T cells'). Others ('T helper cells' or 'CD4$^+$ T cells') have important supporting functions for the development and regulation of T-dependent B cell responses (see Box 2.3). T cells have a particular mode of detecting the presence of foreign antigens (see Box 2.6).

Box 2.6 Antigen recognition in T cell responses

While antibodies patrol extracellular spaces in the body for the presence of pathogens, T cells control the intracellular stages of infections and have mechanisms to clear infected cells. Similar to B cells, each T cell expresses a unique receptor on its cell surface. The immune system creates billions of different T cell clones, each with a unique receptor and antigen specificity. When recognising a protein antigen, T cells are stimulated and start dividing and differentiating, strongly influenced by ongoing innate immune responses. T cells become either effector cells (mediating functions such as producing cytokines) or memory cells (rapidly reacting and being activated by subsequent antigen encounters).

Whereas B cells recognise proteins as whole intact antigens, T cells only react to proteins once they are chopped up by proteases inside antigen presenting cells and exposed as a short linear peptide epitope (size range of 8–11 amino acids) bound to a molecule of the major histocompatibility complex (MHC) at the outer surface of those cells.

Each MHC gene locus has numerous variants in the population. This polymorphism has consequences for the peptide binding preferences of the MHC molecules, resulting in highly individual sets of peptide epitopes presented via the inherited MHC alleles of a single person. T cells from a single person are selected to only recognise foreign peptides in the context of the person's own MHC molecules, called MHC-restricted T cell recognition of antigen. Different peptide epitopes of a single protein antigen can be presented on antigen presenting cells, in the context of different MHC molecules or even of a single one. While at the level of the individual, antigen recognition may consist of completely unique T cell clones responding to a personal MHC-presented peptide repertoire, at the population level protein antigens from pathogens or vaccines will be presented by the majority of MHC molecules and trigger T cell immunity. Certain MHC alleles or sets of alleles may predispose for disease, such as susceptibility for or resistance to infectious diseases, or autoimmunity. Low-responsiveness to certain vaccines (e.g., hepatitis B vaccine) may also have an MHC-related aetiology.

2.4 Systemic and mucosal immunity

The humoral and cellular immune responses just described can be systemic, meaning that they take place in normally sterile sites throughout the body, where cells and molecules are transported by the blood and lymphatic circulation system. They can also take place in certain compartments of the body, for example in a particular organ, in the skin or in one of the body's mucosae and associated lymphoid tissues. Mucosae are mucous tissues lining the respiratory, gastrointestinal and urogenital tract, as well as the inner ear, the eye conjunctiva and ducts of endocrine glands. Since most infections start at and are propagated from mucosae, immune processes leading to mucosal immunity are key mechanisms against infection and infectiousness.

Mucosal immunity is generated essentially independently from the systemic immune response. It is for an important part derived from the local production of a specific form of IgA ('secretory IgA'), which is exclusively present on mucosae and has special properties to be functional there (Holmgren & Czerkinsky, 2005). Locally produced IgA and IgG antibodies also contribute to mucosal immunity, while IgG may also arrive at mucosae by a process called transudation from serum. The IgG concentration in serum is a main determinant of the IgG concentration on mucosae, whereby IgG transudation is more effective in respiratory and urogenital than in gastrointestinal mucosae. Cellular mucosal immunity mainly consists of B, T helper and cytotoxic T cells.

Mucosal immunity can be induced by vaccines irrespective of their mode of delivery. However, vaccines directly administered at a mucosal site ('mucosal vaccines'), for example by administering them in the nose or mouth, are especially capable of inducing mucosal immunity. Licensed mucosal vaccines are by far outnumbered by vaccines that need to be injected. However, as explained above, the latter can also induce mucosal immunity by transudation of IgG. Human papillomavirus (HPV) vaccination, for example, induces such high IgG concentrations that sufficient IgG concentrations are formed in the vaginal mucosa to clear HPV viruses targeted by the vaccine. Live-attenuated viral vaccines, such as oral polio vaccine (OPV) but also measles, mumps and rubella (MMR) vaccine (that needs to be injected), are particularly able to induce secretory IgA, which explains why they generally are highly efficacious. Importantly, mucosal vaccines generally work less well in developing rather than affluent country settings, owing to mechanisms not entirely understood.

2.5 Implications of mucosal and systemic immunity to prevent infection and infectiousness

As mentioned above, most infections start at one of the body's mucosal sites, where (potentially) pathogenic microbes can colonise, may replicate or produce toxins. When there is insufficient mucosal immunity, microbes can invade through the mucosae, eventually reaching the blood circulation system and, through this, their preferential sites of infection. Poliovirus, for example, having invaded through the intestinal mucosae, may lead to viremia after which it can specifically attack the nervous system.

By interfering at different stages of these pathogenic processes, vaccine-induced immunity may prevent, limit, clear or modify infection. When a vaccine is able to induce sufficient levels of mucosal immunity, it has the potential not only to block infection of the vaccine recipient, but also to prevent replication and shedding of the pathogen from the mucosal surfaces, and by doing so prevent the pathogen from being transmitted to others. Through this mechanism, vaccination can cause indirect protection (also known as 'herd immunity', see Chapter 4).

Some pathogens colonise the mucosa of healthy individuals in their microbiomes (the community of micro-organisms in certain body sites such as the nasopharynx), and this is seldom followed by invasive infection. Examples of this are pneumococci and meningococci. For these pathogens, the capability of a vaccine to induce mucosal immunity is of special public health relevance, as it may prevent carriage and thereby reduce the reservoir and hence transmission of pathogens in the population. This can induce a strong herd-immunity effect, as the prevalence of carriage in unvaccinated individuals can be considerable. Another implication of mucosal immunity is, however, that through effectively depleting the microbiome of certain microbes, it may cause others to fill in the niche (see 'serotype replacement' in Chapter 5).

Vaccine-induced systemic immunity works by attacking the pathogen once it has reached normally sterile sites – either by invading through a mucosal lining or by penetrating the skin. Systemic immunity may lead to complete clearance of the pathogen from the body, which then also contributes to indirect protection of others. It may also modify the course of infection, for example by preventing severe disease or complications. In this situation, it is less likely to provide indirect protection, as propagation of the pathogen may still occur.

The different effects of vaccines on preventing infection and modifying disease may be assessed by laboratory studies measuring different mediators of immunity (e.g., antibodies and lymphocytes) at different body sites. Epidemiologic studies of vaccine effectiveness may provide an understanding of the particular type of protection a vaccine affords in real life. The main end points of these studies are the protection against colonisation, infection, clinical disease, progression to severe disease and infectiousness. Further information can be found in Chapter 12.

2.6 Persistence of immunity

Long-term vaccine-induced immunity arises when sustained antibody levels are present in serum and other body fluids or when immunological B and T cell memory is induced to reconstitute immunity. The latter mechanism can take some time and as a result its effectiveness depends on the targeted pathogen's incubation period (see Box 2.7).

Box 2.7 Long-lasting protection induced by vaccination

There are two main mechanisms through which the immune system can generate long-lasting protection following vaccination: by sustaining protective levels of antibodies in serum (by long-lived plasma cells) and by the inducement of immune memory (through long-lived B and T cells). Whether both are necessary for protection depends mainly on the length of the incubation period of the specific infection.

Meningococcal disease is an example of an infection with a relatively short incubation period, which, if left untreated, involves very rapid bacterial growth and extremely fast and often fatal disease progression. In this instance, vaccine-induced immune protection relies on the presence of adequate levels of specific antibodies in serum, since reconstituting these through immunological memory would be too slow: the memory immune response against the group C meningococcus takes between 5 and 7 days to develop while most invasive meningococcal disease occurs within a few days after exposure to the bacterium (Plotkin et al., 2018).

In contrast, hepatitis A and B viruses are pathogens with relatively long incubation periods of up to 50 and 150 days, respectively. Hepatitis A and B vaccines induce such a rapid and effective immune response that protection against infection by vaccination can even be achieved by post-exposure vaccination, provided it is given soon after exposure. Long-lasting protection against infectious diseases often requires the combination of both sustained levels of antibodies and the presence of immunological memory.

The inducement of immune memory enables the adaptive immune system to respond more rapidly and better (e.g., with antibodies of higher affinity; see Box 2.5) when it is exposed to a pathogen it has encountered previously. This memory response is antigen specific and is based on long-living B and T cells. It is the reason why the immune response to a second dose of a vaccine (the 'secondary response') differs in speed, quantity and quality from that elicited by the priming dose (the 'primary response') (see Box 2.8).

Box 2.8 Priming and boosting

The antibody response to primary and subsequent vaccine doses follows a generic pattern for most vaccines (with the exception of live-attenuated viral vaccines), as displayed in Figure 2.1. Key differences between the primary and secondary response are, apart from the ongoing maturation of antibodies (see Box 2.5), that upon a secondary antigen exposure, titres rise much faster and do not return to baseline levels. This is called a 'booster' response. A prerequisite for the inducement of an optimal booster response is that there is sufficient time between the first exposure ('priming') and the booster dose.

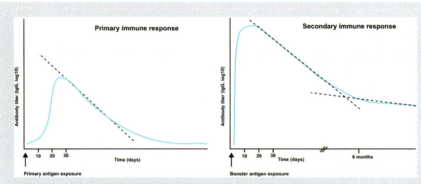

Figure 2.1 **Development of antibody titres over time since the primary exposure to an antigen (left panel) and since a booster exposure (right panel).**
Source: Adapted from Siegrist (2017).

2.7 Determinants of the immune response to vaccination and its persistence

The outcome of the immune response to vaccination is determined by the antigen(s) included in the vaccine, the vaccine's potency, included adjuvants, the vaccine delivery platforms, the route and vaccination schedule of administration and characteristics of the recipient (host factors). Host factors can be further classified as intrinsic factors (such as age, sex and genetic polymorphisms in the immune system), perinatal factors (such as birth weight and gestational age), maternal factors (such as malnutrition and the concentration of maternal antibodies), extrinsic factors (such as concurrent or previous infections), exposome (microbiome), nutritional, environmental and behavioural factors (Zimmermann & Curtis, 2019).

A key host factor determining the immune response to vaccination is age: the quantity and quality of the immune response increases up to a certain age, after which it decreases again. This decrease is due to a process called immunosenescence, which is a gradual alteration of the immune system caused by ageing. The optimal age for immunogenicity may extend into early adulthood, depending on which vaccine is used. The reduced antibody response in young infants can be due to the interference of maternal antibodies (Box 2.4) and the immaturity of the infant's immune system. The optimal age for providing the first dose of a certain vaccine requires balancing optimal immunogenicity against the risk of acquiring the infection, or complications from the infection. A limitation of many vaccines is that they are least immunogenic in the age range for which the consequences of infection are most severe. Influenza is a key example of this. For further information see Chapter 3 on vaccination schedules.

Determinants of the persistence of immunity include many of the determinants of immunogenicity listed at the start of this section. Nearly all vaccines require multiple doses for a long-lasting immune response. Important determinants of a persisting immune response are the type of antigen, the number of doses and the time between them, which relate to priming and boosting of particular adaptive B and T cell clones.

The steering role of innate immune stimuli in vaccines should not be underestimated. Live-attenuated viral vaccines can induce immunity lasting for decades while polysaccharide antigens provide only short-lived protection (see Box 2.3). For inactivated vaccines, a longer period between doses generally induces better persistence of immunity than shorter periods.

2.8 Assessing the immune response to vaccination

The immune response to vaccination in an individual can be assessed by various laboratory assays. These are used to assess, for example, immunogenicity in vaccine trials. From the point of view of evaluating vaccination programmes, these assays are mostly relevant for seroepidemiology (Chapter 9).

The most widely used tests to assess immunity are antibody assays used on serum, since this is a body material that has a relatively constant concentration of components compared to, for example, mucosal secretions that can be more or less diluted. Oral (subgingival) fluid is another material often used for antibody testing. To assess the antibody response to a vaccine, three different types or laboratory tests are available (see Box 2.9).

Box 2.9 Antibody tests: antibody-binding, avidity and functional assays

The presence and functionality of antibodies can be assessed by different types of laboratory assays. In general, functional antibody tests and avidity tests are more labour intensive and difficult to standardise than antibody-binding tests. Antibody-binding tests assess the serum concentration of an isotype or a subclass of antibodies directed against a specific antigen. This concentration can be interpreted as an indicator of immunity when a correlate for protection has been established (see Chapter 9). Examples include the enzyme-linked immunosorbent assay (ELISA or EIA) and the multiplex immunoassay (MIA), an antigen-multivalent bead-based form of ELISA.

Avidity tests measure the strength of the binding of antibodies to antigens, by adding different concentrations of an agent (such as thiocyanate or urea), which elutes the antibody from the antigen (see also Box 2.5).

Functional antibody tests provide an indication of the level of antibodies mediating a particular function, induced by the vaccine. They include neutralisation, serum bactericidal and opsonophagocytic assays:

- *Neutralisation* tests assess an antibody response by measuring how well a toxin or virus gets neutralised.
- *Serum bactericidal* assays measure to what extent bacteria are killed when different dilutions of serum are added.
- *Opsonophagocytic* assays also assess how well a serum kills bacteria. The difference with bactericidal assays is that in the opsonophagocytic assay the killing of bacteria occurs not directly by antibodies, but by certain

> immune cells (phagocytes) that require antibodies to facilitate (opsonise) this process.
>
> In addition to these, there are many more systems serology assays (see Box 2.5).

Assays for cell-mediated immunity include, for example, T cell stimulation tests. Since these are labour intensive, require antigens to be presented via MHC-restriction, and as standards and correlates of protection are lacking, they are not yet widely used to assess levels of population immunity.

A complicating factor in the assessment of vaccine-induced immunity is that for most vaccines used in humans, vaccine-induced immunity cannot be distinguished from immunity induced by natural infection (see Box 2.10 and also Chapter 9).

> ### Box 2.10 Differentiating vaccine-induced immunity from immunity induced by natural infection
>
> For most vaccines, antibodies arising from vaccination are indistinguishable from those induced by natural infection. Especially when there are no specific antibodies resulting only from either vaccination or infection, the interpretation of seroepidemiological studies is complicated (see Chapter 9). An exception to this is tetanus. Antibodies against tetanus toxin can only be induced by vaccination; they do not arise after tetanus infection. This does not hold for diphtheria, where anti-toxin antibodies are induced by both vaccination and natural infection.
>
> At a population level, the concentration of antibodies together with information on the history of vaccination and the incidence of the infection, may give an indication as to whether the immunity in certain birth cohorts is likely to be vaccine induced or the result of natural infection.
>
> For animals, where proof of vaccination is often a legal requirement for trade across countries, so-called differentiating infected from vaccinated animals (DIVA) vaccines are used that induce antibodies that can be differentiated from those induced by natural infection.

2.9 Vaccine failure

Vaccine failure is defined as the occurrence of a vaccine-preventable disease in a person who is appropriately and fully vaccinated, taking into account the incubation period and the normal delay for protection to be acquired as a result of immunisation (CIOMS, 2012). Vaccine-failure monitoring requires this definition to be adapted to local vaccine recommendations and the specific vaccine involved. There are two general types of vaccine failure: primary and secondary vaccine failure, defined in Box 2.11.

Box 2.11 Vaccine failure types

- *Primary vaccine failure*: occurrence of infection in a person who never responded to the receipt of a dose of vaccine targeted against that infection.
- *Secondary vaccine failure*: occurrence of infection in a person who responded to a vaccine but in whom immunity waned over time.

According to these definitions, the distinction between primary and secondary vaccine failure can seldom be made with certainty, since it requires an immune-response test result obtained soon after vaccination (which is usually not available).

Evidence pointing towards the type of vaccine failure can be obtained through specific laboratory testing following infection (see Box 2.12). However, this is usually not routinely done as part of diagnosing the infection, so information is unlikely to be available for surveillance purposes.

Box 2.12 Laboratory testing to differentiate between primary and secondary vaccine failure

Serological tests assessing the avidity and other characteristics of the antibody response can help to distinguish primary and secondary vaccine failure in vaccinated cases of a vaccine-preventable disease.

Low avidity of specific IgG and a slow IgG response combined with IgM positivity indicates that the case did not have an immunologic response to the vaccine prior to infection and hence suggests primary vaccine failure.

In contrast, detecting high-avidity antibodies, with a fast and strong IgG response and low or absent IgM levels, are suggestive of a previous immunological response to the vaccine, indicating secondary vaccine failure.

In addition to serological tests, the amount of virus excreted by the person with vaccine failure (as expressed by the 'viral load' in, for example, a throat swab) can also help to identify the type of vaccine failure: a high viral load suggests primary vaccine failure.

Monitoring the type and incidence of vaccine failure is important, since it may require immediate public health action. For example, a higher than expected rate of primary vaccine failure calls for an investigation into the reasons for it (see Chapter 11 on outbreak investigation). Occurrence of severe disease in cases of vaccine failure may indicate vaccine-associated enhanced disease (VAED) (see Chapter 17).

The expected frequency of secondary vaccine failure is likely to increase by time since vaccination. The assessment of the incidence of secondary vaccine failure therefore requires long-term follow-up studies. The occurrence of an unacceptable number of cases of secondary vaccine failure in a population may require a modification of the vaccination schedule, for example by including a different vaccine or (more) booster doses (see Chapter 3). Some of the methodological issues involved in assessing waning vaccine effectiveness are discussed in Chapter 16.

Summary

- Vaccines induce protection against infectious diseases by interacting with the body's immune system. The effect of the immune response can be to prevent or clear the infection, or modify it.
- Most current vaccines provide protection by stimulating the immune system to produce specific antibodies. This is called the 'humoral' immune response.
- Antibodies mature over time, which means they become better at binding antigens and acquire a particular function. Maturation is expressed by avidity, affinity and isotype or subclass.
- Cell-mediated immunity, operating through T cells, is also relevant for the protection induced by most vaccines, but more difficult to measure by laboratory assays than humoral immunity.
- The immune response can be systemic (taking place throughout the body) or take place at mucosae and associated lymphoid tissues.
- Mucosal immunity is of special relevance to the protection against infection and infectiousness, as most infections start at and are propagated from a mucosal site.
- Long-term vaccine-induced immunity results from the presence of sustained antibody levels in serum and/or when immunological memory in the form of vaccine antigen-specific memory B and T cells is present to reconstitute immunity.
- Immune memory allows the immune system to respond more rapidly and better when it is exposed to an antigen it has encountered previously. This is the main mechanism leading to vaccine-induced immunity.
- The quality of the immune response to vaccination is determined by the vaccine's composition, potency, platform, its administration (schedule) and characteristics of the recipient (particularly age).
- Antibody assays are the most widely used tests to assess the immune response to vaccination. For most vaccines, antibodies induced by vaccination cannot be distinguished by antibodies resulting from infection. Functional antibody assays are key in predicting protective qualities of antibodies.
- Vaccine failure is the occurrence of infection (or disease) in a person who received one or more doses of a vaccine according to the recommended schedule, with a defined time between the last dose and onset of disease.
- Vaccine failure can be primary or secondary. From a vaccination programme evaluation point of view, it is important to assess the type and frequency of vaccine failure since it determines the type of response needed.

References

Council for International Organizations of Medical Sciences (CIOMS). (2012). *Definition and application of terms for vaccine pharmacovigilance*. Retrieved from https://cioms.ch/wp-content/uploads/2017/01/report_working_group_on_vaccine_LR.pdf.

Holmgren, J., & Czerkinsky, C. (2005). Mucosal immunity and vaccines. *Nature Medicine, 11*(4 Suppl.), S45–S53. doi:10.1038/nm1213.

Lu, L. L., Suscovich, T. J., Fortune, S. M., & Alter, G. (2018). Beyond binding: Antibody effector functions in infectious diseases. *Nature Reviews Immunology, 18*(1), 46–61. doi:10.1038/nri.2017.106.

Plotkin, S. A., Orenstein, W. A., Offit, P. A., & Edwards, K. M. (Eds.) (2018). *Plotkin's vaccines* (7th ed.). Philadelphia, PA: Elsevier.

Siegrist, C. A. (2017). Vaccine immunology. In S. A. Plotkin, W. A. Orenstein, P. A. Offit, & K. M. Edwards (Eds.), *Plotkin's vaccines* (7th ed., pp. 16–34). Philadelphia, PA: Elsevier.

Waaijenborg, S., Hahné, S. J., Mollema, L., Smits, G. P., Berbers, G. A., van der Klis, F. R., ... Wallinga, J. (2013). Waning of maternal antibodies against measles, mumps, rubella, and varicella in communities with contrasting vaccination coverage. *Journal of Infectious Diseases, 208*(1), 10–16. doi:10.1093/infdis/jit143.

World Health Organization (WHO). (2020). The immunological basis for immunization series. Retrieved from http://apps.who.int/iris/.

Zimmermann, P., & Curtis, N. (2019). Factors that influence the immune response to vaccination. *Clinical Microbiology Reviews, 32*(2). doi:10.1128/CMR.00084-18.

Chapter 3

Vaccination programmes
Aims and strategies

The public health goal of vaccination is to reduce suffering and death from vaccine-preventable diseases and to improve equity in health. To achieve these aims, a programmatic approach is much more effective, efficient and safe than merely making vaccines available in a population. Such a programmatic approach is characterised by clearly defined and agreed upon aims of the vaccination programme, which determine the required strategy and characteristics of the programme and how it should be monitored and evaluated. Vaccination programmes are most effectively implemented when delivered free of charge to the target population through concerted public health policy, including guidelines, vaccination coverage and/or disease control targets, and a systematic approach to monitoring the programme's implementation and evaluation of its safety and effects. The term 'vaccination programme' can refer to programmes including multiple vaccines or just one. The latter is sometimes referred to as a vertical vaccination programme. Vaccination programmes are usually, except in some emergency situations, the responsibility of governments and can be implemented at national or regional level.

This chapter provides an introduction to vaccination programmes, and sets the context for the epidemiologic methods for monitoring and evaluating them. These methods are presented later in this book. This context provides the reader with a sense of the options available for disease control through vaccination programmes, and how and by whom decisions about such programmes are made. Knowing this context helps to understand the type of evidence from surveillance, outbreak investigations and dedicated epidemiological studies that may be needed. The context is also important for understanding to whom this evidence needs to be delivered, in order to support optimal decision-making for vaccination programmes.

We start this chapter with a brief overview of the history of programmatic vaccination. We then provide a theoretical background of the overall aims of vaccination programmes, and what determines an appropriate aim to be set. Subsequently, we describe different vaccination programme types and strategies, and how decisions about

DOI: 10.4324/9781315166414-4
This Chapter has been made available under a CC-BY-NC-ND license.

vaccine policy and adjustments to vaccination programmes are generally made. We then discuss the rationale for monitoring and evaluation of vaccination programmes and provide an overview of the roles of different stakeholders and international networks in this. We conclude this chapter by providing an overview of the options for modifying vaccination programmes.

3.1 History of vaccination programmes

The first programmatic use of vaccination appears to have been for military purposes in the 18th century, aiming to prevent the occurrence of smallpox epidemics among military troops. Some subsequent vaccination programmes were also first implemented among the military (see Box 3.1).

Box 3.1 Variolation and vaccination programmes for military purposes

Programmatic vaccination appears to have had a military origin. In the American Revolutionary War (1775–1783), army recruits were variolated after an order by George Washington. In the Franco-Prussian War in Europe in 1870, the German army was vaccinated against smallpox, which proved effective when a smallpox epidemic broke out. During the Boer War in the late 19th century in South Africa, an attempt was made to vaccinate British troops with a killed typhoid vaccine, the effectiveness of which was later demonstrated in a trial. Subsequently, this typhoid vaccine was again used for British troops in the First World War (Plotkin, Orenstein, Offit, & Edwards, 2018). In 2020, the first COVID-19 vaccination programme was implemented among military personnel in China (Lewis, 2020).

The first vaccination programmes for the general public rather than the military also targeted smallpox, and started in the early 19th century in Europe and North America (Hennock, 1998). Much later, during the 1950s, routine vaccination programmes against poliomyelitis, diphtheria and tetanus were initiated in many Western countries, which may be marked as the start of their national vaccination programmes. With new vaccines becoming available, most countries had nine or more vaccine antigens in their national schedules by 2018 (Cherian & Mantel, 2020).

An international vaccination programme is required when the aim of disease eradication has been set (see Section 3.2). To date, smallpox is the only human vaccine-preventable disease that has been eradicated (see Box 3.2). The second international programme aiming to eradicate a disease by vaccination targets poliomyelitis. This programme is ongoing (see Box 3.3).

Box 3.2 The smallpox eradication programme

When during the 1950s methods were optimised to produce large quantities of heat-stable smallpox vaccine, eradication of smallpox became a possibility. In 1966, the World Health Assembly (WHA), the decision-making body of World Health Organization (WHO), attended by delegations of all WHO member states, called for and sponsored the establishment of a smallpox eradication programme.

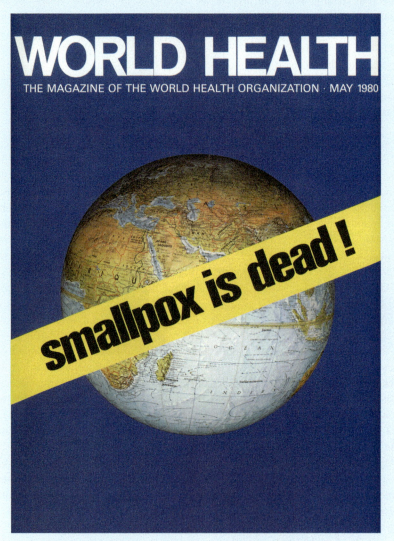

Figure 3.1 Cover of the May 1980 edition of *World Health*.
Source: Reproduced with permission from WHO (1980).

This programme was supported by vaccine donations from the United States and the Union of Soviet Socialist Republics (USSR), and was implemented with the help of many international and national organisations and individuals.

The basic strategy of the programme consisted of mass vaccination campaigns aiming to achieve protection for 80% of the population, weekly reporting of the number of cases with rapid containment of outbreaks by ring vaccination (see also Section 3.4 and Chapter 12) and the dissemination of regular and frequent surveillance reports to key stakeholders. In India and Bangladesh, the most challenging countries for smallpox eradication, intense surveillance in the form of house-by-house searches for cases was implemented (Henderson, 2011).

After 10 years of the programme and 2 years of certification processes, the WHA concluded on 8 May 1980 that smallpox had been eradicated and smallpox vaccination should cease in all countries (Figure 3.1).

Box 3.3 The programme to eradicate poliomyelitis

Poliomyelitis, caused by any of three poliovirus serotypes (1, 2 or 3), was in the pre-vaccine era a predominant cause of permanent disability. Two types of polio vaccines exist: oral polio vaccine (OPV, a live-attenuated vaccine) and inactivated polio vaccine (IPV).

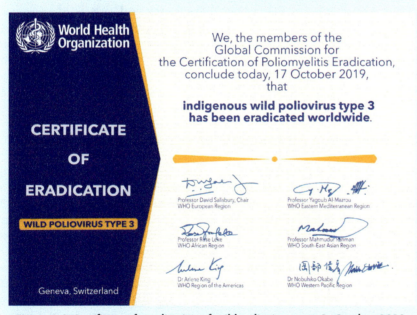

Figure 3.2 Certificate of eradication of wild poliovirus type 3, October 2019.
Source: Reproduced with permission from GPEI (2019).

In 1988, the WHA agreed to the goal of eradication of poliomyelitis and the Global Polio Eradication Initiative (GPEI), a public–private partnership, was established. Since then, there has been a decrease of over 99% in the worldwide number of poliomyelitis cases, while two of the three serotypes have been eradicated. The last case of poliomyelitis due to wild poliovirus type 2 (WPV2) occurred in India in 1999 and global eradication of WPV2 was certified in 2015. In 2019, wild poliovirus type 3 (WPV3) was certified as eradicated (Figure 3.2). The last case of WPV3 infection was detected in northern Nigeria in 2012. Endemic wild poliovirus type 1 is present in only two countries (Pakistan and Afghanistan).

Key elements of the GPEI 2019–2023 strategy for the eradication of poliomyelitis are polio immunisation campaigns (see Box 3.9) and routine polio vaccination, withdrawal of OPV and its replacement with IPV, surveillance of acute flaccid paralysis and environmental surveillance (see Chapter 8) and containment of polioviruses.

Major challenges impeding the progress towards eradication of poliomyelitis are the disruption of polio vaccination due to competing priorities and political turmoil with armed conflicts and insecurity of vaccination teams, resulting in 'inaccessible areas'. Another challenge is the emergence of vaccine-derived polioviruses (see Chapter 17), which may cause outbreaks of paralytic poliomyelitis.

In addition to these vertical international vaccination programmes aimed at eradication of a single disease, WHO established in 1974 an international vaccination programme targeting multiple diseases: the Expanded Programme on Immunization (EPI). At the time of the creation of the EPI, less than 5% of infants in low-income countries were receiving vaccinations. WHO tried to remedy this by expanding the delivery of vaccines against six life-threatening and disabling diseases (tuberculosis, diphtheria, tetanus, pertussis, poliomyelitis and measles) (Cherian, Eggers, Lydon, Sodha, & Okwo-Bele, 2019).

3.2 Goals, aims and targets of vaccination programmes

As mentioned in the introduction to this chapter, the overall goal of vaccination is to reduce the burden of disease and death in a population and to improve its equity in health. When establishing a vaccination programme, an essential first step is to specify a more precise aim of the programme, since this determines the programme's strategy, the coverage needed and the design and intensity of monitoring and surveillance required.

In terms of programme aims, two options are available: a vaccination programme can aim to reduce the burden of disease in the entire population, or it can be focused on protecting a particular population subgroup. From a disease control perspective, protecting the entire population is preferable. However, when the burden of disease is concentrated in a well-defined population subgroup, focusing on protecting this group may be more acceptable from a benefit–risk, ethical, societal and economic perspective. The epidemiology of the targeted infection and disease, and characteristics of available vaccines, are most relevant for choosing the most appropriate aim for the vaccination programme.

When aiming to protect the entire population, three subsequent choices in disease control targets are available: eradication, elimination or containment. Definitions of these are provided in Box 3.4. When the overall aim is to focus on protecting a particular subgroup of the population, containment is the only achievable target for disease control.

Box 3.4 Eradication, elimination or containment: definitions

- A disease is *eradicated* when its causal agent is exterminated from nature, as a result of deliberate control efforts.
- A disease is *eliminated* when in a defined geographic area new cases of the disease caused by sustained indigenous transmission of its causal agent no longer occur, as a result of deliberate control efforts, while it continues to be transmitted elsewhere. Limited transmission from imported cases may still arise.
- A disease is *contained* when it no longer constitutes a significant public health problem, as a result of deliberate control efforts.

The difference between the different vaccination programme targets lies primarily in the expected impact, which is much enhanced in programmes aiming for eradication or elimination as they involve generating herd immunity. The concept of herd immunity is explained in Chapter 4, while its implications are discussed in Chapter 5. Eradication and elimination are highly desirable targets of any public health programme, since they offer a maximum reduction in the burden of disease and in inequities in health. In practice, however, eradication or elimination are seldom feasible. Factors favouring the possibility of elimination and eradication are listed in Box 3.5.

Box 3.5 Factors favouring the possibility of elimination and eradication

- *Biological* factors include characteristics of the pathogen and the infection it causes. Conditions favouring the possibility of eradication are the absence of non-human hosts and of environmental reservoirs of the pathogen, low infectivity of the infection and when infection causes an easy-to-recognise disease without infectious subclinical phases.
- *Vaccine-related factors* include characteristics of the available vaccines: their costs, effectiveness, safety and duration of protection. Regarding effectiveness, the key characteristic is to what extent the vaccine reduces transmission of infection (by reducing the risk of infection and the infectiousness

> of infected individuals) and is hence able to generate herd immunity (see Chapters 2, 4 and 12).
> - *Public health infrastructure and process factors* include the presence of an effective infrastructure to deliver vaccines to the target population, adequate surveillance to detect cases (and ultimately certify the extermination of the pathogen) and adequate response capacity to control spread of infections.
> - *Societal/political factors* include the availability of sustained funding for the vaccination programme and public health infrastructure, and political/societal 'appetite' for the aim of eradication or elimination in the light of competing health and other priorities. It also includes the degree of acceptance by the target population to get vaccinated.

The conditions specified in Box 3.5 were met to a large degree for smallpox, but are clearly not met, for example, for tetanus, which is caused by a bacterium with spores that survive in the environment and in animals such as horses. Therefore, for tetanus, containment is the highest aim achievable for a vaccination programme.

To document eradication and elimination, high-quality surveillance is needed, for example to distinguish cases arising from indigenous transmission from imported cases (see Chapter 8). For poliomyelitis, measles and rubella, WHO has established definitions (see for an example Box 3.6) and a structure of committees for certification (of eradication) and verification (of elimination) to assess the progress in disease control.

> **Box 3.6 WHO Regional Office for Europe definitions for the elimination of measles (WHO, 2014)**
>
> - *Elimination*: the absence of endemic measles in a defined geographical area for a period of at least 12 months, in the presence of a well-performing surveillance system. Regional elimination can be declared after 36 months or longer of absence of endemic measles in all member states of the region.
> - *Endemic transmission*: continuous transmission of indigenous or imported measles virus that persists for a period of 12 months or longer in a defined geographical area.

When an infection is eradicated, the decision to cease the vaccination programme should take into account the risk of (deliberate or accidental) release of the pathogen from laboratories, and the risk of emergence of related pathogens against which the vaccine may or may not provide protection. When an infection has been eliminated or contained, vaccination programmes always need to be continued to prevent re-emergence.

In theory, the aim and disease control target set for a vaccination programme determine its vaccine coverage target (see Chapter 4 on the critical vaccination threshold).

However, in practice the target is usually, from an equity and logistical point of view, to approach 100% coverage. The realisation of this is limited by what is achievable given available resources and acceptance by the population.

3.3 Vaccination programme strategies: universal or selective vaccination

Vaccination programmes can be categorised as universal or selective, depending on whether they aim to reduce the burden of disease in the entire population or are focused on protecting a particular population subgroup, respectively. Universal vaccination programmes are also called 'mass' vaccination programmes, while selective programmes are also known as 'targeted' vaccination programmes.

In universal vaccination programme, all individuals in the population within a certain age range (well before natural infection typically occurs) are offered vaccination, thereby (eventually) protecting the entire population. For communicable infections, immunising a sufficient part of the population may lead to elimination or even eradication of the infection. Selective vaccination programmes aim mainly to protect a certain population subgroup by targeted vaccination of those at increased risk of getting infected or those at increased risk of severe consequences when infected (see Box 3.7).

Box 3.7 Indications for selective vaccination programmes

Increased risk of exposure

Vaccination programmes targeted at travellers is an example where the increased risk of exposure is the rationale behind the targeting. Apart from travel, higher than average risk of infection can also be related to certain risk behaviours or occupations. Examples of selective vaccination programmes based on this rationale include hepatitis B vaccination programmes for men who have sex with men, injecting drug users, commercial sex workers and healthcare workers. For most infections, individuals who are at increased risk of exposure are usually also at higher risk of infecting others. Hence, selective vaccination based on this indication is important for both direct protection of the vaccinee and indirect protection of others (see Chapter 4).

Increased risk of severe consequences of infection when infected

Target groups for this type of selective vaccination programme include individuals who are at increased risk of severe disease, complications and death following infection. Certain conditions or chronic illnesses can predispose for this. Examples include pneumococcal vaccination of people with asplenia and influenza vaccination for those with chronic respiratory disease. For several infectious diseases, such as influenza and COVID-19, advanced age is a risk factor for severe disease and death. Hence, advanced age can also be the indication for selective vaccination.

The aim of protecting those at increased risk of severe consequences of infection can in some situations be best achieved by vaccinating their contacts, particularly when the persons at high risk have a contraindication for vaccination or when it works less well in them. Examples include influenza vaccination for contacts of immunocompromised individuals and pertussis vaccination of new parents to protect newborn infants (a strategy called 'cocooning').

Maternal vaccination, which means the vaccination of pregnant women, is an exception in that it can be considered both a universal and a selective vaccination strategy, depending on the vaccine provided (see Box 3.8).

Box 3.8 Maternal vaccination

Vaccination of pregnant women ('maternal vaccination') is based on a particular paradigm of disease prevention: the possibility of protecting infants through passively acquired maternal antibodies, induced by vaccination of pregnant women. For some infections, for example pertussis, it also works by minimising exposure after birth ('cocooning'). Since the aim is to protect all infants, it can be considered as a form of universal vaccination. Since the targeting is based on a characteristic ('pregnancy') rather than an age, it can also be considered selective vaccination.

Maternal vaccination is an attractive option since it protects young infants whose immune systems are unable to respond adequately to vaccination. There may also be important benefits for the pregnant woman herself. An example of this is influenza where pregnancy is a risk factor for severe disease. Maternal vaccination is currently in use for pertussis, tetanus and influenza, and is likely to be used for additional vaccines in the future.

As shown in Box 3.8, the distinction between selective and universal vaccination programmes is not always clear-cut. Furthermore, even though it is not their primary aim, selective vaccination programmes may well contribute to reducing the burden of disease in non-targeted individuals. Conversely, high-risk groups may be better protected by herd immunity generated in a universal programme than by a selective vaccination programme. This is why, for example, universal rubella vaccination programmes are preferable to selective vaccination programmes for adolescent girls, provided sufficient coverage can be achieved. It is also the rationale for universal influenza vaccination programmes for children, aiming to reduce the incidence of influenza in older people. Chapter 4 provides further information on the relevance of population transmission dynamics for vaccination strategies.

3.4 Delivery of universal vaccination programmes: routine, supplemental and ring vaccination

Vaccines included in a universal vaccination programme are most effectively delivered on an ongoing basis through routine vaccination of children when they reach a certain age, according to a vaccination schedule (see Section 3.5). To accelerate disease control, 'supplementary immunisation activities' (SIAs) or 'pulse vaccination campaigns', may be added to routine vaccination. SIAs are vaccination campaigns targeting all individuals within a set age range, usually irrespective of their vaccination status. SIAs generally target wider age ranges than routine vaccination. SIAs can be delivered nationally or subnationally, and are, for example, used to accelerate disease control of measles and poliomyelitis. Pulse vaccination campaigns involve repeated SIAs; they have been an important feature of the polio eradication campaign in India.

A specific form of SIA is the so-called catch-up campaign, indicating a broad age-range SIA implemented at the start of a new universal routine vaccination programme. The main advantage of this is that it can provide immunity to children who would have otherwise remained susceptible by missing out on both the routine vaccination as well as natural infection. The importance of this for disease control is outlined in Chapter 5. Successful catch-up programmes may quickly stop circulation of the pathogen in the population. However, this may mask inadequate vaccine effectiveness for a certain period (see Chapter 5).

SIAs organised on a single day are called national immunisation days (NIDs) or subnational immunisation days (SNIDs) (see Box 3.9 for an example).

Box 3.9 Role of national or subnational immunisation days in the eradication of poliomyelitis

In addition to including polio vaccination into routine national vaccination programmes, SIAs in the form of national or subnational immunisation days (NIDs or SNIDs) continue to be a key element to achieve sufficient immunity.

The eradication of poliomyelitis in the two remaining endemic countries (Afghanistan and Pakistan) is hampered by armed conflict. To deliver a NID, 'days of tranquillity' can be negotiated in conflict areas.

From a biological point of view, vaccinating a large group of children on a single day with OPV can achieve relatively rapid control of wild poliovirus due to the boosting of population immunity, particularly mucosal immunity due to inducement of IgA (see Chapter 2), and also since OPV vaccine strains are transmitted and can immunise others. There are, however, also particular risks associated with OPV (see Chapter 17).

The optimal timing, frequency and age range of SIAs depend on factors including the prevalence of vaccine-induced immunity resulting from routine vaccination and previous campaigns, the prevalence of immunity due to natural infection, population density and contact patterns, the infectiousness of the pathogen and the effectiveness of the vaccine.

Advantages of SIAs include that they require efforts during a short period of time. This may be the only feasible option in areas of armed conflict. Furthermore, it may be appealing to politicians, funders and executers, who may struggle to plan and support ongoing routine vaccination. Disadvantages of SIAs include that administered vaccines are often not recorded, and that there is a risk of reaching the same children multiple times and missing out others.

SIAs that are targeted at a restricted geographic area or age group thought to have been missed out by vaccination and/or natural infection are called 'follow-up' and 'mopping-up' campaigns (see Box 3.10).

Box 3.10 Eliminating measles from the Americas: 'catch-up, keep-up, follow-up'

To achieve elimination of measles from the Americas (an aim set in 1994), the Pan American Health Organization (PAHO) recommended a three-pronged vaccination strategy:

1. A one-off 'catch-up' campaign during the season with low incidence, targeting all children in a relatively broad age range (1–14 years of age).
2. A 'keep-up' component, indicating the establishment of a routine vaccination programme achieving high coverage in all districts.

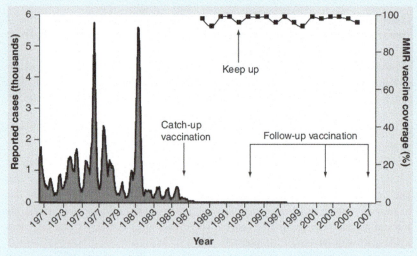

Figure 3.3 Reported measles cases by month and annual MMR coverage, Cuba, 1971–2007*.

Source: Adapted with permission from de Quadros, Andrus, Danovaro-Holliday, and Castillo-Solorzano (2008).

Note: *Coverage data not available.

3. A 'follow-up' component, indicating a campaign in which all children in a relatively narrow age-range (1–4 years of age) are vaccinated, irrespective of previous vaccination, to offer a 'second' opportunity to become immune. This step can include 'mopping-up' campaigns in districts that have not achieved 95% coverage in the follow-up campaigns.

Cuba was the first country to implement this strategy, which lead to elimination of measles in the late 1980s (Figure 3.3). Subsequently, measles was eliminated from the Americas.

Note that there is a certain window of opportunity for the 'PAHO strategy' to be successful, since this also depends on high levels of natural immunity in older generations (by having had measles). If adequate vaccination coverage achieved in any part of the three-pronged approach is not achieved sufficiently fast, susceptibles will accumulate, which may (at some point) sustain measles virus transmission (see Chapter 5).

Ring vaccination is, in addition to routine and supplemental vaccination, a third method of vaccine delivery. It involves the identification of infected individuals, after which their contacts are offered vaccination (Box 3.11). The purpose of ring vaccination is to limit the spread of infection by creating immunity around an infected individual.

Box 3.11 Ring vaccination

In ring vaccination, contacts of infected individuals are offered vaccination as soon as possible. Contacts targeted for vaccination include people who have had direct contact with the infected individual. It may also include secondary and tertiary contacts. The entire group of contacts may be visualised in rings around the index case. In addition to pre-exposure immunisation, for some vaccines (such as measles vaccine), ring vaccination may also work by protecting already infected contacts through post-exposure vaccination.

There are several factors which determine the likelihood that a strategy of ring vaccination will be successful to control transmission of the infection:

Vaccine-related factors

- Effective vaccine available.
- Short period between vaccination and presence of immunity.
- Single dose required for immunity.

Infection-related factors

- Typical clinical features.
- High proportion of infected individuals who develop symptoms.
- Accurate laboratory test available.

Disease surveillance

- High sensitivity and timeliness to detect cases of infection.

Setting

- Feasible to vaccinate a high proportion of contacts within days of identification of the index case.

Ring vaccination was an essential part of the smallpox eradication campaign (see Box 3.2) and is used, for example, in the control of Ebola virus outbreaks. Vaccination of close contacts is routinely recommended for several infectious diseases, including meningococcal disease, measles and hepatitis A and B. A strategy of ring vaccination is unlikely to be successful when a large proportion of those infected have no symptoms of the disease (e.g., poliovirus and SARS-CoV-2 infection).

3.5 Vaccination schedules

A vaccination schedule specifies the recommended number of doses and their age at administration of one or more vaccines. An overview of recommended vaccination schedules in all countries is maintained by WHO (2020). Figure 3.4 provides an example of the recommended schedule in a national immunisation programme.

Ideally, vaccination provides protection as soon as infants are susceptible. This can be at birth, or at the moment maternal immunity has waned. Vaccination schedules need to fill this susceptibility gap as soon as possible, while also taking into account at what age the vaccines have optimal immunogenicity, efficacy and the fewest side effects. The age-specific immunogenicity may depend on the presence of maternal antibodies and the extent of immunological maturation of the vaccine recipient. In children, older age at vaccination and longer intervals between doses are generally associated with higher immunity levels, and for most antigens boosters administered over the age of 12 months are crucial for long-term protection (see Chapter 2).

In addition to these biological factors, an optimal vaccination schedule should also take into account programmatic factors (indicating at what age highest coverage can be achieved and considering the limited number of injections that can be given at a single visit) and epidemiological factors (particularly the age-specific incidence of the targeted infection). The implementation of maternal vaccination (see Box 3.8) may necessitate changing the vaccination schedule for infants, as maternal antibodies may interfere with the infant's response to vaccination.

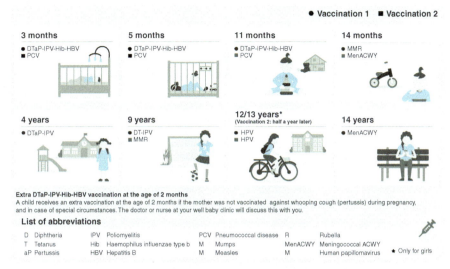

Figure 3.4 Recommended vaccination schedule for children, the Netherlands, 2019.
Source: Adapted with permission from RIVM (2020).

Since most vaccines are delivered as part of combination vaccines, the vaccination schedule for these needs to be a compromise of the optimal schedules of the separate vaccines.

The number of vaccine doses required for optimal protection is assessed in clinical trials as part of the generation of evidence needed for licensure of the vaccine (see Chapter 1). However, post-implementation of a vaccination programme, evidence may be generated suggesting the number of doses can be reduced in certain settings (see Box 3.12) or an extra dose needs to be added.

Box 3.12 Reducing the number of doses in pneumococcal and HPV vaccination schedules

Pneumococcal vaccines were first licensed to be given in a four-dose schedule (three doses in the initial priming series and a booster dose in the second year of life). For human papillomavirus (HPV) vaccine, three doses were recommended. Research carried out after implementation of pneumococcal and HPV vaccination programmes provided evidence that the number of doses could be reduced, with little reduction in protection.

For pneumococcal vaccines, mathematical modelling and immunogenicity studies have supported limiting the number of doses to two in certain settings (Choi, Andrews, & Miller, 2019; Goldblatt et al., 2018).

For HPV, immunogenicity studies conducted subsequent to its implementation in national vaccination programmes provided evidence that two doses provide adequate protection in children below the age of 15 years (WHO, 2017).

3.6 Vaccine policy

Vaccination programmes are usually financed, initiated and adapted by national, federal or regional governments, except for humanitarian emergencies, when non-governmental organisation (NGOs) may have this role. In low- and middle-income countries (LMICs), the United Nations (through its agencies WHO and UNICEF) has been instrumental in improving access to vaccination. This started with the smallpox eradication programme and was expanded to include six other vaccines in the EPI in 1974 (see Section 3.1).

In many countries, scientific advice for vaccine policy is provided by multidisciplinary expert groups called National Immunization Technical Advisory Groups (NITAGs). In order for evidence generated in the evaluation of vaccination programmes to contribute to achieving their public health goals, epidemiologists generating this evidence need to be aware of how, when and in what form evidence is considered by the NITAG in the country they are working in. Reports produced by NITAGs are made accessible by the global NITAG network (GNN, 2020).

Evidence-based policy and strategy recommendations on the use of vaccines in national programmes is provided by the WHO Strategic Advisory Group of Experts (SAGE) for immunisation, which was established in 1999. Important outputs from SAGE are the 'Vaccine Position Papers' (see Box 3.13).

Box 3.13 The WHO Strategic Advisory Group of Experts and the Vaccine Position Papers

The Strategic Advisory Group of Experts (SAGE) for immunisation was established in 1999. Its principal task is to advise WHO on vaccine policy and strategies. SAGE is comprised of 15 members, who serve in a personal capacity rather than representing institutions.

SAGE meets at least twice a year, and working groups are established to review specific vaccine-preventable diseases or relevant methodologies (such as Ebola and quality and use of global immunisation and surveillance data). Working group results are presented to SAGE for discussion and to formulate recommendations for the use of vaccines in national programmes.

These recommendations, together with current evidence on the disease and effects of vaccination, are summarised in the Vaccine Position Papers, which are valuable resources. They are published in the *Weekly Epidemiological Record* (www.who.int/wer) and are available at www.who.int/teams/immunization-vaccines-and-biologicals/policies/position-papers.

The first global vaccination policy was established in 1977, with a goal of universal access to immunisation for all children by 1990. In response to stagnating vaccine coverage and underuse of new vaccines in developing countries, a public–private partnership, the Global Alliance for Vaccination and Immunisation (GAVI), was established in 2000 (see Box 3.14).

Box 3.14 The Global Alliance for Vaccination and Immunisation

In 2000, the Global Alliance for Vaccination and Immunisation (GAVI) was established by four founding member organisations (the Bill and Melinda Gates Foundation, WHO, UNICEF and the World Bank) as a public–private partnership to improve access to vaccination for children in low-income countries. GAVI financially supports countries to implement vaccination programmes for new and under-used vaccines and provides expertise for this. Countries with a gross national income (GNI) per capita below a certain threshold are eligible for GAVI support to implement vaccination programmes or for strengthening health systems. Once the GNI exceeds the threshold, countries start a 'graduation' process, which includes the phasing out of GAVI support and the establishment of plans to sustain their vaccination programmes.

3.7 Monitoring and evaluation of vaccination programmes

Vaccination programmes can have a multitude of effects at individual and population level, and have proven to be enormously beneficial for human health. However, undesirable effects may also occur. Benefits and risks of mass vaccination programmes are further described in Chapters 5 and 17. Since effects may occur immediately after implementation of the programme but may also become apparent over time, monitoring benefits and risks of vaccination programmes remain important throughout their lifetime. The key areas and tools for this are summarised in Box 3.15. This aims to generate evidence to sustain the programme or adapt it to enhance its benefits and reduce any risks. All of these areas and tools are addressed in separate chapters of this book.

Box 3.15 Monitoring and evaluation of vaccination programmes: key areas and tools

The key areas to be studied:

- attitudes towards vaccination;
- vaccine coverage;
- impact of the vaccination programme;
- vaccine effectiveness;
- safety.

> The key tools for this are:
> - surveillance;
> - outbreak investigation;
> - (sero)epidemiological research.

Evidence of the impact of vaccination programmes is of particular importance to prevent programmes from becoming victims of their own success: when diseases are no longer present, the funders, target population and other key stakeholders of the programme may lose sight of the rationale for the programme and cease supporting it or participating in it. Methods to assess impact are discussed in Chapter 10 of this book.

The main stakeholders involved in monitoring and evaluation of vaccination programmes are governments and public health authorities, medicines regulatory authorities and vaccine manufacturers. Their roles and responsibilities are briefly outlined in what follows. To safeguard the (real and perceived) quality of evidence, it should be generated independently from commercial or other interests. It is good practice when presenting results to provide full transparency about any potential conflict of interest.

Governments and public health authorities are usually responsible for implementing and funding vaccination programmes and they spend public money to do so. They therefore have a 'duty of care' to make sure these programmes are as safe and effective as possible. To assess this, they have a leading role in surveillance, outbreak investigations and dedicated studies, resulting in evidence to sustain or improve vaccination programmes and policy.

Medicines regulatory authorities such as the European Medicines Agency (EMA) and the US Food and Drug Administration (FDA) are responsible for the market authorisation of vaccines (see Chapter 1) and also have a responsibility for the post-marketing assessment of the benefits and risks of vaccines. In case of a safety concern, regulators can order vaccine manufacturers to conduct safety studies. Regulators also have a role in assessing the pharmacovigilance (safety monitoring) and risk management plans produced by vaccine manufacturers.

Vaccine manufacturers, also known as vaccine marketing authorisation holders (MAHs) (see Chapter 1) are also involved in monitoring benefits, safety and benefit–risk profiles of vaccines. They may be legally obliged to monitor the effectiveness and safety of their licensed vaccines and report suspected adverse reactions to medicines regulatory authorities.

Academic epidemiologists, often acting independently of manufacturers and public health authorities, play a key role in undertaking epidemiological studies to evaluate vaccines and vaccination programmes. Typically, evaluations rely on data collected in several studies, often in different countries. To aid this process, international collaborative networks are playing an increasingly important role, ensuring, for example, that comparable data are collected in different locations, using standard protocols.

3.8 Modifying vaccination programmes

Modifications to enhance the benefits and/or reduce risks of vaccination programmes can be grouped into three categories: terminating or suspending the programme, adjusting the strategy and modifying its implementation. Surveillance, outbreak investigations and research performed as part of evaluating vaccination programmes contribute to providing evidence for these modifications.

Terminating a vaccination programme may be justified when the targeted disease is eradicated. So far, this has been achieved for only one human vaccine-preventable disease: smallpox. Also, when the risks of a vaccination programme outweigh its benefits, stopping the programme may be required. Alternatively, it may be suspended while more research is undertaken. More information on methods for benefit–risk assessment is available in Part V of this book. An example of a vaccination programme that was terminated is provided in Box 3.16.

Box 3.16 Ceasing the RotaShield rotavirus vaccination programme in the United States

In mid-1998, RotaShield, a live-attenuated rhesus rotavirus tetravalent vaccine, was recommended for use in the United States for the prevention of rotavirus disease. Post-implementation surveillance by the Vaccine Adverse Event Reporting System (VAERS) detected 15 cases of intussusception (a potentially fatal bowel obstruction caused by the bowel folding into itself) among infants who had received RotaShield, with similar findings from three other surveillance systems, upon which the implementation of the programme was suspended in July 1999. Based on additional surveillance data and results of case-control and other studies, it was concluded that there was a significantly increased risk of intussusception following RotaShield vaccination, after which the programme was stopped and the manufacturer withdrew the vaccine from the market, even though a formal benefit–risk analyses had not been done. Although cases of intussusception were observed in pre-licensure trials, an increased risk was not identified as clinical trials are too small in size to detect rare events, highlighting the importance of large-scale post-marketing surveillance of safety (see Chapter 18) (CDC, 1999; Delage, 2000; Vesikari, 2012).

Potential adjustments to vaccination programmes include the use of a different vaccine, changing the age at administration of vaccines and/or the number of doses (see Box 3.12), or adding supplementary vaccination (see Section 3.4).

Modifying the implementation of a vaccination programme may be required when the uptake is inadequate or not achieving targets. Ideally, such modifications are informed by evidence about reasons for the suboptimal uptake, so that these can be addressed. Potential interventions to increase uptake include improving communication to the target population, making vaccination a visa requirement (for travel vaccination) or otherwise compulsory, implementing target payments for vaccine providers or withholding child benefits or school admission when children are not vaccinated. Further discussion of these methods is beyond the scope of this book.

Summary

- From a public health perspective, the main aims of vaccination are to reduce suffering and death from vaccine-preventable diseases and to reduce health inequity in a population. To achieve this, a programmatic approach to vaccination is much more effective, efficient and safe than merely making vaccines available.
- The overall aim of a vaccination programme can be to reduce the burden of disease in the entire population or to only reduce it in a population subgroup.
- In universal vaccination programmes, all individuals in the population within a certain age range are offered vaccination. Selective vaccination programmes aim to protect high-risk population subgroups by targeting them directly for vaccination. Maternal vaccination can be considered both as a selective and universal strategy.
- Disease control targets for universal programmes include eradication, elimination and containment, while selective programmes can only achieve containment. The vaccination programme's overall aim and disease control target determine its strategy, the coverage needed and the design and intensity of monitoring and evaluation required.
- Universal vaccination programmes can be delivered routinely on an ongoing basis to all individuals reaching a certain age, by an SIA and by ring vaccination targeting contacts of a case.
- A vaccination schedule specifies the recommended number of doses and their age at administration. Ideally it should be based on age-specific evidence about susceptibility and immunogenicity of vaccines, as well as programmatic and epidemiological factors.
- Vaccination programmes are usually financed, initiated and adapted by governments, except for humanitarian emergencies, when NGOs may have this role. Vaccine policy can be set at (sub)national or international level.
- Since benefits and risks of vaccination programmes may occur immediately after the implementation of the programme but may also become apparent over time, monitoring benefits and risks of vaccination programmes remain important throughout their lifetime.
- Stakeholders involved in monitoring and evaluation of vaccination programmes include governments and public health authorities, medicines regulatory authorities and vaccine manufacturers.
- Interventions to enhance the benefits and/or reduce risks of vaccination programmes include ceasing the programme, adapting the strategy and adapting its implementation.

References

Centers for Disease Control and Prevention (CDC). (1999). Withdrawal of rotavirus vaccine recommendation. *Morbidity and Mortality Weekly Report*, *48*(43), 1007. Retrieved from www.ncbi.nlm.nih.gov/pubmed/10577495.

Cherian, T., Cutts, F., Eggers, R., Lydon, P., Sodha, S. V., & Okwo-Bele, J. -M. (2019). Immunization in developing countries. In S. A. Plotkin, W. A. Orenstein, P. A. Offit, & K. M. Edwards (Eds.), *Plotkin's vaccines* (7th ed., pp. 1486–1511). Philadelphia, PA: Elsevier.

Cherian, T., & Mantel, C. (2020). National immunization programmes. *Bundesgesundheitsblatt Gesundheitsforschung Gesundheitsschutz*, *63*(1), 16–24. doi:10.1007/s00103-019-03062-1.

Choi, Y. H., Andrews, N., & Miller, E. (2019). Estimated impact of revising the 13-valent pneumococcal conjugate vaccine schedule from 2 + 1 to 1 + 1 in England and Wales: A modelling study. *PLoS Med*, *16*(7), e1002845. doi:10.1371/journal.pmed.1002845.

Delage, G. (2000). Rotavirus vaccine withdrawal in the United states: The role of postmarketing surveillance. *Canadian Journal of Infectious Diseases and Medical Microbiology*, *11*(1), 10–12. doi:10.1155/2000/414396.

de Quadros, C. A., Andrus, J. K., Danovaro-Holliday, M. C., & Castillo-Solorzano, C. (2008). Feasibility of global measles eradication after interruption of transmission in the Americas. *Expert Review of Vaccines*, *7*(3), 355–362. doi:10.1586/14760584.7.3.355.

Global NITAG Network (GNN). (2020). Network. Retrieved from www.nitag-resource.org/.

Global Polio Eradication Initiative (GPEI). (2019). Two out of three wild poliovirus strains eradicated. Retrieved from http://polioeradication.org/news-post/two-out-of-three-wild-poliovirus-strains-eradicated/.

Goldblatt, D., Southern, J., Andrews, N. J., Burbidge, P., Partington, J., Roalfe, L., ... Miller, E. (2018). Pneumococcal conjugate vaccine 13 delivered as one primary and one booster dose (1 + 1) compared with two primary doses and a booster (2 + 1) in UK infants: A multicentre, parallel group randomised controlled trial. *Lancet Infectious Diseases*, *18*(2), 171–179. doi:10.1016/S1473-3099(17)30654-0.

Henderson, D. A. (2011). The eradication of smallpox: An overview of the past, present, and future. *Vaccine*, *29*(Suppl. 4), D7–D9. doi:10.1016/j.vaccine.2011.06.080.

Hennock, E. P. (1998). Vaccination policy against smallpox, 1835–1914: A comparison of England with Prussia and imperial Germany. *Social History of Medicine*, *11*(1), 49–71. doi:10.1093/shm/11.1.49.

Lewis, D. (2020). China's coronavirus vaccine shows military's growing role in medical research. *Nature*, *585*(7826), 494–495. doi:10.1038/d41586-020-02523-x.

National Institute for Public Health and the Environment (RIVM). (2020). *The national immunisation programme in the Netherlands: Surveillance and developments in 2019–2020*. Bilthoven, the Netherlands: RIVM. Retrieved from www.rivm.nl/bibliotheek/rapporten/2020-0077.pdf.

Plotkin, S. A., Orenstein, W. A., Offit, P. A., & Edwards, K. M. (Eds.) (2018). *Plotkin's vaccines* (7th ed.). Philadelphia, PA: Elsevier.

Vesikari, T. (2012). Rotavirus vaccination: A concise review. *Clinical Microbiology and Infection*, *18*(Suppl. 5), 57–63. doi:10.1111/j.1469-0691.2012.03981.x.

World Health Organization (WHO). (1980) *World Health: The Magazine of the World Health Organization*, May. Geneva, Switzerland: WHO.

World Health Organization (WHO). (2014). *Eliminating measles and rubella: Framework for the verification process in the WHO European region*. Retrieved from www.euro.who.int/__data/assets/pdf_file/0009/247356/Eliminating-measles-and-rubella-Framework-for-the-verification-process-in-the-WHO-European-Region.pdf.

World Health Organization (WHO). (2017). Human papillomavirus vaccines: WHO position paper, May 2017. *Weekly Epidemiological Record*, *92*(19), 241–268. Retrieved from www.ncbi.nlm.nih.gov/pubmed/28530369.

World Health Organization (WHO). (2020). *WHO vaccine-preventable diseases: monitoring system*. Retrieved from http://apps.who.int/immunization_monitoring/globalsummary/schedules.

Chapter 4

Dynamics of vaccine-preventable infectious diseases

In this chapter we discuss aspects of the population transmission dynamics of communicable infectious diseases that are relevant to vaccination programmes. Our focus is primarily conceptual rather than technical, though some key quantitative relationships that apply in important special cases will be presented.

We begin in Section 4.1 by discussing the concepts of infectious contacts, transmission and herd immunity. In Section 4.2 we introduce the idea of a reproduction number, and how this relates to the critical immunisation threshold. Then in Section 4.3 we describe how these quantities may be estimated in a simple situation known as homogeneous mixing. In Section 4.4 we discuss the complexities that arise in more realistic scenarios with heterogeneous mixing, and finally in Section 4.5 we describe how models may be used to represent such heterogeneities and to evaluate the likely impacts of vaccination programmes. Key references on the dynamics and control of infectious diseases include Anderson and May (1992), Vynnycky and White (2010) and Keeling and Rohani (2007).

4.1 Contact, transmission, herd immunity and epidemic cycles

For simplicity, we restrict attention to communicable infections that are transmitted directly from person to person, though most of the ideas developed in this chapter also apply to vector-borne infections.

Our starting point is the notion of a contact between two people. This is an event that might result in the infection of interest being communicated from one individual to the other. What counts as a contact depends predominantly on the transmission route of the infection under consideration. Some of the main routes of transmission are detailed in Box 4.1 (the list is not exhaustive and note that often infectious diseases have multiple routes of transmission).

> **Box 4.1 Routes of transmission of infectious diseases**
>
> - *Respiratory:* pathogens are expelled from the respiratory system of one person and enter that of another; examples include measles, whooping cough, influenza, tuberculosis.
> - *Faecal-oral:* pathogens are excreted by one person and swallowed by another; examples include cholera, rotavirus, hepatitis A, polio.
> - *Sexual:* pathogens are transferred between sexual partners during sexual intercourse; examples include HIV, syphilis, chlamydia.
> - *Blood-borne:* pathogens are transferred directly from the blood of one individual to that of another by needles, transfusions, etc.; examples include hepatitis B, hepatitis C, HIV.
> - *Vertical:* pathogens are transferred from mother to baby through the placenta, during childbirth or via breast milk; examples include HIV, hepatitis B, syphilis.

For a given type of contact, the contact rate is the number of contacts per unit time that an individual makes with others. Contact rates usually vary between individuals according to their circumstances and behaviour, and reflect the environment and social customs of the population. In contrast, the transmission probability (per contact) is the probability that infection is transmitted during a contact between an infected and a susceptible individual. The transmission probability depends on the pathogen, as well as the type of contact involved. Note that the focus here is on transmission of the infection, not the presence of disease caused by the infection. Similarly, we are concerned with the effect of vaccination on transmission of infection.

Suppose that an individual makes contacts at rate θ, and that the transmission probability during a contact between them is π. The product

$$\beta = \theta \times \pi$$

is called the effective contact rate. It is the rate (per unit time) at which an individual makes contacts of such a nature that, if one were infected and the other susceptible, then transmission of the infection would occur. The effective contact rate thus influences the rate at which susceptible individuals are infected, which is called the force of infection.

Infection control measures aim to reduce the effective contact rate β. They may do so by reducing the contact rate θ (e.g., by quarantine, closing schools or recommending that infected persons stay at home), or by reducing the transmission probability π (e.g., by promoting clean water, safe sex or washing hands). Immunisation through vaccination lies within the latter category: it lowers the transmission probability by reducing the chance of infection and, for some vaccines, by reducing the infectiousness of a vaccinated infected person.

A key feature of infectious diseases is that infection control measures can also protect individuals indirectly: this effect is called herd immunity. There are many synonyms for the term 'herd immunity', including community immunity, herd effect, indirect effect and indirect protection. For example, unvaccinated individuals may be protected by vaccinating those most likely to make contact with them. Box 4.2 illustrates how such indirect protection may arise.

Box 4.2 Indirect effect of vaccination

The transmission of an infection through a population may be represented by a directed network, a portion of which is shown in Figure 4.1.

If **P** is immunised and as a result can no longer transmit the infection, then **B** and **C** are protected even if they are unvaccinated because (in this network) they can only acquire infection from **P**.

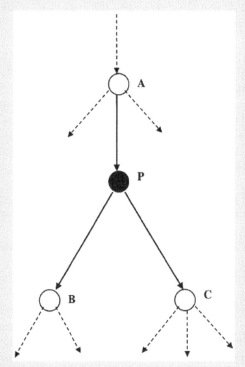

Figure 4.1 **Part of a transmission network.**
Note: The circles represent individuals, the connecting links represent effective contacts and the arrows represent the direction of transmission.
Source: Reproduced with permission from Farrington (2003).

The scenario shown in Figure 4.1 of Box 4.2 is a particularly simple one: individuals B and C can be completely protected by immunising P. In general, it is not practicable to immunise all individuals likely to make contact with a particular person. However, reducing the effective contact rates in the wider population by mass vaccination increases the chance that susceptible individuals will escape infection. If a sufficiently high proportion of the population is immunised, then transmission of an otherwise endemic infection may no longer be self-sustaining: endemic transmission is then said to have been eliminated in this population.

The indirect effects of vaccination are particularly important in providing a degree of protection for individuals who, for medical or other reasons, cannot be vaccinated. Vaccination programmes thus may carry a wider social benefit in addition to the direct protection afforded to vaccinated individuals. Herd immunity also protects vaccinated individuals in whom the vaccine did not work.

Note also that herd immunity (and the potential for vaccination to exhibit indirect effects) arises only for communicable infections, including vector-borne diseases. It does not arise for infections acquired from a natural environmental or animal reservoir, like tetanus or Lyme disease. More generally, the magnitude of the indirect effect of vaccination depends on a range of factors, described in Box 4.3.

Box 4.3 Factors affecting the magnitude of the indirect effect of vaccination

Fine, Eames, and Heymann (2011) list the following factors that affect the magnitude of the indirect effect of vaccination:

- the transmissibility of the infectious agent;
- the nature of the immunity induced by the vaccine;
- the pattern of mixing and infection transmission in the population;
- the distribution of the vaccine and immunity in the population.

For example, a vaccine that only protects against disease, and has no effect on transmission of infection (so that it reduces neither the risk of infection in susceptibles nor the infectiousness of infected individuals), will not generate herd immunity. Conversely, a vaccine that reduces the risk of infection in susceptibles or the infectiousness of infected individuals can have a large indirect effect. This is the case with conjugate vaccines against pneumococcal and *Haemophilus influenzae* type b infections, which protect against nasal carriage and hence reduce infectiousness. This in turn reduces infection rates in unvaccinated individuals. Some of these issues are addressed further in Chapter 12.

Transmissible infections that cause immunity and have short latency and infectious periods typically display epidemic cycles. This is the case, for example, with measles, mumps, rubella and whooping cough. This pattern is caused by the interplay between the increasing prevalence of infection-induced immunity in the population, the accrual of susceptible individuals through births and immigration and the fact that epidemics only start when the proportion of susceptibles reaches a threshold level sufficient to sustain transmission. These dynamics are described in Box 4.4.

> ## Box 4.4 Epidemic cycles for directly transmitted immunising infections
>
> Figure 4.2 displays in schematic form the cyclical pattern in the incidence of many highly infectious, immunising infections over time.
>
>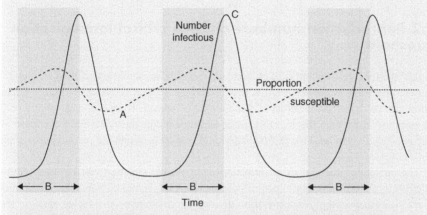
>
> *Figure 4.2* Schematic representation of the incidence of a highly infectious immunising infection (full line) and the proportion of the population that is susceptible to it (dashed line), over time. Features at A, B and C and the horizontal line are described in the text.
>
> Individuals who are susceptible to infection accumulate within the population due to births and immigration, leading to a rise in the proportion susceptible (from point A onwards on the dashed line in Figure 4.2). These individuals make contact with others in the population, some of whom may be infectious (whether through transmission within the population or via infection acquired from outside the population). When the proportion susceptible exceeds a certain threshold (indicated by the horizontal line), an epidemic begins and the number of newly infectious persons rises sharply (period B). Since the infection confers immunity, the proportion susceptible is eventually reduced and falls below the threshold, at which point the incidence of infection begins to drop (point C). The process is then repeated, giving rise to regular epidemics.

Many infections do not display epidemic cycles (notably, infections that do not confer lasting immunity, or with long infectious periods or a carrier state). However, in other respects the transmission dynamics are similar. Thus, from first principles based on the description given in Box 4.4, the key determinants of the dynamics of infection at a population level include the birth rate, the infectiousness of the pathogen, the frequency of contacts between individuals and the extent and duration of immunity conferred by the infection. Many other factors may affect the dynamics, including, for example, age effects and patterns of seasonal contact.

A vaccination programme typically perturbs the transmission process by removing individuals from the susceptible pool (it may also reduce the infectiousness of vaccinated individuals). If enough individuals are removed in this way, the infection may no longer be self-sustaining within the population. The key factors in determining how vaccination affects the dynamics of infection at the population level are the vaccine coverage, the effectiveness of the vaccine and at whom the vaccine programme is targeted.

4.2 Reproduction numbers and the critical immunisation threshold

In this section we develop the key concepts relating transmission to herd immunity. Our starting point is the observation that the progress of an infection through a population can be described in terms of generations of spread. If an outbreak begins with N_0 primary cases, then the N_1 individuals they infect constitute the first generation of spread. They in turn might infect N_2 individuals, who constitute the second generation, and so on.

The epidemic potential of an infection in a specific situation can be assessed by calculating the effective reproduction number at each generation, which is the number of infected cases in the next generation divided by the number of infected cases in the current generation. At generation 1 it is N_1 / N_0; at generation 2 it is N_2 / N_1, and so on. The effective reproduction number R up to generation k is the weighted average of these quantities:

$$R = \frac{N_1 + N_2 + \cdots + N_k}{N_0 + N_1 + \cdots + N_{k-1}}.$$

The effective reproduction number is thus the average number of cases infected by one case. If $R > 1$ at some generation, the number of cases increases from one generation to the next and the outbreak will grow. If, on the other hand, $R \leq 1$ then the outbreak will eventually peter out. (If R is exactly equal to 1, the outbreak will also end eventually.) An example is presented in Box 4.5.

Box 4.5 Outbreak of measles in healthcare workers

In 2014 an outbreak of measles occurred among healthcare workers in a hospital in the Netherlands. The outbreak originated from two primary cases in patients, and spread to eight healthcare workers, six of whom had previously been twice vaccinated (Hahné et al., 2016). Cases were swabbed and their measles virus

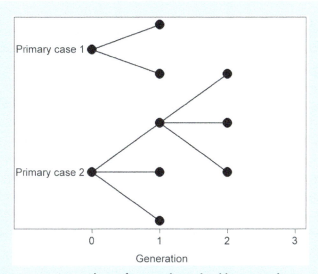

Figure 4.3 Transmission chains for measles in healthcare workers.

strains were characterised by genomic analyses, allowing transmission chains to be identified. These are shown in Figure 4.3.

In this outbreak, $N_0 = 2$, $N_1 = 5$, $N_2 = 3$ and $N_3 = 0$. Thus, the effective reproduction number at the first generation is $R = 5/2 = 2.5$, and the effective reproduction number for the outbreak as a whole (up to generation 3, when it peters out as there are no further cases) is

$$R = \frac{5+3+0}{2+5+3} = 0.8.$$

The authors comment that intense exposure, or a particularly pathogenic strain of measles, may have contributed to this outbreak.

In the measles example of Box 4.5, the spread of infection among healthcare workers in this hospital is limited by their natural immunity and vaccination.

Of special interest is the value of R in a completely susceptible population, in which (initially, at least) the spread of infection is not hindered by natural or vaccine-induced immunity. This quantity is called the basic reproduction number of the infection and is represented by the symbol R_0. More formally, R_0 is the average number of persons that one typical infectious person will infect during their infectious period, when the entire population is susceptible. The term 'typical infectious person' in this definition is to allow for possible heterogeneities in the population, to be discussed in Section 4.4. Some values of R_0 for various infections obtained in a range of different studies are given in Box 4.6.

Box 4.6 Ranges of values of R_0 for selected infections

For any infection, the basic reproduction number R_0 reflects the frequency and intensity of contacts made in the population, and so varies between infections and populations. Some ranges of values estimated in different populations are shown in Table 4.1.

Table 4.1 Low- and high-range estimates of R_o for selected infections

Infection	Basic reproduction number R_o	
	Low range	High range
Measles	5–6	16–18
Mumps	7–8	11–14
Rubella	6–7	15–16
Pertussis	7–8	16–18
Polio	5–6	6–7
Varicella	7–8	10–12
HIV	2–5	11–12

Source: Values obtained from Anderson and May (1992).

R_0 is a quantity of fundamental importance in the epidemiology of infectious diseases and vaccination. It is related to the effective contact rates; for example, when all individuals in the population share the same effective contact rate β, then

$$R_0 = \beta \times D$$

where D is the duration of the infectious period.

Reducing the effective contact rates by some constant factor also reduces R_0 by the same amount. Suppose now that, over a long period, a randomly selected proportion p of newborns are fully immunised at birth. The effective contact rate is then reduced by the factor $1-p$, and so the effective reproduction number in this partially vaccinated population is

$$R = R_0 \times (1-p).$$

Since outbreaks eventually come to an end when $R \leq 1$, there is a threshold value of p, called the critical immunisation threshold and denoted p_c, such that $R \leq 1$ when $p \geq p_c$. This value of p is

$$p_c = 1 - \frac{1}{R_0}.$$

This threshold exemplifies a key aspect of herd immunity: sustained endemic transmission within the population can be interrupted by immunising a (usually high) proportion of the population; the unimmunised within the population are then protected by herd immunity.

Box 4.7 provides an illustration. Further details of this relationship between p_c and R_0 will be discussed in Chapter 12 in the context of vaccine effectiveness.

Box 4.7 The basic reproduction number and critical immunisation threshold

The left panel of Figure 4.4 provides a schematic illustration of an infection with $R_0 = 3$.

The critical immunisation threshold is $p_c = 1 - 1/3 = 2/3$. Suppose that this proportion of newborns is vaccinated at birth (with a vaccine that provides full immunity). This reduces the effective reproduction number to 1, as shown in the right panel of Figure 4.4. The infection can no longer cause an epidemic. If, for example, the vaccine provides immunity to only 75% of vaccinees, the coverage required to reach p_c is $p_c / 0.75$ (which is 89% in the present illustration).

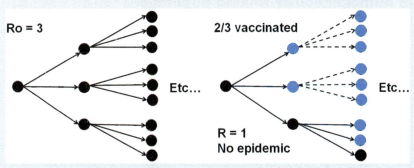

Figure 4.4 Schematic representation of an infection with $R_0 = 3$ soon after the introduction of one infectious individual (the index case).

Note: Black dots represent infected individuals, blue dots uninfected individuals. Left panel: in an entirely susceptible population, the index case infects three people, each of whom goes on to infect three others on average. Right panel: if two out of three of the population are immunised, each case infects at most one other individual on average.

The value of R_0 depends both on the infectious agent, and on the pattern of mixing within the population. For example, measles virus is more infectious than rubella virus; and both infections will spread more rapidly, and require a higher level of immunity to control it, in a densely populated city than in a sparsely inhabited region. For an infection with $R_0 = 20$, such as measles in a dense urban setting, the critical immunisation threshold is 0.95, or 95%. This means that 95% of the birth cohort must be immunised as soon as they become susceptible (after maternal antibodies have waned), in order to achieve full herd immunity for the remaining 5%.

However, vaccines seldom confer complete immunity. The critical vaccination threshold p_v is the vaccine coverage required to interrupt transmission of the infection. The relationship between the critical immunisation threshold p_c and the critical vaccination threshold p_v is as follows:

$$p_v = p_c / VE.$$

VE is the vaccine effectiveness, that is, the level of protection against infection induced by the vaccine. Vaccine effectiveness is discussed in Chapter 12; a more general version of this relationship between critical immunisation and vaccination thresholds applies when the vaccine also reduces the infectiousness of infected vaccinees.

The critical immunisation and vaccination thresholds are primarily of conceptual importance. They seldom provide a hard target for universal vaccination campaigns, the aim of which is usually to achieve 100% coverage of the target population. However, the threshold concept is important in formulating the aims of a vaccination programme, as it allows elimination and global eradication to be envisaged even in the absence of 100% coverage (see Chapter 3).

4.3 Estimating R_0 and the critical immunisation threshold p_c in homogeneously mixing populations

Estimating R_0 and the critical immunisation threshold is relatively straightforward for an endemic immunising infection within a homogeneously mixing population close to equilibrium. An infection is said to be immunising if, once infected, an individual is never again susceptible; homogeneous mixing means that all individuals in the population have the same effective contact rate β; the population and the infection are in equilibrium when the population is of fixed size and the infection rates are (at least roughly) constant.

The calculation is based on the observation that, when an infection is close to equilibrium, the effective reproduction number is 1 on average since otherwise the number of cases would change over time, and therefore the infection would not be in long-term equilibrium. So the average proportion S of the population susceptible (i.e., not having been infected) must satisfy the equation

$$R = R_0 \times S = 1.$$

It then follows that

$$R_0 = \frac{1}{S}.$$

Substituting $1/S$ for R_0 in the formula for the critical immunisation threshold obtained above, namely $p_c = 1 - 1/R_0$, results in a simple formula for p_c:

$$p_c = 1 - S.$$

In homogeneously mixing populations, the critical immunisation threshold is sometimes also referred to as the herd-immunity threshold. This equation exemplifies the equivalence; for example, the horizontal line in Figure 4.2 of Box 4.4 represents the susceptibility threshold S in this case.

The next step is to derive S, the proportion of the population susceptible at equilibrium. This may be done by a serological survey (see Chapter 9). However, in some circumstances, S can be estimated straightforwardly from the quantities L and A, where L is the life expectancy at birth and A is the average age at infection, as shown by Dietz (1975).

Suppose first that that virtually everyone in the population dies around age L (the age structure being roughly rectangular) and that most individuals get infected before they die. The proportion susceptible in the population is then

$$S = \frac{A}{L}.$$

This identity is illustrated in Box 4.8. It then follows that

$$R_0 = \frac{L}{A} \quad \text{and} \quad p_c = 1 - \frac{A}{L}.$$

If not everyone gets infected before they die, then other expressions apply. For example, if infant mortality is high (the age structure being roughly exponential) then

$$S = \frac{A}{A + L}.$$

and in this case

$$R_0 = 1 + \frac{L}{A} \quad \text{and} \quad p_c = 1 - \frac{A}{A + L}.$$

These relationships are illustrated graphically in Box 4.8.

Box 4.8 Proportion susceptible in a homogeneously mixing population

Suppose first that everyone in the population dies at age L, and that everyone becomes infected during their lifetime, at age A on average. This is represented in the left panel of Figure 4.5.

In this population, individuals on average spend A years susceptible out of their L years of life, and so the proportion of the population that are susceptible is $S = A/L$.

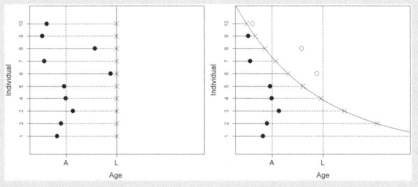

Figure 4.5 **Schematic representation of ages at infection (dots) and death (crosses) for 10 individuals.**

Note: A is the average age at infection. Left: all persons die at the same age L. Right: exponential deaths, with average age at death L; the circles are censored ages at infection.

In contrast, the right panel of Figure 4.5 shows a population with the same average age at infection A and life expectancy L. However, the lifetime distribution is exponential: some individuals live much longer than others. In this situation, some persons die before they are infected: this is the case for individuals 6, 8 and 10 in Figure 4.5. Thus, the proportion susceptible is reduced by censoring. When the times to infection and death both have an exponential distribution in the population it turns out that $S = A/(A+L)$; this is because the duration of susceptibility for each person is the minimum of time to infection and time to death.

These simple formulas for R_0 and p_c based on A and L are often useful in providing rough orders of magnitude. For example, they may provide convenient starting points for assessing possible vaccination strategies. A practical example of their application is described in Box 4.9.

Box 4.9 R_0 and critical immunisation threshold for hepatitis A in Bulgaria

This study was undertaken after the World Health Organization (WHO) classified Bulgaria as a region of intermediate endemicity for Hepatitis A (Tsankova, Todorova, Ermenlieva, Popova, & Tsankova, 2017). Individuals newly infected with hepatitis A reported in five regions of eastern Bulgaria between 2008 and 2014 were studied. The age distribution for 2,589 cases is shown in Table 4.2.

Table 4.2 Number of cases by 5-year age group 0–4, 5–9 ... 55–59 years, with age-group midpoints (years). The final age group is 60+ years, represented by the value 65 years

Age	2	7	12	17	22	27	32	37	42	47	52	57	65
Cases	258	609	383	237	125	166	169	161	136	130	104	73	38

The modal age of the cases is the 5–9-year age group (midpoint 7 years). The average age of the 2,589 cases may be calculated from Table 4.2:

$$A = \frac{2 \times 258 + 7 \times 609 + \cdots + 65 \times 38}{258 + 609 + \cdots + 38} = 21.6 \text{ years.}$$

The life expectancy at birth in Bulgaria in 2015 was 74.5 years. The low number of cases reported in the 60+ years age group suggests that few individuals remain uninfected.

So, assuming that contact rates are homogeneous and that the population and the infection are in equilibrium (both of which are big assumptions), we have

$$R_0 = \frac{74.5}{21.6} = 3.4$$

and the critical immunisation threshold is

$$p_c = 1 - \frac{21.6}{74.5} = 0.71.$$

Thus, it is necessary to immunise over 71% of the population at or close to birth in order to interrupt the endemic transmission of hepatitis A infection in this population.

The calculations in Box 4.9 are based on two main assumptions: that the population mixes homogeneously (i.e., all individuals have the same effective contact rate) and that the population is in equilibrium (constant size and constant average infection rate). These assumptions, particularly the first, are seldom strictly or even approximately true. In particular, the presence of heterogeneity greatly complicates the estimation of the basic reproduction number and of the critical immunisation threshold. Some common sources of heterogeneity are discussed in Section 4.4.

4.4 Heterogeneity

Homogeneous mixing means that all individuals in the population make contacts with others at the same constant rate. This is clearly highly unlikely: most human populations are heterogeneous with regard to most types of contacts. A few of the key variables likely to influence the propensity to make contacts with others via the respiratory route are set out below:

- *Age*: close social contacts are likely to be more frequent during the years of school age, and are usually assortative, that is, individuals tend to mix preferentially within age groups.
- *Location*: contact rates might be expected to vary with population density and are likely to be higher in urban and lower in rural areas.
- *Occupation*: individuals in occupations involving frequent interactions with others might be expected to have higher contact rates than those involved in less interactive occupations.
- *Behaviour*: individuals vary according to their sociability and lifestyle, and contact rates are likely to reflect such individual variation.

The impact of heterogeneity on the basic reproduction number R_0 and the critical immunisation threshold is usually to increase their values compared to those obtained assuming homogeneous mixing. An illustration involving two subgroups is provided in Box 4.10.

Box 4.10 Effect of heterogeneity of contacts on R_0

Suppose that the population comprises two subgroups. The effective contact rates for individuals in group 1 are high; those for individuals in group 2 are low. The contact rates between individuals in different subgroups are also assumed to be low. The situation is represented in Figure 4.6.

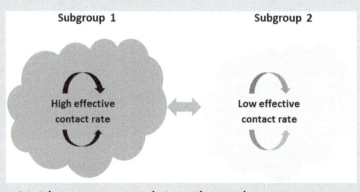

Figure 4.6 A heterogeneous population with two subgroups.

> This simple scenario might be appropriate, for example, for distinguishing between children (high contact rates) and adults (low contact rates), or people living in urban (high contact rates) and rural (low contact rates) communities.
>
> The average effective contact rate over the entire population is lower than that for subgroup 1. So, if a population-wide value of R_0 were calculated based on this average value, it would be lower than the value corresponding to subgroup 1. If the critical immunisation coverage p_c were based on this average value, it would also be too low for subgroup 1. Thus, the transmission of infection would not be interrupted in subgroup 1, and hence nor would it be in the overall population.

The presence of heterogeneities in the pattern of mixing in the population should also inform vaccination strategies. For example, if an identifiable subgroup within the population experiences higher contact rates, then targeting that subgroup may be appropriate. This is the logic underpinning the strategy to control influenza by vaccinating schoolchildren, for example (see also Box 4.13).

Prioritising vaccination of subgroups in which transmission is highest may be beneficial if the vaccine is effective in reducing transmission and if sufficient vaccine coverage to achieve this is realistic. If, on the other hand, the vaccine is effective in reducing clinical symptoms, but does not have a big impact on transmission, prioritising vaccination of subgroups most at risk from disease may be indicated. The different concepts of vaccine effectiveness involved are discussed in Chapter 12. Prioritising vaccination in certain subgroups is likely to be of particular relevance when dealing with emerging infections, such as SARS-CoV-2, when supplies of vaccines are limited.

A further complication for universal vaccination programmes is that vaccine uptake is likely to vary according to socio-demographic variables, with some hard-to-reach subpopulations having lower than average vaccine coverage. Such localised heterogeneities in vaccine uptake may produce pools of susceptible individuals in whom circulation of the infection is more easily maintained, thus tending to increase opportunities for the spread of infection more widely.

Choosing an optimal vaccination strategy requires information about the relevant subgroups in the population, their relative sizes and the effective contact rates within and between each subgroup. Such information is usually difficult to obtain. Box 4.11 describes one approach, based on contact surveys. Alternatively, subgroups at high risk of infection can be identified using serological surveys, as described in Chapter 9.

Box 4.11 Contact surveys for close-contact infections

Surveys were undertaken in eight European countries to obtain data from which to estimate contact rates (Mossong et al., 2008). Some 7,290 participants recorded the characteristics of the contacts they made with others during a day, including age, sex, location, duration, frequency and occurrence of physical contact. Data

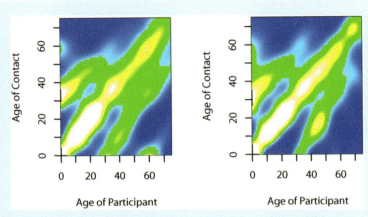

Figure 4.7 **Age of participants and their contacts for Belgium (left) and Germany (right). Darker shades correspond to lower contact rates.**
Source: Reproduced from Mossong et al. (2008).

for young children were obtained by their parents. The results for two countries are shown in Figure 4.7.

Figure 4.7 shows that contacts tend to be assortative, that is, occur preferentially between people of a similar age, as indicated by the strong diagonals. The sub-diagonals represent contacts between parents and children. Broadly similar results were obtained for all eight European countries. The types of contact documented in this study are likely to be relevant to the transmission of infections via the respiratory route that involve close social contacts, such as measles, rubella, influenza, varicella zoster virus and SARS-CoV-2 infection.

Data from surveys such as those described in Box 4.11, together with serological surveys, may be used to estimate R_0 and p_c, taking into account the heterogeneities surveyed. However, in the presence of heterogeneity it is seldom possible to encapsulate the dynamics of infection transmission in one or two numbers. Most usefully, information about patterns of mixing such as described in Box 4.11 can be used to parameterise mathematical models of the transmission of infection, to explore the effect of different vaccination strategies and their long-term consequences.

4.5 Infectious disease models

Infectious disease models are used to explore what might be the potential effects of different vaccination strategies on the dynamics of transmission of infections in a specific population. This can help to decide which population subgroups should be targeted with the highest priority, and what coverage should be aimed for. An infectious disease model is a conceptual framework incorporating what is known about the mechanisms of transmission, often expressed in mathematical language (hence their frequent designation as mathematical models). Such models are used to project forward in time (and sometimes also spatially) the dynamical behaviour of disease transmission and the impact of vaccination programmes. Note that infectious disease models differ from statistical models, which are used to estimate the parameters (such as effective contact rates, or the basic reproduction number R_0) that feature in infectious disease models.

A commonly used infectious disease model is the susceptible–infected–recovered (SIR) model. In this model, the population is partitioned into three compartments: susceptible, infectious and recovered (the latter including previously infected individuals who are no longer susceptible). The model also specifies the rates at which individuals transit between compartments. The SIR and related models are illustrated in Box 4.12.

Box 4.12 The SIR and other compartmental models

Compartmental models were first proposed in the early 20th century; a seminal paper in their development is Kermack and McKendrick (1927). The SIR model involves three compartments. These are represented graphically in Figure 4.8.

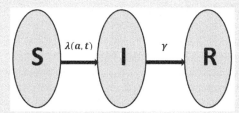

Figure 4.8 **The SIR compartmental model.**

Individuals are born susceptible (S), then become infected (I) at a rate $\lambda(a,t)$, where a denotes age and t denotes time. They recover (R) at a rate γ, which is the reciprocal of the average infectious period D. The rate $\lambda(a,t)$ is the force of infection: it depends on the contact rates within the population, and the numbers of infectives at age a and time t.

The basic SIR model can be elaborated to include additional compartments, for example to represent newborn babies with maternal immunity (compartment M), or individuals infected but not yet infectious (compartment E, for exposed): this leads to the MSEIR model.

For infections that confer no immunity, the R compartment is replaced by the S compartment, indicating that individuals return to the susceptible state after infection: this is the susceptible–infectious–susceptible (SIS) model. Infections that confer some short-term immunity may be represented by a SIRS model, in which individuals in the R (recovered) compartment are returned to the S (susceptible) compartment as their immunity wanes.

Further elaborations are possible, notably to incorporate vaccination programmes, which may be achieved by including one or several compartments comprising vaccinated individuals. Once the structure of the model has been selected, rules for moving individuals from one compartment to another are specified. These take the form of mathematical equations, which may be stochastic (i.e., involving random processes) or deterministic (involving no randomness). Deterministic models are only appropriate for large populations, in which randomness may be ignored. These equations are then solved at each time step using suitable computer-based methods. The details of these procedures lie outside the scope of this book; a practical guide is Vynnycky and White (2010).

Mathematical models can incorporate great biological and epidemiological complexity, such as heterogeneity in individual behaviour, social stratification, the effects of multiple disease strains, imperfect vaccines and real-world vaccination programmes. They can provide new qualitative, and occasionally quantitative, knowledge about the implications and impacts of different vaccination and other infection control policies. An example is in Box 4.13.

Box 4.13 Impact of childhood vaccination on influenza in the elderly

Children have long been known to play an important role in the transmission of influenza, in particular to elderly people who are most at risk from influenza-related disease. This modelling study was undertaken to quantify the direct and indirect impact of vaccinating children on influenza in the United States (Weycker et al., 2005).

The authors implemented a stochastic SIR model within a simulated population. This population realistically replicated key features of the US population, including its age distribution and contact structure within neighbourhoods,

Table 4.3 Baseline US values and percentage reduction (compared to baseline 5% vaccine coverage in children) in hospitalisations and deaths due to influenza at different childhood vaccine coverage levels

Coverage in children	Hospitalisations			Deaths		
	0–18 years	19–64 years	65+ years	0–18 years	19–64 years	65+ years
5% baseline	26,458	50,935	42,844	341	3,516	34,422
20%	−48%	−43%	−43%	−50%	−44%	−42%
40%	−79%	−72%	−71%	−78%	−73%	−71%
60%	−90%	−82%	−81%	−90%	−83%	−81%
80%	−94%	−86%	−85%	−95%	−85%	−85%

households, playgroups, day-care units, schools and workplaces. Influenza vaccine effectiveness values were also based on empirical data.

The model was run using contemporaneous vaccination coverage for influenza vaccine, which in the 6 months to 18 years age group stood at 5%, and calibrated against data for the US population as a whole. This established baseline levels for numbers of influenza cases, hospitalisations and deaths attributable to influenza. The model was then run for a range of different vaccine coverage levels in the 6 months to 18 years age group. The results are in Table 4.3.

Table 4.3 suggests that increasing influenza vaccine coverage in children aged 6 months to 18 years from 5% to 20% would result in a reduction of 42% in influenza-related mortality among persons aged 65 years or older. In the United States as a whole, this corresponds to a reduction from 34,422 to 19,841 deaths. Increasing childhood coverage to 80% would result in an 85% drop in influenza deaths in this age group (to 5,324). Similar effects are observed for hospitalisations.

The example presented in Box 4.13 illustrates how infectious disease models can help to inform vaccination strategies, taking into account the complex dynamics involved. They can also be used to study which aspects of the transmission process are most important, using a procedure known as sensitivity analysis: by varying the inputs to the model, or the assumptions upon which it is based, it is possible to assess which inputs and assumptions really make a difference. Effort can then be put into obtaining evidence in those areas of uncertainty where it matters most.

Summary

- The transmission of an infection within a population is governed by the contact rates between individuals and the transmission probability of the infection. These depend on the transmission route of the infection.
- Herd immunity is the indirect protection of susceptibles resulting from reduced transmission, owing to the presence of immune individuals. If a sufficiently high proportion of the population are immunised, endemic transmission of the infection can be interrupted.
- A key quantity determining this threshold is the basic reproduction number R_0. This is the average number of persons that one typical infectious person will infect during their infectious period, when the entire population is susceptible. The critical immunisation threshold (for immunisation at birth) is $p_c = 1 - 1/R_0$.
- Simple expressions involving the average age at infection and the life expectancy at birth are available for estimating R_0 when the population mixes homogeneously and is close to equilibrium. In practice, heterogeneity in the population may increase the critical immunisation threshold for interrupting endemic transmission.
- Compartmental infectious disease models, such as the SIR model and its extensions, may be used to represent complexities in the transmission of infectious diseases, provide insights into different vaccination policies and highlight those areas of uncertainty that matter most.

References

Anderson, R. M., & May, R. M. (1992). *Infectious diseases of humans: Dynamics and control.* Oxford: Oxford University Press.

Dietz, K. (1975). Transmission and control of arboviruses. In D. Ludwig & K. L. Cooke (Eds.), *Epidemiology* (pp. 104–121). Philadelphia, PA: Society for Industrial and Applied Mathematics.

Farrington, C. P. (2003). On vaccine efficacy and reproduction numbers. *Mathematical Biosciences, 185*, 89–109.

Fine, P., Eames, K., & Heymann, D. L. (2011). 'Herd immunity': A rough guide. *Vaccines, 52*, 911–916.

Hahné, S. J., Nic Lochlainn, L. M., van Burgel, N. D., Kerkhof, J., Sane, J., Bing Yap, K., & van Binnendijk, R. S. (2016). Measles outbreak among previously immunized healthcare workers, the Netherlands, 2014. *Journal of Infectious Diseases, 214*, 1980–1986.

Keeling, M. J., & Rohani, P. (2007). *Modeling infectious diseases in humans and animals.* Princeton, NJ: Princeton University Press.

Kermack, W. O., & McKendrick, A. G. (1927). A contribution to the mathematical theory of epidemics. *Proceedings of the Royal Society A, 115*(772), 700–721.

Mossong, J., Hens, N., Jit, M., Beutels, P., Auranen, K., Mikolajczyk, R., ... Edmunds, W. J. (2008). Social contacts and mixing patterns relevant to the spread of infectious diseases. *PLoS Medicine, 5*(3), e74.

Tsankova, G. S., Todorova, T. T., Ermenlieva, N. M., Popova, T. K., & Tsankova, D. T. (2017). Epidemiological study of hepatitis A in eastern Bulgaria. *Folia Medica, 59*(1), 63–69.

Vynnycky, E., & White, R. (2010). *An introduction to infectious disease modelling.* Oxford: Oxford University Press.

Weycker, D., Edelsberg, J., Halloran, M. E., Longini, I. M., Nizam, A., Ciuryla, V., & Oster, G. (2005). Population-wide benefits of routine vaccination of children against influenza. *Vaccine, 23*, 1284–1293.

Chapter 5

Impact of mass vaccination programmes

Vaccination programmes are often categorised as selective or universal, as discussed in Chapter 3, Section 3.3. An important distinction lies in the ultimate aim of the programme. Selective (or targeted) programmes seek, primarily, to protect the individuals targeted. Universal (or mass) vaccination programmes share this aim, but also seek to reduce the burden of disease in the entire population.

In this chapter we restrict attention to mass vaccination programmes and the changes they induce in the epidemiology of the infection, and in the population more widely. Such changes occurring at the population level are called impacts. Mass vaccination programmes with a safe and effective vaccine will produce enormous short- and long-term benefits for population health. However, as with any intervention applied on a large scale, they can also have more complex and sometimes counter-intuitive consequences, some of which may decrease population health or increase health inequalities. In this chapter, we describe the different kinds of impacts of vaccination programmes and how they arise.

5.1 Reductions in the burden of disease

Mass vaccination programmes have been spectacularly successful. Box 5.1, which details the epidemiology of whooping cough in England and Wales, provides a typical example of the impact of vaccination programmes. Part of the drop in whooping cough notifications after the introduction of vaccination may of course be due to other improvements in public health. However, the specific role of mass vaccination in reducing the burden of disease is demonstrated by the sudden upsurge in notifications coinciding with the dramatic fall in vaccine coverage in the mid-1970s, followed by a decline in cases as vaccine coverage recovered.

Box 5.1 Pertussis vaccination in England and Wales

Vaccination against *Bordetella pertussis*, the bacterium that causes whooping cough, was introduced in the United Kingdom in 1957.

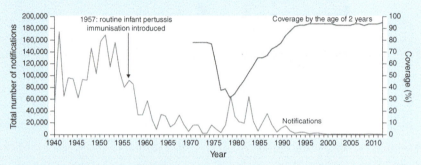

Figure 5.1 Notifications of whooping cough (England and Wales, 1940–2012), and percentage coverage by the age of 2 years (England only, 1970–2012).
Source: Reproduced with permission from Amirthalingam et al. (2013).

Figure 5.1 shows a sharp decline in whooping cough notifications after the introduction of vaccination in 1957. By the early 1970s, vaccine coverage had reached 80%. In 1974, concerns were expressed about the safety of the whole-cell diphtheria, tetanus and pertussis (DTP) vaccine in use at the time. Vaccine coverage dropped to under 40%, before gradually climbing back to over 90% as confidence in the vaccine returned (Amirthalingam, Gupta, & Campbell, 2013).

Vaccination programmes can have impacts across the age range. They may arise both as a result of the direct effects of vaccination (through the individual protection conferred on vaccinated individuals) and from its indirect effects (by altering contact rates with infectious individuals). Thus, in order to fully assess the impact of a vaccination programme on the burden of disease, monitoring should take place across all age groups and not be restricted to the age groups in which the vaccine is administered. Box 5.2 illustrates this point in the case of rubella vaccination in China, which was introduced nationwide in 2008.

Box 5.2 Rubella vaccination in China

China introduced rubella vaccination nationwide in 2008, with a two-dose schedule at 8 and 18 months. Prior to this, some provinces had their own vaccination programmes. By 2012, vaccine coverage for each dose was more than 95%, after which the rubella incidence declined to very low levels.

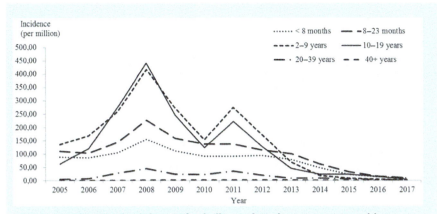

Figure 5.2 Reported incidence of rubella in China by age group and by year, 2005–2017.
Source: Reproduced with permission from Su et al. (2018).

Figure 5.2 shows that, since the nationwide introduction of rubella vaccination in 2008, the incidence of rubella declined in all age groups (the decline in the 40+ age group is not apparent on the graph, as the incidence is so low in that age group). This provides reassurance that the vaccination programme is working as intended.

Note, however, that observing a decline in incidence over a given period does not mean that the incidence will remain low in all age groups thereafter, even if vaccine coverage is maintained at a constant level. Such rebound effects will be described in Section 5.3.

5.2 Herd immunity and elimination of endemic transmission

Vaccination on a large scale within a given population may indirectly confer a degree of protection to unvaccinated individuals: this is known as herd immunity (see also Chapter 4). The magnitude of the herd-immunity effect depends on the incidence of infection, the vaccine coverage and the degree and duration of immunity that vaccination confers. It also depends on whether the vaccine reduces infectiousness of infected individuals, and by how much. Herd immunity is a consequence of the drop in transmission of infection following the introduction of mass vaccination: unvaccinated individuals are less likely to make contact with infectious individuals, and so are more likely to escape infection.

Herd immunity is an important benefit of vaccination, as certain people cannot be vaccinated. For example, vaccination may be inappropriate for newborns or infants, or for individuals with contraindications to vaccination such as immunodeficiency. This is illustrated in Box 5.3.

Box 5.3 Protection of unvaccinated children against cholera by herd immunity

Killed whole-cell cholera vaccines are increasingly used alongside sanitation and hygiene measures to control and prevent cholera in endemic areas. However, the vaccines currently in use are not licensed for use in infants and very young children.

In one study in Bangladesh, cholera vaccines were administered to a random sample of adults and children aged over 2 years, and the authors looked for evidence of herd immunity among children aged less than 2 years (Ali et al., 2008). To do this they calculated 1-year incidence rates (per 1,000 children aged less than 2 years) within geographically defined family clusters, ranked in quintiles according to vaccine coverage. The incidence was highest (18.9) in the quintile with the lowest coverage (<28%), and lowest (8.6) in the quintile with the highest coverage (>51%). Furthermore, protection of children aged less than 2 years was strongly associated with vaccination of adult women (and not with vaccination of older children).

The study builds on earlier findings that cholera vaccination confers herd immunity to unvaccinated adults and older children. In addition to demonstrating herd immunity in infants and young children who are not eligible for vaccination, the study suggested that adult women play a prominent role in the transmission of cholera to this group. This finding can help inform vaccination strategies in this population.

Importantly, herd immunity also protects vaccinated people in whom the vaccine did not work. In this way, herd immunity may even mask inadequate vaccine effectiveness for some time, as illustrated in Box 5.4.

Box 5.4 Herd immunity masking vaccine failure of Hib vaccine

In 1992, *Haemophilus influenzae* type b (Hib) vaccine was introduced in the United Kingdom in a routine three-dose schedule at 2, 3 and 4 months of age, combined with a catch-up programme for children up to 4 years of age. After the introduction of this programme, Hib carriage prevalence in preschool children dropped from around 4% to very low levels, and the incidence of Hib was much reduced (Figure 5.3).

From 1999, however, Hib incidence increased, particularly in children below 4 years of age. This increase is believed to be due to the decreasing impact of the catch-up programme implemented at the time of introduction of the programme in 1992. This catch-up had been particularly effective since it involved vaccinating

IMPACT OF MASS VACCINATION PROGRAMMES 79

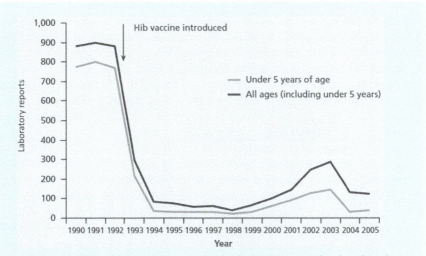

Figure 5.3 **Number of laboratory reports of Hib disease in England and Wales (1990–2005).**
Source: Adapted from PHE (2017).

children at an older age, when the vaccine effectiveness was relatively high. The subsequent removal of the Hib bacterium from the population by herd-immunity effects had masked the relatively low Hib vaccine effectiveness when administered to younger children. The incidence was reduced again after the implementation of a booster Hib vaccination campaign in 2003 and the introduction of a booster dose in the second year of life in 2006 (PHE, 2017).

The impact of herd immunity increases as the vaccination coverage increases, as illustrated in Box 5.5. In fact, a threshold effect may come into play at high vaccination coverage levels. This occurs when the proportion of the population immunised in a given area exceeds the critical immunisation threshold (see Chapter 4), and endemic transmission of the infection within that area is interrupted. This state is known as elimination (see also Chapter 3). It differs from global eradication (worldwide removal of the pathogen from circulation) in that infections may still be imported from endemic areas.

Box 5.5 Herd immunity and human papillomavirus vaccination

From 2007, vaccination with human papillomavirus (HPV) vaccines was introduced in many countries. The primary aim of this vaccination programme is to protect women against those strains of HPV that cause cervical cancer; some vaccines also protect against strains that cause anogenital warts. In many countries, following cost–benefit evaluations, the vaccination programme was restricted to women. An important issue is whether men benefit from this selective vaccination strategy, through the indirect effects of herd immunity.

A meta-analysis based on 20 studies conducted in nine high-income countries summarised the evidence, by comparing the incidence of anogenital warts in pre-vaccination and post-vaccination periods (Drolet et al., 2015). The study found that, where HPV vaccination coverage in women exceeded 50%, there was a 61% drop in the incidence of anogenital warts in girls aged 13–19 years.

Significant drops in men under 20 years of age, and in older women not targeted by the vaccination programme, were also found.

These results suggest that herd effects in men and older women are present when HPV vaccine coverage in women is high. In countries where the vaccine coverage in women was low (under 50%), a significant drop in anogenital warts was observed in vaccinated women, but there was little evidence of herd-immunity effects.

The elimination state is reached in a given community or country when the number of susceptibles is insufficient to sustain transmission of the infection. Cases may still occur, through importations from outside the community, but only limited spread from these importations can arise: the infection can no longer take off and re-establish sustained transmission in this community.

As explained in Chapter 4, the critical vaccination threshold to achieve elimination is directly related to the basic reproduction number R_0 of the targeted pathogen and the vaccine effectiveness. This is illustrated in Box 5.6 for a number of vaccine-preventable infections.

Box 5.6 Ranges of values of R_0, vaccine effectiveness and the critical immunisation and vaccination threshold for selected infections

Estimates of R_0 and of vaccine effectiveness can be used to calculate the critical immunisation and vaccination thresholds for elimination. These are shown in Table 5.1 for a range of infections. A critical vaccination threshold >100% indicates that vaccine effectiveness is too low to achieve herd immunity.

Table 5.1 Low and high estimates of R_0 (from Anderson & May, 1992), the critical immunisation threshold, vaccine effectiveness estimates and the critical vaccination threshold, for selected infections

Infection	R_o Low	R_o High	Critical immunisation threshold (%) Low	Critical immunisation threshold (%) High	Vaccine effectiveness (%)*	Critical vaccination threshold (%) Low	Critical vaccination threshold (%) High
Measles	5	18	80	94	97	82	97
Mumps	7	14	86	93	80	>100	>100
Rubella	6	16	83	94	99	84	95
Pertussis	7	18	86	94	82	>100	>100
Polio	5	7	80	86	99	81	87
Varicella	7	12	86	92	95	87	96

* Derived from WHO vaccine position papers (see Chapter 3) for illustration.

The values in Box 5.6 are purely illustrative, as R_0 and vaccine effectiveness vary both within and between different populations. Thus, while the elimination state might be reached at given vaccine coverage in one area, it may not be in another with the same coverage.

Local variations in vaccine uptake and the degree to which herd immunity is achieved may require the introduction of supplementary immunisation activities, described in Chapter 3, as well as tackling the underlying social inequalities that give rise to these sources of heterogeneity.

5.3 Delayed impacts: changing patterns of susceptibility

Usually, mass vaccination programmes are implemented by vaccinating a particular age group within the population. Provided the vaccine is effective, this immediately reduces levels of susceptibility, and hence infection rates, within this age group. However, over time, other types of impact of the vaccination programme may become apparent. In this section, we discuss delayed impact due to three main causes: the presence of pools of susceptible individuals, reduced boosting of antibody levels and waning of vaccine effectiveness.

When a childhood vaccination programme is introduced, individuals older than those included in the vaccination programme remain unvaccinated. This means they do not receive any direct protection from the vaccine. In addition, some who would have become infected through contact with younger children no longer do so, as younger children have been vaccinated. Thus, a pool of susceptible individuals may develop within some age groups. This creates the potential for outbreaks of infection at some later stage, when these individuals mix at higher rates, for example at school, college or in other contexts.

In consequence, the introduction of vaccination may lead to a period of low incidence after which an outbreak occurs, resulting from the build-up of a susceptible pool. This type of outbreak is sometimes called a post-honeymoon outbreak (see also Chapter 11). An example is described in Box 5.7.

Box 5.7 A post-honeymoon outbreak of measles in Muyinga, Burundi

Vaccination against measles was introduced in 1981 in Burundi, a densely populated country of East-Central Africa. Vaccination was targeted at children aged 9–23 months. In 1988, an outbreak of measles occurred in the Muyinga district of Burundi, despite reasonably good vaccine coverage in this area (Chen et al., 1994).

Figure 5.4 shows the annual incidence of measles and chickenpox over the period 1980 to 1988.

Figure 5.4 shows that, following the introduction of routine measles vaccination in 1981, the annual incidence of measles was more than halved in 1982–1987. But in 1988 the incidence suddenly returned to pre-vaccination levels.

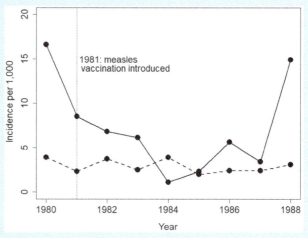

Figure 5.4 Annual incidence (cases per 1,000) of measles (full line) and chickenpox (dashed line) in Muyinga, 1980–1988.
Source: Adapted from Chen et al. (1994).

> This upsurge in measles incidence does not appear to be due to a change or bias in the way the incidence is calculated, as the chickenpox incidence remains constant. This is as expected since no special measures to control chickenpox were taken over this period.
>
> Further investigations show that the measles vaccine coverage increased steadily in Muyinga between 1982 and 1988, reaching over 60% at age 1 year in 1988. The measles vaccine effectiveness in 1988–1989 was about 73%. Thus, failure to vaccinate or primary vaccine failure do not appear to be the main causes of the 1988 outbreak. The majority (63%) of outbreak cases were aged less than 9 or more than 23 months. The authors concluded that the outbreak was primarily attributable to a build-up of unvaccinated susceptibles from the pre-vaccination era.
>
> As a result, the vaccination policy in Burundi was changed to include vaccination of unvaccinated children over 2 years of age whenever they come into contact with the healthcare system.

A post-honeymoon outbreak such as that described in Box 5.7 may undermine a vaccination programme by suggesting that it has been ineffective. Thus, it is important to estimate vaccine coverage and vaccine effectiveness during the outbreak. In the study described in Box 5.7, it was possible to demonstrate that low vaccine coverage or primary vaccine failure were not the primary cause of the outbreak. Rather, the outbreak resulted from a build-up of susceptibles among older children, who were too old to receive the vaccine when it was first introduced, and who would have been infected at a younger age had the vaccine not been introduced.

To eliminate such susceptible pools, catch-up vaccination programmes in older age groups are often implemented at the start of a mass vaccination programme. However, such programmes usually have an upper age limit, so the potential for a susceptible pool to develop is always there. This issue may be compounded by insufficiently high vaccine effectiveness. An example is described in Box 5.8.

> ### Box 5.8 Mumps vaccination in England and Wales
>
> Mumps vaccination was introduced in the United Kingdom in 1988 as part of the measles, mumps and rubella (MMR) programme. The recommended schedule was a single MMR dose at 12–15 months of age. A catch-up programme was also implemented for children aged 2–4 years.
>
> The numbers of confirmed cases of mumps in 1995–2001 are shown in Figure 5.5. By the early 1990s, the MMR vaccine coverage reached over 90%, and the incidence of mumps was low. However, from the mid-1990s, outbreaks began to occur, predominantly in secondary schools, in children aged 12–17 years, who were too old to have been vaccinated in the catch-up campaign.

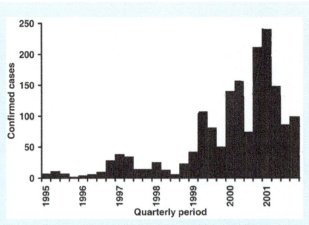

Figure 5.5 Laboratory-confirmed cases of mumps in England and Wales by quarter, 1995–2001.
Source: Adapted from Vyse et al. (2002).

Earlier modelling had predicted this effect and had led to the conclusion that mumps could not be eliminated with a single dose of vaccine. A second routine MMR dose was introduced in 1996 for preschool children (Vyse et al., 2002).

Changes in the pattern of susceptibility by age in the population require careful monitoring, for example through serological surveillance, described in Chapter 9.

The presence of pools of susceptible individuals resulting from cohort effects related to the introduction of mass vaccination, as illustrated in Boxes 5.7 and 5.8, is most often a transient effect. The other effects to be described here are long-lasting.

The first of these is the impact of mass vaccination on opportunities for boosting naturally acquired protection. In an unvaccinated population, the antibody levels of persons who have already been infected may be boosted when they come into contact with infectious people (these will often be younger people). After universal vaccination is introduced, particularly when vaccine coverage is high, the circulation of the infection within the population may be much reduced. Thus, there are fewer opportunities for boosting of immunity. This affects both individuals whose immunity derives from natural infection, and those who have been vaccinated. Susceptibility to infection may increase among individuals whose immunity has waned, notably in older age groups, resulting in outbreaks or higher incidence. Other more complex effects may also arise, as described in Box 5.9.

Box 5.9 Chickenpox vaccination and shingles

Vaccination against varicella zoster virus (VZV), which causes chickenpox, has been available since the early 1990s. However, mass vaccination with this new vaccine has not been adopted by some countries owing to concerns that, by reducing the circulation of VZV, opportunities for boosting antibody levels in elderly persons will be reduced. Concerns have been expressed that this may lead to an increase in cases of shingles (herpes zoster), which is caused by the reactivation of latent VZV which, after primary infection, persists within the nervous system.

Accordingly, different countries have chosen different vaccination strategies. Some have introduced universal childhood VZV vaccination. Others have introduced targeted vaccination of susceptible adolescents or have focused on the prevention of shingles in the elderly. The issues and uncertainties that help to explain the diversity of vaccination policies are discussed in Carrillo-Santisteve and Lopalco (2014).

The example described in Box 5.9 illustrates the fact that impacts of mass vaccination can be delayed, and that detailed understanding of the biological and epidemiological mechanisms involved may be insufficient to predict what is likely to happen.

The final instance of a delayed impact resulting from changes in susceptibility levels within a vaccinated population relates to waning vaccine effectiveness. If the protection afforded by the vaccine declines with age, or with time since vaccination, then childhood vaccination may not confer indefinite protection. Thus, the incidence of infection may rise in older age groups, even with vaccination programmes that have been in place for decades, as illustrated in Box 5.10.

Box 5.10 Adult pertussis in the Netherlands

Universal pertussis vaccination was introduced in the Netherlands in 1953, and for many years whooping cough was well controlled. Then from 1996, an increase in incidence in all age groups was observed, as shown in Figure 5.6.

A booster vaccination was introduced in 2001 for 4-year-olds, and other changes were made to the vaccination programme. The incidence of pertussis in children dropped, but remained high in adolescents and adults. Serological evidence suggests that *Bordetella pertussis* is circulating in these age groups and may limit the impact of the vaccine in children. These observations are believed to result in part from waning effectiveness of the vaccine in older people (de Greeff et al., 2010).

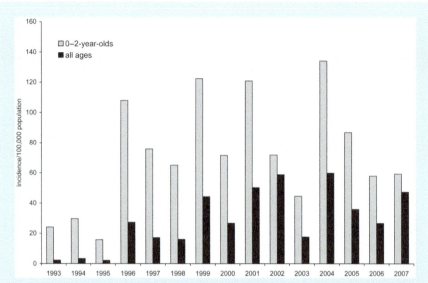

Figure 5.6 Incidence of reported pertussis in the Netherlands, 1993–2007, for children aged 0–2 years, and in all age groups.
Source: Reproduced from de Greeff et al. (2010).

Waning vaccine effectiveness may be addressed, in principle, by introducing booster vaccine doses, or by improving the vaccine. As illustrated in Box 5.10, its impact may only be felt decades after the vaccination programme was introduced, when individuals vaccinated in childhood reach adulthood. Waning of vaccine effectiveness will be discussed further in Chapter 16.

5.4 Epidemiological shifts: age at infection and inter-epidemic period

Mass vaccination programmes have long-term impacts on the epidemiology of the infection. These may or may not be beneficial. In this section we consider two such impacts: shifts in the age at infection and changes in the periodicity of epidemics.

Mass vaccination generally reduces the incidence of infection in the population. As a result, any infections that still arise will typically do so later in life than if no mass vaccination were present. This is because a susceptible individual will take longer to make contact with an infectious individual, such individuals having been depleted by vaccination. This phenomenon results in an increase in the average age at infection in the population. It is a feature of most mass vaccination programmes that do not achieve an immunisation level sufficient to interrupt circulation of the infection in the population.

The consequences of an increase in the average age at infection vary according to the infection. If the clinical severity of disease resulting from infection increases with age at infection, as is the case with mumps and rubella, for example, this might mean that, while the overall number of cases drops (because of the decrease in incidence of infection), the cases that do occur may be more severe. Some implications are illustrated in Box 5.11.

Box 5.11 Impact of mass vaccination on the average age at infection in the United States

Fefferman and Naumova (2015) estimate the impact on disease severity in unvaccinated cases of measles, chickenpox and rubella in the United States, resulting from the increase in the average age at infection following the introduction of mass vaccination against these infections. They found that negative outcomes are 4.5 times worse for measles, 2.2 times worse for chickenpox and 5.8 times worse for rubella than would have been expected in the pre-vaccine era in which the average age at infection was lower.

The authors note that vaccines protect those who accept them. But additional risks may be incurred by those who refuse vaccination when coverage is not high enough to interrupt transmission.

In the case of rubella, infection in pregnancy may result in congenital rubella syndrome (CRS) in the child. Rubella vaccine is highly effective: a single dose provides life-long immunity in over 95% of vaccinees, and hence the elimination of rubella is achievable with high vaccine uptake. However, when implemented at coverage levels that are insufficient to achieve elimination, a universal rubella vaccination programme could result in the persistence of CRS incidence at an appreciable level because the increase in the age at infection means that relatively more infections occur in pregnancy. An example is discussed in Box 5.12.

Box 5.12 Persistence of CRS cases in Greece following mass rubella vaccination

Childhood rubella vaccination was introduced in Greece in the mid-1970s, but vaccine coverage remained consistently under 50% until the 1990s. A review of the available data has suggested that the average age at infection had increased over this period (Panagiotopoulos, Antoniadou, & Valassi-Adam, 1999). This is illustrated in Figure 5.7.

Figure 5.7 shows a rise in the average age at rubella infection between 1986 and 1993, both of which were epidemic years. The proportion of pregnant women susceptible to rubella, assessed in successive serological surveys, also increased over the 1980s.

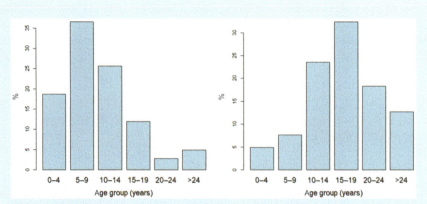

Figure 5.7 Shift in the age distribution of rubella cases presenting at outpatient departments of hospitals within the Athens region. Left: 1986 data; right: 1993 data.

The study gives details of the large 1993 rubella epidemic in Greece, including 25 documented CRS cases. Historical comparisons of CRS incidence with earlier periods are complicated by a lack of directly comparable data (Giannakos, Pirounaki, & Hadjichristodoulou, 2000). However, it is apparent that CRS remained an ongoing public health problem in 1993 under the vaccination policy in operation in Greece at the time. The rubella vaccination programme has since been reinforced.

Many immunising infections with short latent and infectious periods display regular epidemic cycles, resulting from the dynamics of infection transmission (see also Chapter 4). Following a rapid rise in the number of infections, a shortage of susceptibles causes the incidence to drop until the susceptibles are sufficiently replenished by births, at which point the incidence rises again. The time interval between successive peaks is called the inter-epidemic period.

Mass vaccination, with coverage below the level required for elimination, reduces the incidence of infection and thus inhibits transmission. This in turn results in a lengthening of the inter-epidemic period. Box 5.13 provides examples of this phenomenon.

Box 5.13 Impact of vaccination on the dynamics of measles and whooping cough in Senegal

Data on measles and whooping cough have been collected since 1983 in Niakhar, a rural area of Senegal. Mass vaccination against both infections began at the end of 1986. Vaccine coverage in the whole population of this area is around 38% for measles and 40% for whooping cough, and both infections remain endemic. The present study uses data available up to 2001 (Broutin et al., 2005).

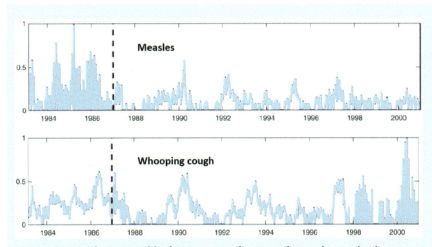

Figure 5.8 Relative weekly frequencies of cases of measles and whooping cough over time in Niakhar, Senegal. The vertical dashed lines mark the beginning of mass vaccination.
Source: Reproduced with permission from Broutin et al. (2005).

The average age at infection for measles prior to mass vaccination was 4.6 years. It rose to 7.2 years after mass vaccination was introduced. The corresponding figures for whooping cough are 4.7 years pre-vaccination and 6.2 years post-vaccination. The weekly time series of relative frequencies of cases (weekly count divided by maximum weekly count over the period) are shown in Figure 5.8.

Prior to the introduction of mass vaccination at the end of 1986, both time series in Figure 5.8 show roughly annual epidemic peaks. After the introduction of mass vaccination, the inter-epidemic periods for both infections increased. For measles, epidemics occurred every 2 years on average, with some variation. For whooping cough, the inter-epidemic period increased to about 3 to 4 years until 1997. After 1997, whooping cough epidemics became more frequent, following a drop in vaccination coverage.

5.5 Ecological shifts: pathogen adaptation and serotype replacement

The reduction in the incidence of infection through mass vaccination may also affect the ecology of the infective pathogen, by altering selection mechanisms. Thus, the pathogen targeted by vaccination may adapt to the new environment of mass vaccination: a phenomenon called pathogen adaptation. This may affect the effectiveness of the vaccine, and the impact of the vaccination programme. An example is presented in Box 5.14.

Box 5.14 Pertussis in the Netherlands

In Box 5.10 we described the changing epidemiology of pertussis in the Netherlands, where adult pertussis has emerged as a new epidemiological problem after decades of mass immunisation.

While waning vaccine effectiveness, discussed in Box 5.10, is likely to be an issue, it is also believed that pathogen adaptation is a contributory factor. Thus, the strains of *Bordetella pertussis* circulating since the late 1990s have been shown to contain a mutation that may enhance the infection of primed hosts (de Greeff et al., 2010).

A further ecological impact of vaccination is serotype replacement, which is particularly problematic for infections with multiple serotypes when only some of these are included in the vaccine. Such a vaccine may not provide cross-protection against all of the serotypes that are not included in the vaccine formulation. This may lead to serotype replacement, where previously minor serotypes become dominant after the introduction of mass vaccination. Furthermore, the replacing serotype may be more resistant to antibiotics, or have a different case–carrier ratio (i.e., the proportion of carriers who develop disease). This is an issue, for example, with pneumococcal vaccination, as outlined in Box 5.15.

Box 5.15 Pneumococcal vaccination and serotype replacement

The bacterium *Streptococcus pneumoniae* is commonly carried in the nasopharynx. There are over 90 serotypes, some of which may cause invasive disease, in some cases leading to pneumonia, sepsis or meningitis. The World Health Organization (WHO) recommends the routine use of conjugate pneumococcal vaccines for childhood immunisation. However, these vaccines only contain a relatively small proportion of the serotypes.

Weinberger, Malley, and Lipsitch (2011) reviewed the impact of the heptavalent pneumococcal conjugate vaccine (PCV7). This vaccine was very widely used before it was replaced by vaccines that include more serotypes, and significantly reduced the burden of pneumococcal disease. However, it was found that among asymptomatic carriers, the prevalence of non-vaccine serotypes had increased substantially since the introduction of PCV7, to the extent that there had been little change in the prevalence of bacterial carriage. The study also found that while serotype replacement had been virtually complete in carriage, it had been only partial in pneumococcal disease. Thus, in this 2011 study, mass vaccination was found to have led to a net reduction in disease. Incomplete serotype replacement in disease was attributed, in part, to the lower invasiveness of the replacement serotypes.

Serotype replacement in pneumococcal disease essentially results from a vaccine-induced change in the population of microbes inhabiting the nasopharynx, also called its 'microbiome'. The effects of changes in the microbiome may extend to other bacterial species than those targeted by the vaccine, and can also result from vaccination against viral diseases. An overview of such generalised herd effects is provided by Mina (2017).

5.6 Wider public health impacts of vaccination programmes

Reducing the population burden of disease is a key aim of public health programmes. A further important aim is to reduce health inequalities. Vaccination programmes can also contribute to this, especially when the vaccine uptake is highest in groups at highest risk of infection or complications. However, the impact of vaccination on health inequalities may vary according to circumstances, as illustrated in Box 5.16.

Box 5.16 Contrasting socio-economic impacts of rotavirus vaccination

Free monovalent rotavirus vaccination was introduced in the United Kingdom in 2013, with two doses at 2 and 3 months of age. A study in Merseyside, England, found that, prior to the introduction of vaccination, the most socio-economically deprived communities suffered the greatest risk of hospitalisation due to acute gastroenteritis (Hungerford et al., 2018). The most deprived communities also had the lowest rotavirus vaccination rates. However, the greatest impact (in terms of hospitalisations averted per 1,000 first doses of vaccine) was achieved in these same communities, in spite of the lower vaccine uptake. The authors conclude that prioritising vaccine uptake in socio-economically deprived communities is likely to deliver the greatest health benefit.

These conclusions contrast somewhat from those obtained in Quebec and Sweden. Free monovalent rotavirus vaccination was introduced in Quebec in 2011. However, the vaccine effectiveness was found to be lower in neighbourhoods with more deprived households than in more affluent areas (Gosselin, Genereux, Gagneur, & Petit, 2016). A Swedish study found that, following the introduction of free rotavirus vaccination in Stockholm, the reductions in outpatient paediatric care utilisation due to viral gastroenteritis benefited primarily those from more socio-economically affluent backgrounds (Schollin Ask, Liu, Gauffin, & Hjern, 2019).

Clearly, vaccinations that are not free of charge to the target population may actually increase health inequalities, as relatively affluent subgroups of the population are likely to benefit most from them. However, Box 5.16 shows that free vaccination may not automatically reduce health inequalities. This example serves to emphasise the need for greater understanding of how socio-economic inequalities influence the impact of vaccination programmes.

Another important public health benefit of vaccination programmes may arise in the context of limited availability of emergency and hospital care. This is common in low- and middle-income countries, but also arises in winter in high-income countries, when general practitioners and some hospital departments may become overburdened by a peak in healthcare needs due to seasonal infections. By preventing infections that contribute to the peak burden of hospitalisation and emergency care needs (such as rotavirus, influenza and RSV), pressures on the healthcare system can be alleviated. This may improve the quality of care, allow access to hospital care for patients with other diseases and avoid the need to postpone planned interventions. An example is described in Box 5.17.

Box 5.17 Hospital admissions due to rotavirus gastroenteritis in Bangladesh

In Bangladesh, the availability of hospital care for children is inadequate with only 3 beds per 10,000 population compared to, for example, 31 beds per 10,000 population in the United States.

Saha, Santosham, Hussain, Black, and Saha (2018) estimated that in the largest paediatric hospital in Bangladesh, a considerable proportion of admissions (6.5% of 23,064 admissions between November 2015 and October 2016) were children with acute gastroenteritis caused by rotavirus, whereas 5,879 children were refused hospital admission because of unavailability of beds in the study period. The authors estimated that implementation of a rotavirus vaccination programme in Bangladesh could prevent up to 629 rotavirus admissions per year in this single hospital, thus permitting the same number of children to be treated who would otherwise have been refused admission owing to lack of capacity.

5.7 Off-target impacts of vaccination programmes

In addition to impacts resulting from the prevention of the disease at which the vaccine is targeted, vaccination programmes can also have beneficial consequences by reducing morbidity and mortality due to other diseases. There are several mechanisms for this.

The first arises when the vaccine included in the programme is able to induce heterologous protection against other pathogens than those targeted (see also Chapter 2). An example of this is the reduction in gonorrhoea that may occur following introduction of a meningococcal B vaccination programme (see Box 5.18).

Box 5.18 Reduction in gonorrhoea hospitalisation following introduction of meningococcal B vaccination in New Zealand

Some meningococcal B vaccines target proteins present in both *Neisseria meningitidis* and *Neisseria gonorrhoea* and are hence effective against both pathogens. Indeed, a reduction in gonorrhoea after implementation of meningococcal B vaccination has been observed in Cuba, New Zealand and Norway.

To control a prolonged epidemic of meningococcal group B disease in New Zealand, a universal vaccination programme with a strain-specific meningococcal B vaccine was implemented between 2003 and 2006, with a coverage of 81% among 0–20-year-olds. A cohort study among individuals who had been eligible to be vaccinated in the meningococcal B vaccination programme found a vaccine effectiveness of 24% (95% confidence interval (CI) 1–42%) against gonorrhoea hospitalisation (Paynter et al., 2019).

A second mechanism for preventing non-targeted infections by vaccination programmes is when infection with the pathogen targeted by the programme is associated with subsequent opportunistic infection by other pathogens. This is the case for measles, which causes long-lasting immune suppression. It has also been postulated for other viral diseases such as influenza, which may be associated with pneumococcal disease. Through this mechanism, vaccination programmes with an impact on viral infections may also reduce the incidence of the associated bacterial infections. When the targeted infection puts individuals at increased risk of non-infectious diseases, effective vaccination will also reduce the incidence of these. An example of this is diabetes, which in some cases is associated with congenital rubella, and hence is preventable by rubella vaccination.

A further, non-directly targeted impact of vaccination may be the prevention of antimicrobial resistance, as outlined in Box 5.19.

Box 5.19 The impact of live-attenuated influenza vaccine in reducing amoxicillin prescribing for children

Even though influenza cannot be treated by antibiotics, and rarely leads to secondary bacterial infections, it nevertheless is linked to excess antibiotic prescriptions for children.

A study was undertaken to investigate whether influenza vaccination of children was effective against receiving a prescription for amoxicillin in primary care. By using the self-controlled case series method (see Chapter 20), the authors found a 12.8% (95% CI 6.9%–18.3%) to 14.5% (9.6%–19.2%) reduced

> rate of receiving an amoxicillin prescription during periods of influenza vaccine-induced immunity in preschool children in 2013/2014 and 2014/2015, respectively (Hardelid et al., 2018).
>
> Since overuse of antibiotics is a causal determinant of the development of antimicrobial resistance, reducing overuse by vaccination may aid the prevention of antimicrobial resistance. An overview of mechanisms of how vaccination can reduce antimicrobial resistance and its impact is provided by Lipsitch and Siber (2016).

In addition to the effects described above, which arise through the prevention of the targeted (or a related) infection, vaccines may also induce non-specific effects against a wide variety of pathogens, arising through the stimulation of the innate immune system.

It had long been thought that the innate immune system does not retain lasting effects of exposure to antigens (sometimes referred to as 'memory'), but this has recently been disproved: the innate immune system can be 'trained', by a process called 'epigenetics'. The extent to which vaccines induce lasting and broad protective effects through the innate immune system is an area of much scientific debate.

Additional effects of vaccination programmes are likely to be identified in the future, as new causal associations between infections and (infectious and other) sequelae and new immune mechanisms are being discovered.

In conclusion, ongoing surveillance of vaccination programmes is essential in order to evaluate their performance and current and likely future impact. This includes monitoring the disease burden and susceptibility levels in different age groups, and the presence and impact of any epidemiological and ecological shifts including changes in the age at infection, pathogen adaptation or serotype replacement. Studying non-targeted and wider public health impacts of the programme may provide further evidence to sustain or improve it.

Summary

- Mass vaccination programmes are likely to have impacts on the burden of disease in all age groups, not just those routinely vaccinated. These impacts should be carefully monitored.
- Mass vaccination offers the opportunity to protect unvaccinated individuals through herd-immunity effects. Immunisation levels above the critical threshold can even eliminate the infection by interrupting endemic transmission.
- Mass vaccination against certain seasonal infections may alleviate peak healthcare burdens.
- The introduction of mass vaccination may produce delayed effects. One of these is a post-honeymoon outbreak caused by the build-up of pools of susceptibles.
- Other long-term effects of mass vaccination include reduced (natural) boosting of immunity and waning vaccine effectiveness in older age groups.
- Mass vaccination may produce epidemiological shifts, including increased age at infection, which may have negative consequences, and a lengthening of inter-epidemic periods.

- Mass vaccination may also produce ecological shifts such as pathogen adaptation and serotype replacement, and changes in the microbiome.
- Beneficial impact of vaccination programmes may include impacts beyond the targeted infections, such as reductions in non-targeted infections, antimicrobial resistance and sequelae of vaccine-preventable diseases. Wider public health impacts may also arise.
- Ongoing surveillance of vaccination programmes is needed to assess their current and likely future impact.

References

Ali, M., Emch, M., Yunus, M., Sack, D., Lopez, A. L., Holmgren, J., & Clemens, J. (2008). Vaccine protection of Bangladeshi infants and young children against cholera. *Pediatric Infectious Disease Journal*, 27, 33–37.

Amirthalingam, G., Gupta, S., & Campbell, H. (2013). Pertussis immunisation and control in England and Wales, 1957 to 2012: A historical review. *Eurosurveillance*, 18(38), 20587.

Anderson, R. M., & May, R. M. (1992). *Infectious diseases of humans: Dynamics and control.* Oxford: Oxford University Press.

Broutin, H., Mantilla-Beniers, M., Simondon, F., Aaby, P., Grenfell, B. T., Guegan, J. -F., & Rohani, P. (2005). Epidemiological impact of vaccination on the dynamics of two childhood diseases in rural Senegal. *Microbes and Infection*, 7, 593–599.

Carrillo-Santisteve, P., & Lopalco, P. L. (2014). Varicella vaccination: A laboured take-off. *Clinical Microbiology and Infection*, 20(Suppl. 5), 86–91.

Chen, R. T., Weierbach, R., Bisoffi, Z., Cutts, F., Rhodes, P., Ramaroson, S., … Bizimana, F. (1994). A 'post-honeymoon period' measles outbreak in Muyinga sector, Burundi. *International Journal of Epidemiology*, 23(1), 185–193.

de Greeff, S. C., de Melker, H. E., van Gageldonk, P. G., Schellekens, J. F., van der Klis, F. R., Mollema, L., … Berbers, G. A. (2010). Seroprevalence of pertussis in the Netherlands: Evidence for increased circulation of Bordetella pertussis. *PLoS One*, 5(12), e14183. doi:10.1371/journal.pone.0014183.

Drolet, M., Bénard, É., Boily, M. -C., Ali, H., Baandrup, L., Bauer, H., … Brisson, M. (2015). Population-level impact and herd effects following human papillomavirus vaccination programmes: A systematic review and meta-analysis. *Lancet Infectious Diseases*, 15, 565–580.

Fefferman, N. H., & Naumova, E. N. (2015). Dangers of vaccine refusal near the herd immunity threshold: A modelling study. *Lancet Infectious Diseases*, 15(8), 922–926.

Giannakos, G., Pirounaki, M., & Hadjichristodoulou, C. (2000). Incidence of congenital rubella syndrome in Greece has decreased. *British Medical Journal*, 320, 1408.

Gosselin, V., Genereux, M., Gagneur, A., & Petit, G. (2016). Effectiveness of rotavirus vaccine in preventing severe gastroenteritis in young children according to socioeconomic status. *Human Vaccines and Immunotherapeutics*, 12, 2572–2579.

Hardelid, P., Ghebremichael-Weldeselassie, Y., Whitaker, H., Rait, G., Gilbert, R., & Petersen, I. (2018). Effectiveness of live-attenuated influenza vaccine in preventing amoxicillin prescribing in preschool children: A self-controlled case series study. *Journal of Antimicrobial Chemotherapy*, 73, 779–786.

Hungerford, D., Vivancos, R., Read, J. M., Iturriza-Gomara, M., French, N., & Cunliffe, N. A. (2018). Rotavirus vaccine impact and socioeconomic deprivation: An interrupted time-series analysis of gastrointestinal disease outcomes across primary and secondary care in the UK. *BMC Medicine*, 16, 10.

Lipsitch, M., & Siber, G. R. (2016). How can vaccines contribute to solving the antimicrobial resistance problem? *mBio, 7*(3), e000427–16.

Mina, M. J. (2017). Generalized herd effects and vaccine evaluation: Impact of live influenza vaccine on off-target bacterial colonisation. *Journal of Infection, 74*, S101–S107.

Panagiotopoulos, T., Antoniadou, I., & Valassi-Adam, E. (1999). Increase in congenital rubella occurrence after immunisation in Greece: Retrospective survey and systematic review. *British Medical Journal, 319*, 1462–1467.

Paynter, J., Goodyear-Smith, F., Morgan, J., Saxton, P., Black, S., & Petoussis-Harris, H. (2019). Effectiveness of a group B outer membrane vesicle meningococcal vaccine in preventing hospitalization from gonorrhoea in New Zealand: A retrospective cohort study. *Vaccines, 7*, 5.

Public Health England (PHE). (2017). *Immunisation against infectious disease (the green book)*. London: Public Health England.

Saha, S., Santosham, M., Hussain, M., Black, R. E., & Saha, S. K. (2018). Rotavirus vaccine will improve child survival by more than just preventing diarrhea: Evidence from Bangladesh. *American Journal of Tropical Medicine and Hygiene, 98*(2), 360–363.

Schollin Ask, L., Liu, C., Gauffin, K., & Hjern, A. (2019). The effect of rotavirus vaccine on socioeconomic differentials or paediatric care due to gastroenteritis in Swedish infants. *International Journal of Environmental Research and Public Health, 16*, 1095.

Su, Q., Ma, C., Wen, N., Fan, C., Yang, H., Wang, H., … Yang, W. (2018). Epidemiological profile and progress towards rubella elimination in China, 10 years after nationwide introduction of rubella vaccine. *Vaccine, 36*, 2079–2085.

Vyse, A. J., Gay, N. J., White, J. M., Ramsay, M. E., Brown, D. W., Cohen, B. J., … Miller, E. (2002). Evolution of surveillance of measles, mumps and rubella in England and Wales: Providing the platform for evidence-based vaccination policy. *Epidemiologic Reviews, 24*(2), 125–136.

Weinberger, D. M., Malley, R., & Lipsitch, M. (2011). Serotype replacement in disease after peumococcal vaccination. *Lancet, 378*(9807), 1962–1973.

Chapter 6

Vaccination
A societal perspective

In the present chapter we set the issue of vaccination in a broader social context. In particular, we discuss how vaccination programmes as social interventions may be perceived by their target population, and how, in turn, public attitudes can impact on vaccination programmes. These issues are relevant to the acceptability and therefore the success of any vaccination programme. In consequence, monitoring attitudes to vaccination should be integrated within epidemiological surveillance. Methods for this are reviewed in Chapter 7.

In Section 6.1 we discuss some of the contextual features of vaccination programmes that shape public attitudes towards them. In Section 6.2 we illustrate the potential vulnerability of vaccination programmes to changes in risk perception and in Section 6.3 we describe some of the issues relating to vaccine hesitancy. Finally, in Section 6.4 we briefly touch upon some of the difficulties involved in presenting scientific evidence.

6.1 Vaccination programmes in society

Vaccination programmes are large-scale public health interventions targeted at individuals who, for the most part, are in good health, very often children or babies (in which case the decision to vaccinate may lie with parents or guardian). They are undertaken with the purpose of preventing future disease rather than to treat an existing medical condition. And while an individual may decide to get vaccinated, or to get their child vaccinated, primarily for their or their child's benefit, vaccination programmes often have wider purposes: they may provide indirect protection to persons who, for whatever reason (e.g., because they are immunocompromised), cannot be vaccinated. Thus, the interplay between individual and societal risks and benefits is a factor in vaccination programmes, which is not present for most other medical interventions.

As a result, these interventions often come with a powerful institutional pressure to abide by them. Indeed, in some countries, vaccination programmes are associated with elements of overt compulsion. An example is described in Box 6.1.

DOI: 10.4324/9781315166414-7
This Chapter has been made available under a CC-BY-NC-ND license.

Box 6.1 Extension of compulsory vaccination in France in 2018

For several decades, vaccination against diphtheria, tetanus and polio was obligatory in France for children up to 18 months of age. In 2018 mandatory vaccination was extended to a further eight vaccines in children up to age 2 years: against pertussis, *Haemophilus influenzae* type b, hepatitis B, pneumococcal infections, meningitis C, measles, mumps and rubella. The only permitted exemptions are on medical grounds. While the policy will not be enforced by penal sanctions, unvaccinated children will not be admitted to collective state services such as schools and nurseries.

This policy was adopted after public consultation as a temporary measure. Its purpose was to increase vaccination coverage and to promote the public health message that vaccination is important. The public health arguments against the policy were that it may prove to be counterproductive, by entrenching vaccine hesitancy that was already widespread in France (Levy-Bruhl, Desenclos, Quelet, & Bourdillon, 2018).

A consequence of these features is that, beyond benefits and risks to the individual, and to society as a whole, the role of government, state institutions and public health officials in promoting vaccination programmes may also come into play. Perhaps for this reason, vaccination programmes have often become arenas of cultural, ideological or political controversy and, sometimes, protest. As illustrated in Box 6.2, none of this is new: opposition to vaccination is as old as vaccination itself.

Box 6.2 Opposition to smallpox vaccination in the United Kingdom in the 19th century

Widespread vaccination against smallpox was introduced in the United Kingdom in the early 1800s and, as illustrated in Figure 6.1, was immediately controversial. In the mid-19th century, laws were passed to make smallpox vaccination compulsory with heavy penalties for non-compliance, resulting in widespread dissent and protest.

The arguments of the anti-vaccinators, reviewed by Porter and Porter (1988), coalesced around several themes that went far beyond the simple issue of risk. One was distrust of scientific medicine and cherishing of 'natural' methods of treatment, sometimes within a religious context. A second was opposition to compulsion by the state and to the growing power and paternalism of the medical profession. A third dismissed vaccination as a mere palliative and a diversion from the task of tackling the social ills that condemned the poorest in society to live in insanitary conditions.

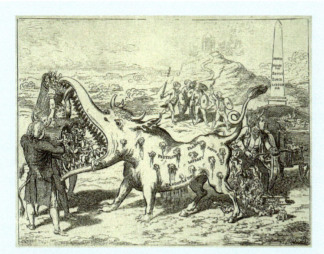

Figure 6.1 A monster, symbolising vaccination and its effects, being fed baskets of infants and excreting them with horns. Etching by C. Williams, 1802.
Source: Wellcome Collection.

Similar arguments against vaccination have been echoed in more recent times (Wolfe & Sharp, 2002). Equally, the challenges facing public health authorities on how to approach opposition to vaccination from individuals and anti-vaccination movements remain highly topical.

While vaccination programmes have been extremely effective in reducing the burden of disease, and indeed are widely recognised as among the most effective medical interventions ever implemented, attitudes to vaccines can be amplified by societal issues well beyond the ambit of medical practitioners. Epidemiology is usually defined as the study of diseases and their determinants in populations. It could be argued that a more appropriate definition, particularly relevant for vaccines and vaccine-preventable infections, is that it is the study of diseases and their determinants in societies, an understanding of which is as important as that of the diseases themselves.

6.2 The vulnerabilities of vaccination programmes

Very occasionally, vaccination programmes may come under sustained critical scrutiny, or even full-scale attack. Such attacks may be fuelled by concerns about perceived risks, but may also chime with other societal concerns, and may be amplified by charismatic opinion formers, the media and on the Internet. Such vaccine scares can result in a sudden loss of confidence in the vaccination programme, with potentially severe public health implications. When the safety of a particular vaccine is challenged, it is seldom possible to substitute an alternative vaccine: withdrawal of a vaccine may leave the entire population unprotected. Added to which, loss of confidence in a particular vaccine may extend to reluctance to vaccinate per se.

It is important to be aware of the history of such episodes, and learn from them. The example in Box 6.3 relates to vaccination against whooping cough with whole-cell pertussis vaccines.

Box 6.3 Whole-cell pertussis vaccine and brain damage

In the early 1970s, diphtheria, tetanus and pertussis (DTP) vaccine coverage (with a whole-cell pertussis component) in England and Wales was around 80%. In 1974 a report was published ascribing 36 neurological reactions to the pertussis component of the vaccine. This was taken up by the print media and TV, leading to widespread concern that the vaccine caused brain damage. The vaccine coverage plummeted, reaching a low of 31% in 1978. The controversy was fuelled by the claims of a prominent public health academic, Gordon Stewart, that the vaccine provided little protection and that the risks of pertussis vaccination outweighed the benefits. Following large whooping cough epidemics in the late 1970s and early 1980s, vaccine coverage gradually recovered to over 90% in the early 1990s, as previously described in Chapter 5, Box 5.1.

Loss of public confidence in whole-cell pertussis vaccines had international repercussions. In Sweden, DTP vaccine coverage dropped from 90% in 1974 to 12% in 1979 following concerns about the safety and lack of effectiveness of the vaccine, at which point the public health authorities abandoned whooping cough vaccination altogether, resulting in a huge increase in the incidence of pertussis and pertussis-related complications. In Japan, public perceptions about the risks of the whole-cell vaccine and the low incidence of pertussis led to abandonment of the pertussis vaccination programme in 1975 after two infants died within 48 hours of receiving DTP vaccine. A pertussis epidemic ensued in 1979 with 41 deaths. In 1981 Japan became the first country to introduce less reactogenic acellular pertussis vaccines. Several other countries, including Australia, Ireland, Italy and the then German Federal Republic, were also affected by anti-vaccine movements.

Subsequent investigations came to the conclusion that, while mild transient local and systemic reactions to whole-cell pertussis vaccine are fairly common, moderate reactions are rare and severe side effects are so rare as to defy measurement (Gangarosa et al., 1998).

Three key factors contributed to the crisis of confidence, described in Box 6.3, that afflicted whole-cell pertussis vaccination programmes from 1974. The first, which provided the trigger for heightened concerns over vaccine risk, was the observation of severe neurological events in infants and young children occurring within 48 hours after DTP vaccination. However, close temporal association does not demonstrate causality, and in this instance these cases were most likely due to chance. Nevertheless, for many people, serious events occurring soon after vaccination are immensely persuasive of a causal link, especially when reported outside of any scientific context. Second, the reduction of pertussis incidence to low levels, largely owing to the success of the vaccination programmes, led to whooping cough no longer being seen as a serious threat. Finally, doubts were expressed, sometimes by public health experts, over the effectiveness of vaccination. Although these doubts were subsequently disproved by the rapid resurgence of pertussis once vaccine coverage dropped, they undoubtedly contributed to a re-evaluation in people's minds of the benefits to be derived from getting their children vaccinated.

The collapse in confidence in whole-cell pertussis vaccine in the mid-1970s exacted a heavy toll in pertussis deaths, disease and complications. However, it also had some positive consequences: the speedier development and testing of acellular pertussis vaccines and, in Austria, Denmark, Japan, New Zealand, Sweden, Switzerland and the United Kingdom, the implementation of no-fault vaccine injury compensation schemes (Looker & Kelly, 2011).

A notable feature of the aftermath of the pertussis vaccine scare was its long duration. In Sweden, universal vaccination against whooping cough was only reinstated in 1996, 17 years after the whole-cell vaccine was withdrawn. This reflects the long time needed to develop and test replacement acellular vaccines. In the United Kingdom, while vaccination coverage gradually recovered after its 31% low point in 1978, it took 12 years to return to pre-scare levels.

The advent of data linkage and computerised administrative databases in the 1990s, along with new analysis methods, enabled health authorities to obtain scientific evidence much more rapidly and thus to respond more effectively to emerging crises of public confidence in vaccines. Nevertheless, such crises may still cause untold damage to vaccination programmes, and thus to the public that the programmes exist to protect. This is illustrated in the next example, relating to measles, mumps and rubella (MMR) vaccine and autism, in Box 6.4.

Box 6.4 MMR vaccine and autism

In 1998 an article by Andrew Wakefield and colleagues in the *Lancet* hypothesised that measles vaccination could lead to developmental regression, an autistic disorder. This hypothesis was based on an uncontrolled, descriptive study of 12 children with pervasive developmental disorder; in eight cases a parent or physician had reported a worsening of behavioural abilities shortly (24 hours to 2 weeks) after receipt of MMR vaccine. Wakefield's article was eventually retracted in 2010 amid evidence of scientific fraud, ethical improprieties and financial conflicts of interest (DeStefano & Shimabukuro, 2019).

Encouraged by Andrew Wakefield, the UK media gave wide publicity to the alleged link between MMR vaccine and autism, and to the theory that combination vaccines presented a special risk owing to overload of the immune system – a wholly unsubstantiated claim. These claims were rapidly rebutted in a series of controlled scientific studies that were published from 1999. These studies made extensive use of the opportunities offered by the availability of computerised vaccination records, health data from administrative databases and population registries in the United Kingdom, Denmark and the United States.

Adverse media publicity about a link between MMR vaccination and autism, which did not reflect the scientific evidence against such a link, nevertheless intensified in 2001. MMR vaccination coverage by age 2 years in England and Wales dropped from 92% in 1995/1996 to a low of 80% in 2003/2004, before recovering. The number of confirmed measles cases increased substantially after 2005, with several deaths. Ireland also experienced a drop in MMR vaccine coverage and subsequent rise in measles deaths. The MMR and autism controversy fuelled anti-vaccine sentiment, together with new but equally unsubstantiated claims of vaccine-related risks of autism in many countries (Gerber & Offit, 2009).

The suggested link between MMR vaccine and autism was, from the start, lacking in scientific credibility, and was rapidly disproved in study after study. However, the plausibility of a link was relentlessly exaggerated in media reports that, at the time, seldom reflected the true balance of the evidence against it, and it gained some purchase in the public imagination. Perhaps thanks to the strength of evidence, the negative impact of the scare on vaccine coverage in England and Wales was much less than that affecting the whole-cell pertussis vaccine in the mid-1970s. However, owing to the much higher infectiousness of measles, its consequences were equally serious and long-lasting.

The MMR vaccine safety scare was to some degree facilitated by the low incidence of the diseases so successfully targeted by this vaccine. The crisis coincided with growing awareness and improved diagnosis of autistic spectrum disorders, which tend to be identified soon after the age at which MMR was administered (in the second year of life), thus reinforcing the semblance of a causal link. Furthermore, public trust in the scientific establishment in the United Kingdom in the late 1990s had been jeopardised by the episode of bovine spongiform encephalitis (BSE). Despite repeated denials that transmission of BSE to humans was likely to occur, a new and fatal BSE-related variant of Creutzfeldt-Jakob disease in humans emerged in 1996. Thus, wider societal issues can also come into play, and may seriously undermine the public's engagement with vaccination programmes, as further illustrated in Box 6.5.

Box 6.5 The northern Nigerian polio vaccine boycott

Between July 2003 and August 2004, five northern Nigerian states suspended the use of oral polio vaccine (OPV), in what was a serious setback to the polio eradication campaign led by the World Health Organization (WHO). The boycott ostensibly was a response to rumours that OPV was a conspiracy from the United States to spread HIV and cause infertility in Muslim girls.

These rumours gained traction owing to special circumstances prevailing in the area, including socio-economic marginalisation, political division, historical neglect of the health infrastructure, suspicion as to why such efforts were being targeted at polio eradication rather than more pressing health needs, past negative experience of clinical trials run by Western companies and the role of prominent opinion formers in endorsing the boycott. Marginalised communities thus asserted their voice by rejecting what was perceived as a government-driven initiative.

Negotiations were undertaken to resolve the issues, involving respected personalities with local access and key international organisations, including leading African and Islamic bodies. These discussions, conducted with due emphasis on the need for respect and sensitivity, eventually persuaded local leaders and the population to support the OPV vaccination campaign, though engagement with key players within the Nigerian scientific community was less successful (Ghinai, Willott, Dadari, & Larson, 2013).

The boycott of OPV in northern Nigeria lasted a year and poliomyelitis cases in Nigeria rose from a low of 56 in 2001 to 1,143 in 2006. The virus spread from Nigeria, leading to polio outbreaks in 15 other sub-Saharan countries. It travelled as far as Indonesia, where 303 polio cases were traced back to Nigeria (Larson, Cooper, Eskola, Katz, & Ratzan, 2011).

As was the case with MMR vaccine and autism in the United Kingdom, the northern Nigerian OPV boycott illustrates how safety evidence emanating from the scientific establishment may not, on its own, be sufficient to convince people of the benefits of vaccination when these are challenged so comprehensively. In order to allay such concerns, a response solely at the scientific level may not properly engage with people's concerns, and may even make matters worse by legitimising those concerns. In such circumstances, a much broader range of expertise may be required. An anthropological perspective on attitudes to vaccination, in particular, provides an insightful critique of categories such as ignorance, risk, trust and rumour, which are commonly employed by the scientific community in an attempt to allay vaccine anxieties, but often to limited effect as described by Leach and Fairhead (2007).

The final example in this section, in Box 6.6, illustrates how careful public health authorities must be in handling matters relating to the potential risks associated with vaccination, for fear of generating counterproductive reactions among the public.

Box 6.6 Thiomersal and autism

Thiomersal (thimerosal in the United States), a compound containing ethylmercury, was once commonly used as a preservative in some vaccines to prevent bacterial contamination. In 1997, the US Food and Drug Administration noted that, because of the increasing number of vaccines recommended, the total dose of ethylmercury in infancy might exceed the level set for methylmercury, a recognised toxicant.

A joint statement was issued in 1999 by the American Association of Pediatricians and the Centers for Disease Control and Prevention (CDC), asking vaccine manufacturers to remove thiomersal from their vaccines as soon as

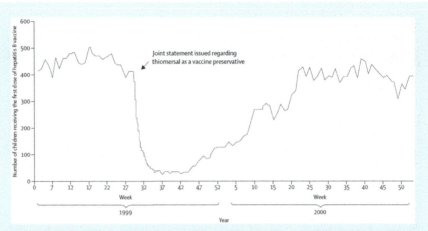

Figure 6.2 **Number of children receiving the first dose of hepatitis B vaccine less than 5 days after birth, United States, 1999–2000.**
Source: Reproduced with permission from Larson et al. (2011).

practicable. This statement was misinterpreted as supporting the suggestion that vaccines were contributing to a rise in autism, and had an immediate impact on the uptake of some vaccines, as shown in Figure 6.2. The 1999 recommendation, which was issued on a purely precautionary basis, also created tension with global vaccine programmes owing to the cost and logistical implications of removing thiomersal from vaccines.

Numerous epidemiological studies undertaken after 1999 have failed to confirm any association between thiomersal and autism, and removal of thiomersal from many vaccines has not been accompanied by a drop in autism frequency (Larson et al., 2011).

6.3 Vaccine hesitancy

In the previous section we described occasions when vaccines became the focus of vocal opposition that had an immediate impact on vaccine uptake. Such vaccine scares, however, are only the more extreme manifestations of a pervasive and long-term problem, which has been labelled 'vaccine hesitancy'.

Vaccine hesitancy is the reluctance or refusal to get vaccinated despite the availability of vaccine services. In 2019, it was listed by WHO as one of the 10 global threats to global health, alongside air pollution and climate change, non-communicable diseases and a global influenza pandemic. Vaccine hesitancy is now a major subject of cross-disciplinary research. Changing attitudes towards vaccination can lead to a decline in coverage and a subsequent increase in the incidence of the targeted disease. The dynamic relationship between disease incidence, vaccine coverage and concern about potential adverse events is described in Box 6.7.

Box 6.7 Vaccine hesitancy and the life cycle of vaccination programmes

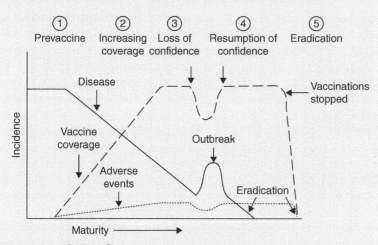

Figure 6.3 Evolution of a vaccination programme.
Source: Reproduced with permission from Chen and Orenstein (1996).

Figure 6.3 displays a schematic representation of vaccine coverage, disease incidence and adverse events after immunisation over the life of a vaccination programme, from its inception to withdrawal of the vaccine after eradication has been achieved. Disease incidence is high before vaccination is introduced. Once the vaccination programme begins, vaccination coverage increases over time and incidence of disease declines. Then, owing to growing concerns about adverse events in a context of low disease incidence, there may be a loss of confidence in vaccination. As a result, vaccine coverage drops and an outbreak occurs. Confidence in vaccination is subsequently restored, vaccine coverage recovers and disease incidence declines.

In reality, matters are often not as simple as suggested in Box 6.7. Vaccine hesitancy may be due to a range of issues, which are context specific and may vary across time and vaccines. It may occur at any stage of the maturity of the vaccination programme and may not be dispelled as rapidly as suggested in Box 6.7.

Vaccine hesitancy threatens to reverse the progress made in tackling vaccine-preventable diseases, some countries already having experienced setbacks in hitherto steady progress. One example is described in Box 6.8.

Box 6.8 Measles vaccination worldwide: one step forward, two steps back?

Live-attenuated measles vaccines are among the most effective available: two doses at 12–15 months and 4–6 years of age confer a protective effectiveness in excess of 95%. The vaccine has an excellent safety record, its most common side effect being transient pain at the injection site and fever. It is credited with preventing many millions of deaths. High vaccination coverage led to WHO verification that measles had been eliminated in many countries in the Americas and in Europe.

These gains, however, are under threat from declining vaccine coverage in some countries, notably within Europe. The number of measles cases increased globally by 31% between 2016 and 2017. In Europe, the number of reported cases in 2018 was 15 times that in 2015. Measles transmission has been re-established in several countries where measles had once been eliminated, and global progress towards the elimination of measles now appears to be elusive.

The loss of herd immunity and the re-establishment of measles transmission resulting from reduced vaccine coverage pose new threats to health, because measles in older people, in pregnant women and in immunocompromised persons carry substantial risks (Paules, Marston, & Fauci, 2019).

It should be stressed that vaccine hesitancy is not the only barrier to achieving high vaccine coverage: cost of vaccines, lack of access to vaccines, poor primary healthcare infrastructure and institutional complacency can also present significant hurdles that inhibit vaccination programmes in many parts of the world. It is also important to emphasise that support for vaccination programmes remains high in most countries, though there is considerable country-to-country variation, as illustrated in Box 6.9.

Box 6.9 Global levels of confidence in vaccines

A global study of trends in vaccine confidence in 2015–2019 was based on 290 surveys in 149 countries involving 284,381 individuals. The analysis focused on three domains: the importance of vaccination, its safety and its effectiveness (de Figueiredo, Simas, Karafillakis, Paterson, & Larson, 2020).

In 2018, most respondents in most countries agreed that vaccines were important for children to have. However, there was much variability between countries and over time. For example, in 2015, 89% in Argentina and 86% in Bangladesh strongly agreed that vaccines are safe, but only 8.9% did so in Japan and France; and while 87% in Ethiopia and 82% in Mauritania strongly agreed that vaccines were effective, only 13% did so in Mongolia and 10% in Morocco.

> Confidence in vaccines was particularly low in Europe, compared to other continents. However, the study identified improvements in several European countries, including France where it had been low since 2015. On the other hand, drops in confidence were identified elsewhere, notably in the Philippines, which the authors suggest may be attributable to safety concerns over dengue vaccination that emerged in 2017. Likewise, confidence levels remained low in Japan, possibly owing to a vaccine scare over human papillomavirus (HPV) vaccination, which was suspended in 2013.

Some of the issues that may underpin vaccine hesitancy were discussed in Section 6.2: typically, they involve a range of personal, socio-economic, cultural and political factors and the interplay between them. The study reported in Box 6.9 found particularly high levels of vaccine hesitancy in some European countries, albeit with some signs of improvement. Box 6.10 describes some of the issues that have been found to be important there.

Box 6.10 Vaccine hesitancy in Europe

A systematic review of studies on attitudes to vaccination in Europe was undertaken, with a focus on risk perception in relation to the benefits of vaccination and individual assessment of the benefit–risk balance (Karafillakis & Larson, 2017).

Some 145 papers published between 2004 and 2014 were selected for review, mainly from the United Kingdom, the Netherlands, France, Germany, Greece and Sweden. As expected, concerns varied between vaccines, between countries and

Table 6.1 Concerns most frequently identified in 145 studies

Concern or viewpoint identified	Number of mentions (out of 145)
Vaccine safety	107
Low risk of vaccine-preventable disease	51
Vaccine-preventable disease is benign	36
Low vaccine effectiveness	32
Lack of information	31
Vaccines are not necessary	24
Insufficient testing of vaccines	21

between categories of respondents (healthcare workers, parents, adults, high-risk groups). However, across all categories, the major factor was found to be the risks associated with vaccination, followed by the perception that vaccine-preventable diseases present a low risk or are of low severity. This suggests that the perception that the risks of vaccination outweigh the benefits is one of the obstacles to maintaining high vaccine coverage. Table 6.1 lists the main concerns identified in the studies reviewed.

There are limits to what can be achieved by purely quantitative studies of vaccine hesitancy. For example, they may be ill-suited for warning of rapid changes in confidence levels and limited in their ability to explore in depth the reasons for people's anxieties about vaccination. Nevertheless, surveys on attitudes to vaccination provide essential information on topics of concern to the public, and provide an evidence base for further, more focused research and for communication strategies. Such surveys should thus be an integral component of the epidemiological surveillance of vaccination programmes; they are discussed further in Chapter 7.

6.4 Communicating scientific evidence on vaccination

In this final section we discuss issues relating to communication about the risks and benefits of vaccination. This is a much-researched topic that we shall only very briefly touch upon, with reference to the MMR and autism scare in the United Kingdom, which was described in Box 6.4.

From a scientific perspective, it is evident that claims about the risks and benefits of vaccination should be underpinned by reliable scientific evidence. However, presenting such evidence can be far from straightforward. Box 6.11 pinpoints some of the stumbling blocks.

Box 6.11 Is the MMR vaccine safe?

The following is an apocryphal interview, based on real experience at the height of the MMR and autism scare. A journalist is interviewing a public health official:

Journalist:	Parents want to know that the MMR vaccine is safe. Can you reassure them on this count?
PH official:	Yes, absolutely, it is a safe vaccine.
Journalist:	So you're saying it's 100% safe.
PH official:	I'm saying it's safe in the usual meaning of the word 'safe'.
Journalist:	What do you mean by that?

PH official:	I mean that serious adverse reactions to the MMR vaccine are very rare indeed.
Journalist:	So you're saying it's not 100% safe.
PH official:	Well nothing is 100% safe, is it.
Journalist:	So first you said the vaccine is safe, now you're saying nothing is safe, what are parents to make of that?

A parent with doubts about the safety of the vaccine, upon hearing the exchange in Box 6.11, may find their doubts reinforced rather than allayed. And yet the public health official being interviewed is being perfectly truthful. Even if zero adverse reactions had been observed up till that point, it would still not be possible to guarantee that none will occur in future or, more to the point, that any given child will not experience a reaction upon being vaccinated. This is so even for vaccines that, by any measure, are deemed to be safe.

Box 6.11 illustrates the very real difficulty of articulating scientific discourse on safety in everyday terms and focuses attention on the disjuncture between what an epidemiologist can truthfully assert, which pertains to populations, and what parents might want to hear, which relates to their own child. This contrast in how scientific questions are framed is central to the anthropological perspective on vaccine anxieties explored by Leach and Fairhead (2007).

Public health authorities sometimes set out the evidence for vaccination as a type of balance sheet in which risks associated with vaccination are contrasted to the risks associated with disease in the absence of vaccination. This is illustrated in Box 6.12.

Box 6.12 Setting out risks and benefits

In response to the claims that MMR vaccine causes autism, the UK Department of Health issued a leaflet in 2001 setting out the comparative risks associated with MMR vaccine and the diseases targeted by the vaccine. These are presented in Table 6.2.

A qualitative study undertaken to evaluate risk communication during the MMR and autism scare reported that parents generally found this information interesting and useful. Parents had little difficulty in conceiving what the data were portraying, though younger parents and those from more deprived backgrounds found the information more difficult to assimilate (Petts & Niemeyer, 2004).

Table 6.2 **Comparison of the serious effects of the disease and reactions to MMR**

Condition	Children affected after the natural disease	Children affected after the first dose of MMR
Convulsions	1 in 200	1 in 1,000
Meningitis or encephalitis	1 in 200 to 1 in 5,000	Less than 1 in a million
Conditions affecting blood clotting	1 in 3,000 (rubella) 1 in 6,000 (measles)	1 in 22,300
SSPE (a delayed complication of measles that causes brain damage and death)	1 in 8,000 (children under 2)	0
Deaths	1 in 2,500 to 1 in 5,000 (depending on age)	0

Source: Health Promotion England (2002), *MMR: The Facts*, reproduced in Petts and Niemeyer (2004).

Such a presentation of the evidence, in as an accessible format as possible, is an essential requirement of risk communication, but has obvious limits. On the positive side, it seeks to build trust by sharing information, and implicitly recognises both the ability of members of the public to make informed decisions and the need to win consent from the public. However, as the authors of the study reported in Box 6.12 point out, this type of official information tends to follow a traditional top-down educational mode, designed to deal with 'misunderstandings' by the public. The authors further suggest that it did not fully engage with the depth and breadth of parental concerns and identified a long list of questions that remained unanswered.

Thus, scientific evidence of the type presented in Box 6.12 is only a starting point. It cannot readily fulfil the requirements of a genuine conversation in which parents are able to formulate and pursue the issues that concern them. A more responsive approach is necessary given that the issues of concern are likely to be diverse, complex and may vary between different individuals and groups of individuals. Tailored public engagement strategies with an effective listening mechanism are required: communication as a one-way process is unlikely to succeed in influencing behaviour.

In Sections 6.2 to 6.4 we have focused on vaccine scares, vaccine hesitancy and the pitfalls of risk communication. However, as shown in Box 6.9, levels of public confidence in vaccination programmes generally remain high. The benefits of vaccination have been brought to the fore by the SARS-CoV-2 pandemic that started in 2019, which has demonstrated just how difficult it is to control respiratory infections through means other than mass vaccination. But the experiences outlined in this chapter demonstrate that such levels of confidence need to be nurtured through effective engagement, and ought never to be taken for granted.

Summary

- Vaccination programmes are large-scale public health interventions that bring into play wider societal considerations and may come under sustained critical scrutiny or loss of public confidence, resulting in vaccine scares.
- Less dramatically, vaccine hesitancy may reduce support for vaccination and thus undermine vaccine coverage. A multidisciplinary approach is required to understand the cultural, economic, social and political issues involved.
- Effective communication about vaccination requires both scientific evidence and engagement with the community. Such engagement will benefit from targeted research and monitoring of attitudes towards vaccination, which should be integrated within the surveillance of vaccination programmes.

References

Chen, R. T., & Orenstein, W. A. (1996). Epidemiologic methods in immunization programs. *Epidemiologic Reviews*, *18*(2), 99–117.

de Figueiredo, A., Simas, C., Karafillakis, E., Paterson, P., & Larson, H. J. (2020). Mapping global trends in vaccine confidence and investigating barriers to vaccine uptake: A large-scale retrospective temporal modelling study. *Lancet*, *396*(10255), 898–908. doi:10.1016/S0140-6736(20)31558-0.

DeStefano, F., & Shimabukuro, T. T. (2019). The MMR vaccine and autism. *Annual Review of Virology*, *6*(1), 585–600.

Gangarosa, E. J., Galazka, A. M., Wolfe, C. R., Phillips, L. M., Gangarosa, R. E., Miller, E., & Chen, R. T. (1998). Impact of anti-vaccine movements on pertussis control: The untold story. *Lancet*, *351*, 356–361.

Gerber, J. S., & Offit, P. A. (2009). Vaccines and autism: A tale of shifting hypotheses. *Clinical Infectious Diseases*, *48*, 456–461.

Ghinai, I., Willott, C., Dadari, I., & Larson, H. J. (2013). Listening to the rumours: What the northern Nigeria polio vaccine boycott can tell us ten years on. *Global Public Health*, *8*(10), 1138–1150.

Karafillakis, E., & Larson, H. J. (2017). The benefit of the doubt or doubts over benefits? A systematic literature review of perceived risks of vaccines in European populations. *Vaccine*, *35*, 4840–4850.

Larson, H. J., Cooper, L. Z., Eskola, J., Katz, S. L., & Ratzan, S. (2011). Addressing the vaccine confidence gap. *Lancet*, *378*, 526–535.

Leach, M., & Fairhead, J. (2007). *Vaccine anxieties: Global health, child health and society*. London: Taylor & Francis.

Levy-Bruhl, D., Desenclos, J. -C., Quelet, S., & Bourdillon, F. (2018). Extension of French vaccination mandates: From the recommendation of the Steering Committee of the Citizen Consultation on Vaccination to the law. *Eurosurveillance*, *23*(17), 18-00048. https://doi.org/10.2807/1560-7917.es.2018.23.17.18-00048.

Looker, C., & Kelly, H. (2011). No-fault compensation following adverse events attributed to vaccination: A review of international programmes. *Bulletin of the World Health Organization, 89*, 371–378.

Paules, C. I., Marston, H. D., & Fauci, A. S. (2019). Measles in 2019: Going backward. *New England Journal of Medicine, 380*(23), 2185–2187.

Petts, J., & Niemeyer, S. (2004). Health risk amplification and communication: Learning from the MMR vaccination controversy. *Health, Risk and Society, 6*(1), 7–23.

Porter, D., & Porter, R. (1988). The politics of prevention: Anti-vaccinationism and public health in nineteenth-century England. *Medical History, 32*, 231–252.

Wolfe, R. M., & Sharp, L. K. (2002). Anti-vaccinationists past and present. *British Medical Journal, 325*, 430–432.

Part II

Field tools for monitoring vaccination programmes

Chapter 7

Monitoring vaccine coverage and attitudes towards vaccination

The progress of a vaccination programme towards achieving its disease control aims depends on three main determinants: the effectiveness of the vaccine used, which population is targeted and the vaccine coverage in that population. Monitoring vaccine coverage is therefore essential to assess progress towards disease control targets, to identify regions or population subgroups where outbreaks may occur and to guide and evaluate interventions to improve the implementation of the programme where necessary.

Furthermore, data on vaccine coverage is used to generate hypotheses about factors affecting vaccine uptake and for studying vaccine effectiveness and vaccine safety. In a broader sense, vaccine coverage data can be used as an indicator of access to healthcare.

Achieving high vaccine coverage in a population depends on three main factors: vaccines being available, effective health services to administer them and demand among (parents of) the target population to get (their children) vaccinated. The demand for vaccination, which encompasses acceptance and taking action to get vaccinated, is strongly related to attitudes towards vaccination. The societal context to this is described in Chapter 6. Problems with any of the three factors may ultimately be identified in vaccine coverage and disease incidence data. However, it is useful also to monitor risk factors for low coverage to detect any problems early. Furthermore, this may help to identify problems affecting specific population subgroups that may not be apparent in overall or regional vaccine coverage or disease incidence data.

In this chapter, we first define vaccine coverage, describe the main methods for monitoring it and how to interpret results. We also include a brief overview of where national vaccine coverage data may be found. We end the chapter by providing an overview of methods to monitor attitudes towards vaccination. The other determinants of coverage (availability of vaccines and health services) are outside the scope of this book.

DOI: 10.4324/9781315166414-8
This Chapter has been made available under a CC-BY-NC-ND license.

7.1 Defining vaccine coverage

Vaccine coverage is defined as the proportion of the target population that has been vaccinated:

$$Vaccine\,coverage = \frac{Number\,of\,vaccinated\,individuals\,in\,the\,target\,population}{Size\,of\,the\,target\,population}$$

Vaccine coverage is also called 'immunisation coverage'. 'Vaccine uptake' refers to the proportion of people vaccinated with a certain vaccine dose in a specified time period (e.g., a year). Since vaccines are usually effective for a long period after administration, vaccine coverage, taking into account all doses received in the past, is most relevant from an epidemiological point of view.

To be able to interpret vaccine coverage estimates, a specific description of what is reported is needed (see Box 7.1).

Box 7.1 Reporting vaccine coverage estimates

For reported vaccine coverage estimates to be useful, it is necessary to be specific by describing the vaccine, the number of doses, the population and the age and time of assessing coverage. A statement such as, for example, 'the coverage of MMR in Finland in 2012 was 96%', is of limited value, as it is not clear what population the percentage refers to. A more useful statement is: 'In Finland, the two-dose MMR coverage of the 2005 birth cohort by the age of 7 years was 96%'. It is important to provide enough detail for the estimate to be reproducible, at least in principle.

Another example of a suitably specific statement is:

> The proportion of surviving infants aged 12–23 months in the West Nile district of Uganda who received three doses of DTP-HepB-Hib vaccine at any time before the 2016 Demographic Health Survey (according to a vaccination card or the mother's report) was 83.1%.
>
> (Uganda Bureau of Statistics, 2016)

7.2 Methods for monitoring vaccine coverage

Vaccine coverage can be monitored by three main methods: administrative methods, repeated surveys and registers. Which of the methods to use depends on a variety of factors, detailed in Box 7.2. Alternatives to vaccine coverage studies, such as health facility surveys or the '100-households survey), can equally provide relevant information for local vaccination programme management and should also be considered (Cutts, Claquin, Danovaro-Holliday, & Rhoda, 2016).

Box 7.2 Monitoring vaccine coverage: register-based, survey and administrative methods

Population-based vaccine registers are the gold standard source of data for vaccine coverage estimation. Hence, if such a register is available in a country, it is likely to be the most appropriate source of data for vaccine coverage estimation.

In many low- and middle-income countries (LMICs), population-based vaccine registers are not available. In many of these settings, multipurpose survey programmes (DHSs and MICS, see Box 7.3) are implemented every 3–5 years, which are sufficient to monitor changes in coverage. Dedicated nationwide vaccine coverage surveys in countries with low coverage are usually not feasible due to lack of resources or conflict. In many high-income countries, nationwide surveys continue to be the main source of data on vaccine coverage (O'Flanagan & Mereckiene, 2012).

In LMICs, dedicated vaccine coverage surveys are mostly used to assess coverage achieved following supplementary immunisation activities (SIAs) for a specific vaccine, in certain regions or after major changes to the vaccination programme.

In countries without nationwide coverage or multipurpose surveys, administrative methods to assess coverage are used, based on routinely available data. This is often considered the least reliable method to assess coverage, as the denominator is often extrapolated from outdated census figures.

Which methods to use depends on what type of data is needed for programme decisions ('actionable data'), which vaccine delivery method was used (routine immunisation and/or SIAs), which existing surveys (demographic health surveys (DHS) or multiple-indicator cluster surveys (MICS)) including vaccine coverage data are present and the resources available.

7.2.1 Administrative methods

Administrative methods to estimate vaccine coverage use routinely recorded data on the number of individuals vaccinated and the size of the target population. The coverage is then calculated using the formula in Section 7.1.

The *numerator* in this formula is obtained from tally sheets or vaccination registers kept at health facilities. In tally sheets, health workers record the number of doses of a particular vaccine administered. An alternative numerator is the number of vaccines distributed, but this overestimates coverage since some vaccines are contained within multi-dose vials and inevitably some vaccines are wasted.

The *denominator* in the formula can be defined as the number of live births in a specific cohort, the number of infants surviving to a specific age or the number of individuals in a specific age range. Data on this is usually obtained from the national statistics office, based on projections from census data or from a population register. Uncertainty in the size of the target population especially affects the precision of vaccine coverage estimates when the true coverage is high (Brown, Burton, Feeney, & Gacic-Dobo, 2014).

Administrative coverage estimates are often considered less reliable than those derived from surveys. They overestimate coverage when the population denominator used is too low, the number of children vaccinated is overestimated or when vaccinations are given outside the target population (e.g., to populations across borders) are counted. They underestimate vaccine coverage when the size of the target population is overestimated, or when vaccination is provided in the private sector and there is no system in place for reporting to public health authorities.

In general, administrative methods tend to overestimate coverage. Therefore, if administrative coverage estimates are low, it is more useful to implement a study assessing determinants for low coverage (for instance a health facility survey) than to perform a vaccine coverage survey to obtain more precise estimates. An exception to this may occur in settings of displaced persons such as refugee camps, where accurate population size estimation is difficult and administrative methods can both over- and underestimate vaccine coverage.

7.2.2 Vaccine coverage surveys

Survey methods to assess vaccine coverage differ from administrative and register-based methods in that a sample rather than the entire target population is studied. In addition to data quality, the quality of the sampling therefore also determines the validity of the coverage estimate. The main advantage of surveys is that they can collect information on vaccines delivered by both routine programmes and by SIAs. Post-SIA surveys require very specific timing, as they have to be conducted soon after completion of the campaign. Therefore, they tend not to be suitable for inclusion within multi-domain household surveys (see Box 7.3). An overview of the role of surveys in vaccine coverage monitoring is provided in Cutts et al. (2016).

Most low-income countries implement multi-domain nationwide surveys using one of two globally operating survey programmes: the demographic and health surveys (DHS) and the multiple-indicator cluster surveys (MICS) (see Box 7.3). When available, these may supersede the need for dedicated nationwide vaccine coverage surveys. However, vaccine coverage surveys continue being used at subnational level in low- and middle-income countries and at national level in many high-income countries.

Box 7.3 Demographic health surveys and multiple-indicator cluster surveys

Globally, two survey programmes exist that provide nationally representative data on a wide variety of indicators, including vaccine coverage, in mainly low-income countries: the demographic and health surveys (DHS) and the multiple-indicator cluster surveys (MICS). The DHS is funded by the US Agency for International Development (USAID) while MICS is led by UNICEF.

Both are based on household surveys and have developed standard methodologies and manuals. The surveys are usually implemented by National Statistics Offices every 3 to 5 years. For further information, see http:www.dhsprogram.com, http://mics.unicef.org/, Hancioglu and Arnold (2013) and Cutts, Izurieta, and Rhoda (2013).

Usually, the sample for a vaccine survey is drawn using cluster sampling, where sampling units are clusters rather than individuals. This allows the fieldwork to be restricted to certain geographical areas, which increases feasibility. Also, it avoids the need for a population register, which is required as a sampling frame to select a simple random sample of individuals.

Cluster sampling is usually done in several stages, for example sampling first clusters (such as geographical units), then households within selected clusters and then individuals within these households. A general principle is that the precision of the coverage estimate is improved more by increasing the number of clusters than by increasing the number of individuals in each cluster. For nationwide surveys, the first step is usually to partition the country into geographic strata of about equal population size. The survey is then performed within each stratum to ensure geographic representativeness. Box 7.4 presents an example.

Box 7.4 Vaccine coverage estimates in Greece

In Greece, childhood vaccinations are administered in a range of settings, including the private sector. They are recorded in home-based records (child health booklets). There is no national vaccine register and those delivering vaccines do not keep detailed records.

Vaccine coverage among children is monitored at national level through population-based surveys. The 2013 survey was a stratified two-stage cluster sample, in which strata were regions (defined by the Nomenclature of Territorial Units for Statistics, Level 3 (NUTS 3)) (Figure 7.1) and nurseries/kindergartens were primary sampling units, sampled randomly proportional to size (Georgakopoulou et al., 2017). In each sampled nursery/kindergarten, parents of all 2–3-year-olds were invited to participate. The sample-size calculation assumed vaccine coverage was 80%, to be estimated within +/− 2.25%, with a response rate of 80% and a design effect (to adjust for within-cluster correlations) of 2.

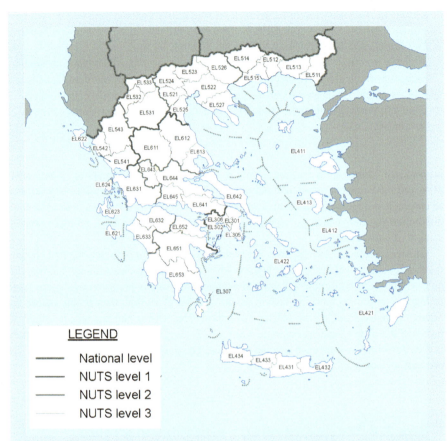

Figure 7.1 Nomenclature of territorial units for statistics (NUTS) – three regions of Greece, 2016.
Source: Adapted from Eurostat (not dated).

The study's results included an estimated vaccine coverage of >95% for three diphtheria, tetanus and pertussis (DTP) doses, three polio doses and two measles, mumps and rubella (MMR) doses. A limitation mentioned by the authors was that immigrants and Greek Roma children were underrepresented in the survey. A subsequent study among Roma children found very low vaccine coverage (<40%) (Papamichail et al., 2017).

Sampling for vaccine coverage surveys can be done in a probabilistic or non-probabilistic manner. In a probabilistic sample, each individual has a known and non-zero chance of being included in the survey. Non-probabilistic sampling may be deterministic or involve an element of discretion on the part of the investigator to determine which clusters, households and/or individuals are included.

Using a standard method for vaccine coverage surveys increases quality and reproducibility, allowing results to be used to assess trends over time. In 1982, the World

Health Organization (WHO) introduced a standard methodology for vaccine coverage surveys referred to as the 'EPI coverage survey method'. Since 2015, this methodology has been superseded by new guidance of which the most important difference is that it recommends only probabilistic sampling (Box 7.5).

Box 7.5 The 'EPI coverage survey' and subsequent WHO guidance for vaccine coverage surveys

The 'Expanded Programme on Immunisation (EPI) coverage survey method', also referred to as the 'EPI 30-cluster survey', was based on experience gained during smallpox elimination (Henderson & Sundaresan, 1982). Since its publication in 1982, the method has been very widely used. It involved a two-stage sampling. First 30 clusters (e.g., villages) were sampled with a probability proportional to size. Then, in each cluster, field workers randomly chose a central starting point from which they selected households to include, in total, seven individuals per cluster. This was not true probabilistic sampling, as it involved an element of choice by the investigator.

In 2015, WHO published new guidance, which was finalised in 2018 (WHO, 2018). Here a range of survey methods is recommended, all based on probability sampling. Three different aims of vaccine coverage surveys are distinguished, which determine optimal methods and sample sizes:

- obtaining a coverage estimate;
- classifying coverage according to certain pre-set standards; or
- comparing coverage in a particular area/time with other estimates.

It is recommended to sample clusters with a probability proportional to size, which means that larger clusters are more likely to be sampled. In addition to maps, global positioning system (GPS) devices and Google Earth can be used for sampling. The new guidance includes an update to the 'lot quality assurance sampling' (LQAS) method, used to classify areas according to their vaccination status rather than estimating coverage.

In a survey, assessing the vaccination status of individuals can be done, in order of decreasing validity, by checking home-based records ('vaccination cards'), health centre records and recall ('verbal history') of vaccination. With the increasing availability of digital photography (by mobile phones), it is good practice to photograph vaccination cards so that information may be accessed at a later stage for data validation.

The usefulness of vaccine coverage surveys can be enhanced by collecting information on reasons for non-vaccination and by adding sampling of biomarkers for infection or immunity.

The validity of vaccine coverage estimates obtained through surveys depends on the magnitude of sampling error, systematic errors, data handling errors and completeness of data. Sampling error is inevitable when studying a sample rather than the entire population, but the precision of an estimate obtained with probabilistic sampling may be quantified. Systematic errors can be introduced by bias. Selection bias occurs, for example, when certain populations are systematically excluded from participation. Since these populations are usually also prone to being missed by routine and supplementary vaccination, selection bias usually leads to overestimating vaccine coverage; an example was given in Box 7.4. Information bias can lead to misclassification of a child's vaccination status due to absence of records or mistakes in parental recall. This can lead to both over- and underestimates of vaccine coverage.

7.2.3 Vaccine registers

In vaccination registers (also called 'immunisation information systems'), individuals are registered with details on vaccines received. An electronic vaccine register that records all vaccinations administered to all individuals targeted for vaccination residing within a certain administrative area is the gold standard to assess vaccine coverage. Ideally, the register is used for operational management (e.g., to issue invitations and reminders) of the programme, since double use of the system increases its quality and sustainability. Representativeness of vaccine registers is optimal when the register is robustly linked to a population register updated with births, deaths and migration, so that information on unvaccinated individuals is also present. Globally, only a few countries, mainly in northern Europe, have such a vaccine register (see Box 7.6).

Box 7.6 A population-based vaccine register in Norway

In 1995, Norway was among the first countries to establish a national population-based vaccine register ('SYSVAK') (Derrough et al., 2017; Trogstad et al., 2012). It is governed by the national Norwegian Institute for Public Health and funded by the national government. It registers data on all administered vaccinations, without restrictions on age or setting of administration.

Outputs of the register include web-based applications providing real-time visualisations of the coverage at desired geographical levels and individual vaccine status information accessible to vaccine recipients or their guardians. The register has been linked to other health databases to study adverse events following immunisation (AEFIs), vaccine effectiveness and attitudes towards vaccination.

Challenges for the implementation of such a vaccine register include ensuring privacy, confidentiality and security of the data, identifying adequate resources and funding for building, implementing and maintaining it and ensuring completeness (e.g., also covering SIAs), accuracy, standardisation and timeliness of the data.

An important advantage of vaccine registers is that they can provide up-to-date vaccine status and coverage data at any given moment. Other uses of vaccine registers include record linkage to health or other data to allow vaccine effectiveness and safety studies (see Chapters 12–16 and 17–20) and the study of determinants of uptake. When the linkage is based on individual characteristics rather than a unique identifier, the interpretation of these linkage studies may be problematic. In particular, absence of linkage may not necessarily signify lack of vaccination.

7.2.4 Innovative approaches to assessing vaccine coverage

In addition to the three main methods to assess vaccine coverage described above, innovative methods using electronic health registers (such as general practitioner (GP) registers) or health insurance data have been explored. The advantage of such methods is that they avoid data entry for the purpose of assessing coverage and that coverage in specific subgroups such as pregnant women or high-risk groups for influenza may be estimated. An example is provided in Box 7.7.

Box 7.7 Monitoring vaccine coverage through health insurance claims data in Germany

In Germany, vaccine coverage data at national level is only available from annual school entrance examinations. At federal state level, vaccine coverage data at an earlier age is available from kindergarten entrance examination. In a study covering birth cohorts 2004–2009, the added value of using health insurance refund claims as data for monitoring nationwide vaccine coverage at preschool ages was studied (Rieck, Feig, Delere, & Wichmann, 2014).

The authors compared coverage estimates at federal state level from kindergarten and school entrance examination data with those based on health insurance data (Figure 7.2) and concluded there was sufficient agreement.

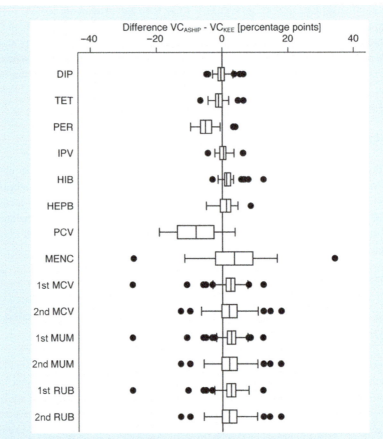

Figure 7.2 Difference between vaccination coverage (VC) estimates based on health insurance claims (ASHIP) and kindergarten entry examination (KEE) data, by vaccine and dose, Schleswig-Holstein, Germany.

Note: Boxes indicate lower and upper quartile while horizontal lines indicate medians. The whiskers span all data points within 1.5 times the range between the upper and lower quartile. Dots indicate further data points. DIP: diphtheria vaccine; TET: tetanus vaccine; PER: pertussis vaccine; IPV: polio vaccine; HIB: *Haemophilus influenzae* type b vaccine; HEPB: hepatitis B vaccine; PCV: pneumococcal conjugate vaccine; MENC: meningococcal C vaccine; MCV: measles vaccine; MUM: mumps vaccine; RUB: rubella vaccine.

Source: Adapted from Rieck et al. (2014).

7.3 Interpretation of vaccine coverage data and indicators

Ideally, public health authorities will have set vaccine coverage targets against which coverage estimates (taking into account precision of the estimates) can be compared. For vaccination programmes where herd immunity plays a role, these coverage targets should ideally be set by taking the critical immunisation threshold into account (see Chapter 4), along with the effectiveness of the vaccine. In countries with high overall coverage, local vaccine coverage targets may be more useful than national ones, since heterogeneity in coverage is an important cause for outbreaks and sustained transmission of infection. In addition to vaccine coverage targets, the proportion of children vaccinated in a timely manner is an important indicator of the quality of the immunisation programme.

Trends in coverage over time are key information to monitor vaccination programmes. To visualise jointly both the coverage and the timeliness of vaccination, the cumulative proportion of the target population that is vaccinated can be displayed by age (e.g., for childhood vaccines) or time (e.g., for influenza vaccines), but this requires vaccination information from all individuals from a vaccine register.

Indicators that are useful in addition to coverage estimates include information on the quality of the vaccination data (whether it is based on records or recall), on vaccine wastage, the pattern of dropout between starting and completing the vaccination series, the timeliness of vaccination and the occurrence of missed opportunities for vaccination. The latter refers to an individual having had an encounter with health services while not receiving all vaccines they were eligible for at that time.

Vaccine coverage data is usually presented at national or subnational level. For programme monitoring, and in particular for monitoring its equity, it is useful to present it also by population subgroup (e.g., migrant children and non-migrant children or by socio-economic class). To assess the risk of outbreaks or ongoing transmission of infection, it is useful to present coverage by social contact networks (e.g., schools or kindergartens) rather than by large geographic areas, since the latter may conceal clusters of unvaccinated individuals. Suitable data for these purposes may be obtained through data linkage of registers (Moore et al., 2018).

Especially when vaccine coverage is estimated to be low or suboptimal, evidence of determinants of uptake can guide targeted strategies to improve it. Descriptive analyses of coverage data by time, place and person may help to generate hypotheses about the reasons for low coverage. However, usually the information on potentially important determinants is too limited to test these hypotheses and dedicated studies are required. This can also be done as part of an outbreak investigation (see Chapter 11).

7.4 Accessing coverage data

Globally, national vaccine coverage estimates are collated annually by WHO in collaboration with UNICEF, and published online as the WHO/UNICEF Estimates of National Immunization Coverage (WUENIC) (see Box 7.8) (Murray et al., 2003). At national level, public health institutes often endeavour to make national and subnational coverage estimates accessible, when available.

Box 7.8 WHO/UNICEF vaccine coverage estimates

WHO considers as 'official' coverage estimates those reported by national public health authorities in the 'WHO/UNICEF Joint Reporting Form' (JRF) on vaccine-preventable diseases. Data collected through the JRF is available at:
 https://apps.who.int/gho/data/node.wrapper.immunization-cov.

Specific data on the most recent coverage estimates for dose 3 of DTP and 12 other vaccines are available at:

http://apps.who.int/immunization_monitoring/globalsummary/timeseries/tswucoveragedtp3.html.

These estimates reflect national authorities' assessment of the most likely coverage, based on any combination of administrative coverage data, survey-based estimates or other data sources and/or adjustments. Since approaches to determine official coverage differ between countries and over time, WUENIC data is based on a range of different methods.

7.5 Monitoring attitudes towards vaccination

Attitudes towards vaccination among the target population (or their parents, if the target population is children) are a key determinant of uptake. They may be influenced by a wide variety of factors, such as knowledge about and past experiences with the diseases and vaccination, socio-economic status, religious convictions, social influences (such as peer pressure) and trust in the safety and effectiveness of vaccines and the organisations and professionals administering them. Attitudes of healthcare workers towards vaccination are also a key determinant of achieving high coverage, as they are an important source of information and advice on vaccination. The societal context of vaccination programmes is discussed in Chapter 6.

Monitoring attitudes towards vaccination among the target population (or their parents in the case of childhood vaccination) and healthcare workers can provide evidence to address information needs, may detect trends of declining trust in vaccination and is a source of data to assess the impact of interventions to increase coverage. It can also help generate hypotheses about reasons for changes in attitudes. Declining trust is a signal for public health action, for example to implement new communication strategies or to initiate further studies into the reasons for the decline. These studies of attitudes towards vaccination are usually of a social, psychological or anthropological nature and are outside the scope of this book.

Two main methods are used for monitoring attitudes towards vaccination: repeated surveys and social media monitoring. An example of the use of repeated surveys is provided in Box 7.9. Questionnaires used in these surveys are most effective when based on prior qualitative research in the target population (e.g., using focus groups).

Box 7.9 Repeated surveys of parental attitudes towards vaccination in England, 2001–2015

Between 2001 and 2008, and in 2010 and 2015, annual surveys to assess views towards vaccination among parents of children under 5 years of age were performed in England (Campbell et al., 2017). These surveys were designed to be representative of all regions and all levels of deprivation. To further ensure representativeness, results were weighted by parents' age, region and social grade. Several themes were addressed in face-to-face structured interviews, including parents' trust in different source of advice on immunisation.

The 2015 survey, based on interviews with 1,792 parents, showed that health professionals were the most trusted sources of advice on immunisation and that trust in this group increased over time (Figure 7.3). These findings suggest that training professionals in delivering vaccines is of continued importance.

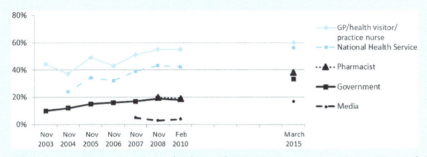

Figure 7.3 Trust in sources of advice about immunisation among parents of 0–2-year-old children by year of survey, 2003–2015.

Note: The y-axis represents the proportion of parents who state they strongly agree with the statement: 'I trust the advice on immunisation given by ...' for each of the listed sources of advice.
Source: Adapted from Campbell et al. (2017).

Social media monitoring of attitudes towards vaccination has developed over the past decade. Social media is a communication form based on participative media applications on the Internet, such as Facebook, Twitter, LinkedIn, YouTube and Instagram. The use of social media is accelerated by the increased use of mobile phones in high- as well as low- and middle-income countries.

An example of a study assessing attitudes towards vaccination by analysing (social) media reports posted on the Internet is provided in Box 7.10. Box 7.11 includes an example of how the number of social media messages referring to vaccination is monitored in the Netherlands.

Box 7.10 Analyses of internet reports to assess public concerns about vaccines

In 2010, the 'Vaccine Confidence Project' adapted an automated online data collection system to assemble a worldwide dataset of online (social) media reports with vaccine-related content, covering May 2011 to April 2012 (Larson et al., 2013). Reviewers assigned whether the content of each report was positive, negative or neutral and awarded a priority status to the report (e.g., 'high priority' when it explicitly mentioned vaccine refusal). This resulted in a global overview of the proportion of online media reports that were positive, neutral or negative. The project also provided insights into country- and vaccine-specific issues, which the authors suggest might be useful to tailor strategies to address public concerns.

Box 7.11 Monitoring of vaccination-related social media messages in the Netherlands

The National Institute for Public Health and the Environment (RIVM) in the Netherlands uses the social media monitoring and analyses tool 'Coosto' to monitor social media messages mentioning vaccination. The tool scans various social media sources (including Facebook, Twitter, LinkedIn and Instagram) for messages related to vaccination, and produces an automated report with information about the volume, source and content of the messages (see Figure 7.4). By using Dutch search terms, messages mostly coming from the Netherlands are found.

The tool allows for monitoring of the number of social media messages regarding vaccination. This can be used to detect sudden changes in attitudes towards specific vaccines, which is especially useful when a new programme is introduced. A peak in the number of vaccine-related messages can be further investigated, for example by word-cloud visualisation (made by a Wordl tool) or generating a list of messages including a certain search term. Importantly, the content and attitude (positive, negative or neutral) cannot be assessed automatically; human review is needed for this. This social media analysis is used to improve information provided by RIVM about vaccination, and to identify issues/themes that require further investigation.

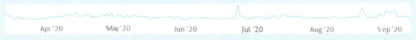

Figure 7.4 Volume of social media messages related to vaccination, April–September 2020.
Source: Coosto RIVM report 16.9.2020. Reproduced with permission from M. Smorenburg.

An example of using Twitter messages to study population attitudes towards vaccination is a study by Lutkenhaus, Janz, and Bouman (2019). In this study, separate communities of individuals posting messages about vaccination were identified (e.g., 'pro-vaccination' and 'anti-establishment'). By also considering Twitter interactions between these communities, an assessment of how much they influence each other was made (Lutkenhaus et al., 2019).

The advantage of monitoring social media is that it provides fast and direct access to digital information on attitudes and opinions of the public. An important limitation of social media monitoring is that it still requires human review of the individual reports to adequately classify their content in terms of a positive, neutral or negative attitude towards vaccination, limiting the volume of data that can be processed. Another important limitation is that those posting social media messages cannot be assumed to represent the general population: social media users are likely to exclude certain population subgroups and may include non-human entities such as trolls and bots. In general, the volume of reports may not be representative of the number of people it represents, with active social media users being overrepresented. Further studies to assess the added value of using social media to monitor attitudes towards vaccination and coverage are needed.

Summary

- Vaccine coverage is a major determinant of the impact of a vaccination programme. Monitoring vaccine coverage is therefore essential for evaluating impact.
- Methods to monitor vaccine coverage include administrative, register-based and survey methods. The choice for which method to use depends on local resources, the availability of multipurpose surveys such as DHS and MICS, the setting and the type of vaccination programme being assessed.
- Vaccine coverage may also be assessed using electronic health records that are collected for other purposes. These are important resources for linkage studies.
- Ideally, vaccine coverage targets exist, against which coverage estimates can be evaluated. Descriptive analyses of coverage data can be used to study trends, identify low-coverage subgroups and generate hypotheses for low uptake.
- Attitudes towards vaccination among (parents of) the target population and healthcare providers are a key determinant of vaccine coverage. These can be monitored by repeated surveys.
- Through automated social media analyses, the number of messages referring to vaccination can be monitored. Further evaluations are needed to assess the added value of this for monitoring population attitudes towards vaccination and vaccine coverage.

References

Brown, D. W. Burton, A. H., Feeney G., & Gacic-Dobo, M. (2014). Avoiding the will-o'-the-wisp: Challenges in measuring high levels of immunization coverage with precision. *World Journal of Vaccines*, *4*, 97–99. doi:10.4236/wjv.2014.43012.

Campbell, H., Edwards, A., Letley, L., Bedford, H., Ramsay, M., & Yarwood, J. (2017). Changing attitudes to childhood immunisation in English parents. *Vaccine*, *35*(22), 2979–2985. doi:10.1016/j.vaccine.2017.03.089.

Cutts, F. T., Claquin, P., Danovaro-Holliday, M. C., & Rhoda, D. A. (2016). Monitoring vaccination coverage: Defining the role of surveys. *Vaccine*, *34*(35), 4103–4109. doi:10.1016/j.vaccine.2016.06.053.

Cutts, F. T., Izurieta, H. S., & Rhoda, D. A. (2013). Measuring coverage in MNCH: Design, implementation, and interpretation challenges associated with tracking vaccination coverage using household surveys. *PLoS Med, 10*(5), e1001404. doi:10.1371/journal.pmed.1001404.

Derrough, T., Olsson, K., Gianfredi, V., Simondon, F., Heijbel, H., Danielsson, N., ... Pastore-Celentano, L. (2017). Immunisation information systems: Useful tools for monitoring vaccination programmes in EU/EEA countries, 2016. *Eurosurveillance, 22*(17). doi:10.2807/1560-7917.ES.2017.22.17.30519.

Eurostat. (not dated). European statistics. Retrieved from https://ec.europa.eu/eurostat/.

Georgakopoulou, T., Menegas, D., Katsioulis, A., Theodoridou, M., Kremastinou, J., & Hadjichristodoulou, C. (2017). A cross-sectional vaccination coverage study in preschool children attending nurseries and kindergartens: Implications on economic crisis effect. *Human Vaccines and Immunotherapeutics, 13*(1), 190–197. doi:10.1080/21645515.2016.1230577.

Hancioglu, A., & Arnold, F. (2013). Measuring coverage in MNCH: Tracking progress in health for women and children using DHS and MICS household surveys. *PLoS Med, 10*(5), e1001391. doi:10.1371/journal.pmed.1001391.

Henderson, R. H., & Sundaresan, T. (1982). Cluster sampling to assess immunization coverage: A review of experience with a simplified sampling method. *Bulletin of the World Health Organization, 60*(2), 253–260. Retrieved from www.ncbi.nlm.nih.gov/pubmed/6980735.

Larson, H. J., Smith, D. M., Paterson, P., Cumming, M., Eckersberger, E., Freifeld, C. C., ... Madoff, L. C. (2013). Measuring vaccine confidence: Analysis of data obtained by a media surveillance system used to analyse public concerns about vaccines. *Lancet Infectious Diseases, 13*(7), 606–613. doi:10.1016/S1473-3099(13)70108-7.

Lutkenhaus, R. O., Jansz, J., & Bouman, M. P. A. (2019). Mapping the Dutch vaccination debate on Twitter: Identifying communities, narratives, and interactions. *Vaccine 10*(1), 100019. doi:10.1016/j.jvacx.2019.100019.

Moore, H. C., Fathima, P., Gidding, H. F., de Klerk, N., Liu, B., Sheppeard, V., ... Group, A. L. I. (2018). Assessment of on-time vaccination coverage in population subgroups: A record linkage cohort study. *Vaccine, 36*(28), 4062–4069. doi:10.1016/j.vaccine.2018.05.084.

Murray, C. J., Shengelia, B., Gupta, N., Moussavi, S., Tandon, A., & Thieren, M. (2003). Validity of reported vaccination coverage in 45 countries. *Lancet, 362*(9389), 1022–1027. doi:10.1016/S0140-6736(03)14411-X.

O'Flanagan, D. C., & Mereckiene, J. (2012). *Vaccination coverage assessment in EU/EEA, 2011*. Retrieved from http://venice.cineca.org/Final_Vaccination_Coverage_Assesment_Survey_2011_1.pdf.

Papamichail, D., Petraki, I., Arkoudis, C., Terzidis, A., Smyrnakis, E., Benos, A., & Panagiotopoulos, T. (2017). Low vaccination coverage of Greek Roma children amid economic crisis: National survey using stratified cluster sampling. *European Journal of Public Health, 27*(2), 318–324. doi:10.1093/eurpub/ckw179.

Rieck, T., Feig, M., Delere, Y., & Wichmann, O. (2014). Utilization of administrative data to assess the association of an adolescent health check-up with human papillomavirus vaccine uptake in Germany. *Vaccine, 32*(43), 5564–5569. doi:10.1016/j.vaccine.2014.07.105.

Trogstad, L., Ung, G., Hagerup-Jenssen, M., Cappelen, I., Haugen, I. L., & Feiring, B. (2012). The Norwegian immunisation register – SYSVAK. *Eurosurveillance, 17*(16). Retrieved from www.ncbi.nlm.nih.gov/pubmed/22551462.

Uganda Bureau of Statistics. (2016). *Uganda demographic and health survey*. Kampala, Uganda: Uganda Bureau of Statistics. Retrieved from https://dhsprogram.com/pubs/pdf/FR333/FR333.pdf.

World Health Organization (WHO). (2018). *World Health Organization vaccination coverage cluster surveys: Reference manual*. Geneva, Switzerland: WHO. Retrieved from https://apps.who.int/iris/handle/10665/272820.

Chapter 8

Surveillance of vaccine-preventable diseases and pathogens

Once a vaccine has been introduced in a vaccination programme, continued assessment of the programme's performance is needed to justify its continuation and to obtain evidence to improve vaccine policy and programme implementation. Surveillance of vaccine-preventable diseases and pathogens is a key tool for this assessment. The first aim of surveillance in this context is to provide data needed to assess the programme's impact on the occurrence and distributions of the targeted infections and pathogens. A second aim is to allow the identification of remaining pockets of susceptible individuals, outbreaks and changes in the epidemiology of the targeted diseases. In addition to its use for vaccination programme evaluation, surveillance is also a direct tool for controlling the spread of certain infectious diseases, through early detection and isolation of cases and quarantining of their contacts – a public health practice dating back to the control of plague in the 14th century and still being used to this day.

As outlined in Chapter 5, mass vaccination programmes can have a multitude of effects, altering the epidemiology of infection and disease among both vaccinated and non-vaccinated individuals. In order to monitor benefits and risks of the programme comprehensively, it is important therefore that surveillance covers the entire population, not just the targeted individuals. To assess, for example, the impact of a pneumococcal vaccination programme for infants, the occurrence of pneumococcal infections among the elderly also needs to be monitored, as much of the benefit of the programme may arise in this age group.

In this chapter, we will first outline the main methods of vaccine-preventable disease surveillance, considering data sources, case definitions, biases and methods for descriptive analyses. These methods are applicable to surveillance at both national and subnational level and are hence also relevant for countries or diseases where national surveillance is lacking. In addition to reducing the incidence of disease, mass vaccination programmes can also impact on the ecology of both targeted and non-targeted micro-organisms. The ecological effects on micro-organisms can include a change in the distribution of subtypes of the pathogen by pathogen adaptation and serotype replacement (see Chapter 5). These changes are important to monitor since they may necessitate changes in vaccine policy, irrespective of whether the changes are induced by the vaccination programme. In the second section of the chapter we provide an overview of methods to monitor changes in pathogen populations.

The methods for surveillance of vaccine-preventable diseases are largely the same as those used in the surveillance of non-vaccine-preventable diseases. A general overview of infectious disease surveillance can be found in (M'ikanatha, Lynfield, van Beneden, & de Valk, 2013; WHO, 2018). In contrast to many other disease control programmes, vaccination can be extremely effective in reducing the incidence of infection. As we will outline in this chapter, the methods for vaccine-preventable disease and pathogen surveillance usually need to be adapted to the different phases of control of the targeted disease.

When a vaccination programme has been successful and the targeted infection is near elimination, vaccine-preventable disease surveillance encounters specific epidemiological challenges while at the same time the requirements of surveillance, in terms of, for example, sensitivity and specificity, are more demanding. In this context, enhanced (pathogen) surveillance and international collaboration are of increasing importance. This is discussed in the last section of this chapter.

8.1 Surveillance of vaccine-preventable diseases

8.1.1 Sources of data

Which sources of data to use in vaccine-preventable disease surveillance depends on several factors including the characteristics of the disease under surveillance, the diagnostic practices in the country, the aims of the vaccination programme and the availability of data. The severity and incidence of the disease under surveillance determine which data sources are most useful. Data obtained from general practitioners, for example, are of limited use for the surveillance of severe and rare infections such as invasive meningococcal or pneumococcal disease (which usually get diagnosed in hospital); while they are useful, for example, for monitoring the incidence of influenza-like illness. When the aim of the vaccination programme is to eliminate a disease, surveillance covering the entire population, rather than sentinel site surveillance, is needed.

To assess impact of vaccination, long-standing sources of data for which data collection methods have remained largely unchanged over several years are most useful. Limitations of individual data sources may to some extent be overcome by considering results from different sources together. This process is referred to as 'data triangulation'. Below we list the most commonly used sources of data for vaccine-preventable disease surveillance.

8.1.1.1 Disease notification

Most countries have a list of infectious diseases of relevance to public health that clinicians or laboratories are legally obliged to report to public health authorities. Since vaccination programmes are one of the main tools in public health, vaccine-preventable diseases targeted by vaccination programmes are usually included in the list of notifiable diseases. The notification ideally includes the date of onset of symptoms, sex, age, place of residence, results of laboratory testing and vaccination status of the patient. Sometimes, information on risk factors is present. The definitive diagnosis of nearly all vaccine-preventable diseases requires laboratory testing. Exceptions to this are tetanus and, to a lesser extent, chickenpox, which can be diagnosed with fairly high certainty based on clinical symptoms alone.

The usefulness of notifiable disease data depends on whether a standardised definition is applied when selecting patients to be notified. Furthermore, it is important to be aware of the validity of the case definition used (see Box 8.1). From a surveillance point of view, the sensitivity and positive predictive value are the most relevant validity indicators for a case definition. These indicate, respectively, how good the definition is at identifying all cases, and, for cases identified, how likely it is that they are true cases of the disease of interest. Often, layered definitions that differ in sensitivity and specificity are used in surveillance (e.g., 'confirmed cases' and 'probable cases'), which allow a subset of cases to be chosen that best fits the aims of the analyses.

Box 8.1 Measures of validity of a case definition: sensitivity, specificity and positive predictive value

The validity of a case definition can be described in terms of sensitivity, specificity and positive predictive value, as for diagnostic laboratory tests.

- The *sensitivity* is the proportion of true cases (i.e., cases caused by the infection of interest) that meet the case definition. It thus indicates how good the case definition is at identifying all true cases.
- The *specificity* is the proportion of true non-cases that do not meet the case definition. It thus indicates how good the case definition is at excluding non-cases.
- The *positive predictive value* is the proportion of cases meeting the case definition that are due to the infection of interest.

Table 8.1 demonstrates the calculation of these indicators.

Table 8.1 Validity of case definition

		True case Yes	True case No
Meeting case definition	Yes	a (60)	b (60)
	No	c (5)	d (875)

Sensitivity = $a / (a + c)$ = 92%
Specificity = $d / (b + d)$ = 94%
Positive predictive value = $a / (a + b)$ = 50%
Prevalence of the disease of interest = $(a + c) / (a + b + c + d)$ = 7%

When a case definition is based only on clinical symptoms, it is likely to be very sensitive but also quite non-specific. The sensitivity of the case definition depends solely on the definition itself. In contrast, the positive predictive value depends on the specificity of the case definition, the prevalence of the disease of interest and, for a clinical case definition, on the prevalence of the clinical syndrome (as used in the definition) caused by other diseases.

For several reasons, case definitions used for surveillance may need to be adapted according to the stage of the vaccination programme. First, a decrease in the incidence of the targeted disease may result in an unacceptably low positive predictive value of a clinical case definition. An example of this is provided in Box 8.2. Second, close to elimination, high sensitivity of surveillance becomes important to detect all remaining cases, coupled with even higher specificity to not waste too many healthcare resources on false positive cases, and case definitions may need to be adapted again (see Section 8.3). Requirements for case definitions used in outbreak investigations and studies of vaccine effectiveness are discussed in Chapters 11 and 13, respectively.

Box 8.2 Clinical case definitions for measles: positive predictive value depends on the level of measles control achieved

In the United Kingdom, the following clinical case definition for measles was used in the past: *rash, fever and cough, coryza or conjunctivitis*. This definition was sensitive but not very specific. When measles was common in the pre-vaccine era, clinical cases had a high chance of being true measles cases, meaning the case definition had a high positive predictive value. However, when measles was nearly eliminated, most clinical cases were due to other causes, of which the incidence had not changed (such as B19 virus or group A streptococcus), which made the positive predictive value decline towards zero (Figure 8.1).

For measles surveillance to remain useful, the case definition had to be made more specific. This can be done by adding the requirement for an epidemiological link or for laboratory confirmation. This is reflected in the World Health Organization (WHO) and European Union (EU) case definition for confirmed measles currently used in the United Kingdom: *Any person not recently vaccinated* and meeting the clinical and the laboratory criteria.***

* Not vaccinated with measles containing vaccine in the 6 weeks prior to specimen collection.

** Clinical criteria: any person with fever, maculo-papular rash and at least one of the following three: cough, coryza, conjunctivitis. Laboratory criteria: at least one of the following four: isolation of measles virus from a clinical specimen, detection of measles virus nucleic acid in a clinical specimen, measles virus-specific antibody response characteristic for acute infection in serum or saliva, detection of measles virus antigen by direct fluorescence antibody in a clinical

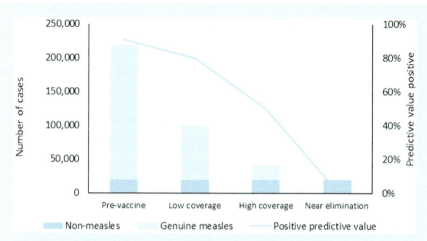

Figure 8.1 The number of reported clinical measles cases by cause (bars) and the positive predictive value of the clinical case definition (blue line), in different stages of measles control in the United Kingdom.
Source: Theoretical example adapted with permission from M. Ramsay.

specimen using measles specific monoclonal antibodies. Laboratory results need to be interpreted according to the vaccination status. If recently vaccinated, investigate for wild virus.

To facilitate comparison of disease surveillance data between countries, international public health organisations propose standardised case definitions. For example, those used by the European Centre for Disease Prevention and Control (ECDC) are available at https://ecdc.europa.eu/en/surveillance-and-disease-data/eu-case-definitions.

A disadvantage of notification data is that it usually represents only the tip of the iceberg of all patients with the notifiable condition. One reason for this is that patients with mild symptoms may not seek healthcare, and if they do are unlikely to undergo laboratory testing, since the results would not alter their clinical management. Furthermore, subclinical infections (infections without symptoms) are not included. This may not be a problem for public health decision-making, depending on how constant, representative and unbiased the reporting is (see Section 8.1.2). To improve the sensitivity of surveillance for public health purposes, less invasive tests (e.g., using oral fluid (saliva)) have been developed. Notification data is also often incomplete in providing information on sequelae or death, since these usually occur after the patient was notified. Assessing the population burden of infection may require more advanced methods. Some of these, notably QALYs and DALYs, are discussed in Chapter 21 in the context of benefit–risk evaluations.

8.1.1.2 Laboratory surveillance

Laboratory surveillance is usually organised by laboratories throughout the country who voluntarily report identifications of pathogens on a regular basis (e.g., weekly) to a central public health authority (see Box 8.3 for an example). The main advantage is that this offers highly specific data, sometimes even including subtypes or genomic information about the pathogen (see also Section 8.2 on pathogen surveillance). The usefulness of laboratory surveillance data is greatly enhanced when data on the number of specimens tested is also provided. This helps clarify whether an observed change in the number of positive tests is due to a genuine change in the incidence or is due to changes in testing (or reporting) practices.

A limitation of laboratory surveillance is that demographic, clinical, epidemiological and vaccine status information are often not available. As with notification data, the sensitivity of laboratory surveillance is low when only a small proportion of patients are tested. Another limitation of laboratory surveillance data is that often the denominator (e.g., the 'catchment population' for the laboratory) is unknown so it is problematic to calculate population incidence rates. However, if the catchment populations are stable, trends over time are meaningful. In general, the usefulness of laboratory surveillance depends on the standardisation and coding of the information, the availability of additional information (or the possibility to link the data to other data sources) and the representativeness of the population under surveillance.

The increased implementation of point-of-care-tests (POCTs) in clinical management of infectious diseases is a challenge from the perspective of laboratory surveillance. The validity of the tests may be lower compared to standard tests, subtyping results are usually not available, and capturing the data in a surveillance system is likely to require additional efforts (Dickson et al., 2020).

Box 8.3 Use of multiple data sources for the surveillance of rotavirus in the Netherlands

Rotavirus infection can cause acute gastroenteritis, which is in most cases short-lived and does not require healthcare visits but can lead to dehydration and death in very young infants.

Rotavirus infection is not notifiable in the Netherlands, and the main source of data for rotavirus surveillance is laboratory surveillance: the weekly reporting of the number of rotavirus diagnoses by a number of virological laboratories to the national public health institute. This system does not capture any additional data such as age, sex, the number of tests and the population under surveillance. The simplicity of the system is likely to have contributed to its sustainability for over 20 years, which is a very important asset for surveillance. A second data source is obtained through sentinel surveillance of acute gastroenteritis in primary care. The incidence of rotavirus infection in the Netherlands has a striking seasonal pattern, with sharp peaks in early spring (Figure 8.2).

The absence of the usual peak in rotavirus detections in early 2014 was surprising. It could reflect a genuine decrease in transmission of rotavirus but also a decrease in how frequently cases of acute gastroenteritis are tested for rotavirus, or some other surveillance artefact. The fact that the usual winter peak was also missing in acute gastroenteritis GP consultations for children under five supported the conclusion that there had been a genuine decline in rotavirus transmission (Hahné et al., 2014). This is an example of data triangulation.

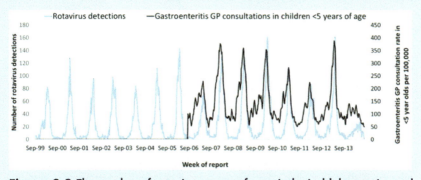

Figure 8.2 The number of rotavirus reports from virological laboratories and the number of GP consultations in <5-year-olds for acute gastroenteritis per 100,000 children, by week, 3-week moving average, the Netherlands, August 1999–August 2014.
Source: Adapted from Hahné et al. (2014).

8.1.1.3 Death registration and verbal autopsy

Mortality statistics are available from vital registration systems in most countries, and can be used to monitor the mortality due to vaccine-preventable diseases. However, late availability of data and incomplete classification and/or misclassification of the cause(s) of death often limit the reliability and usefulness of the data. To overcome the limitations of death registration data, statistical modelling of excess mortality can be used to assess the mortality attributable to infection, as, for example, for influenza (see Box 8.4).

Box 8.4 EuroMOMO: monitoring excess deaths due to respiratory diseases in Europe

EuroMOMO is a collaboration involving several European countries, with the purpose of monitoring excess deaths due to influenza, pandemics and other health threats. It publishes weekly reports comprising analyses by country and age group, available from www.euromomo.eu.

Figure 8.3 shows the time series of deaths in the participating countries for several years up to week 40 of 2020.

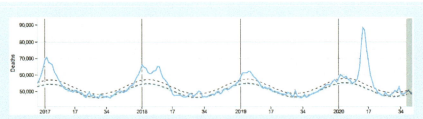

Figure 8.3 Observed weekly deaths (full line), expected deaths (lower dashed line) and upper threshold (upper dashed line), week 49 of 2016 to week 40 of 2020.
Source: Adapted from EuroMOMO (2020).

Expected deaths and the upper threshold (above which deaths may be considered to be in excess of expectation) are obtained using a statistical model. Figure 8.3 shows that, over the participating countries, excesses occurred in the winters of 2017, 2018 and 2019: these excess deaths may be attributed to seasonal influenza. Virtually no excess is observed for the 2020 influenza season. The very large peak in spring 2020 corresponds to the epidemic of SARS-CoV-2 infection that swept the world, detected in late 2019 in China. Data in the grey bar to the right of the graph are estimated by adjusting the numbers of most recent reports for reporting delays (a technique called 'nowcasting').

These methods for calculating excess deaths due to respiratory infections, particularly influenza, go back to Serfling (1963).

In the absence of reliable cause of death registration, data on the number of deaths due to certain vaccine-preventable diseases may also be obtained by interviewing relatives of a deceased person about signs, symptoms and events prior to their death, a method known as 'verbal autopsy'. It is particularly useful in settings with weak death certification systems and when a large proportion of deaths occur outside of a hospital or in facilities with limited diagnostic capability. Verbal autopsy is most reliable when the disease is characterised by a specific set of symptoms, as is the case, for instance, for tetanus (Kyu et al., 2017). Measurement bias is a major problem of verbal autopsy, caused by variations in methods used to collect and analyse the data, and depending on training of interviewers. To avoid this, WHO has developed an instrument for systematic verbal autopsy (WHO, 2016).

8.1.1.4 Sentinel surveillance and clinical surveillance schemes

For common infectious diseases that do not require a public health response for each case, sentinel surveillance is an efficient method to monitor the incidence of disease. It involves only a selection of health service providers or laboratories (sentinel sites) reporting cases. The relatively small number of health service providers contributing data allows for data quality to be improved by training and enhanced by collecting additional information including laboratory test results. Sentinel surveillance is the main surveillance method used for influenza (see Box 8.5).

Box 8.5 Influenza sentinel surveillance in Australia

The Australian Sentinel Practices Research Network (ASPREN) is a national sentinel surveillance system established in 1991. Influenza-like illness (ILI) and a small number of additional infectious diseases are reported weekly by participating practices. Nasal swabs for viral testing are taken from a systematic sample of ILI-patients. Results for 2016 are presented in Figure 8.4, indicating the dominance of influenza virus A in the 2016 season.

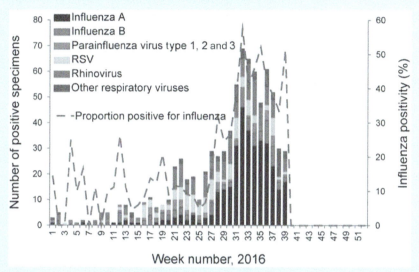

Figure 8.4 Influenza-like illness swab testing results by week, ASPREN, 1 January to 30 September 2016.
Source: Adapted from Chilver et al. (2016).

Data from sentinel influenza surveillance is used to monitor the incidence of influenza and to assess which strains are circulating. The latter information is essential information for the selection of influenza vaccine strains by WHO. Influenza sentinel surveillance networks also serve as a platform for influenza vaccine effectiveness studies (see Chapter 15; Chilver, Blakeley, & Stocks, 2017).

8.1.1.5 Routinely recorded healthcare data

Health service data on medical encounters (also called 'electronic health records') include the routine registration of health events in primary care, hospitals, specialist care, by health insurance companies, death registration and pharmacotherapeutical records. Such data is attractive to use for surveillance since it may be routinely available. This type of data is most useful when information on health events is coded, for example using the International Classification of Diseases (ICD) developed by WHO. An overview of coding systems can be found at www.nlm.nih.gov/research/umls/sourcereleasedocs/#.

Most routine registrations of health events can be classified as syndromic surveillance, indicating that it is based on recording of a certain clinical syndrome while information on laboratory testing of patients is not systematically included. This limits the usefulness of such data for vaccine-preventable disease surveillance. Since the targeted diseases are usually uncommon after the implementation of a successful vaccination programme, highly specific data including laboratory confirmation is needed for surveillance (see Box 8.2). For vaccine-preventable diseases that remain common because there are only selective, relatively ineffective or no vaccination programmes, routinely recorded health service data may be a useful source of data. Examples of this are general practice surveillance data on acute gastroenteritis, which can be used to monitor the incidence of rotavirus (Box 8.3) and influenza (Box 8.5). In addition, electronic health records are an important source of data for surveillance of adverse events following immunisation (AEFIs) (See Chapter 18).

8.1.1.6 Citizen science

The growing use of the Internet by members of the public has enabled new forms of surveillance. One example is 'citizen science', where individuals are invited to report certain health issues online (see Box 8.6).

Box 8.6 'GrippeNet', an example of citizen science-based surveillance in France

GrippeNet.fr is an online platform to which every week ca. 5,000 participants resident in France report the occurrence of signs and/or symptoms suggestive of influenza. It is used to produce estimates of the incidence of influenza. A comparison of results for two influenza seasons suggested good consistency with the French traditional, sentinel influenza surveillance (Guerrisi et al., 2018). Over a third of EU countries run a similar participatory surveillance system to monitor influenza (Guerrisi et al., 2016). Many of these collaborate in the Europe-wide network Influenzanet. In many countries, the online platforms for influenza have been adapted to monitor the occurrence of symptoms related to SARS-CoV-2 infection in the community.

Advantages of citizen science include the rapid availability of data, representing people who have not consulted formal healthcare. Biases may arise since the study population is self-selected and usually relatively well educated and young.

The analysis of disease-related internet search queries or social media messaging (e.g., via Google and Twitter, respectively) can also potentially provide useful data. However, disease-related internet search queries or messages in social media may, of course, be unrelated to the true occurrence of infections.

8.1.2 Biases in surveillance of vaccine-preventable diseases: the surveillance pyramid

To understand biases and underreporting in surveillance, it is helpful to consider the so-called surveillance pyramid. This represents a stratification of persons with an infection according to the data source they may be registered in (Figure 8.5).

Individuals in a certain level of the pyramid are not necessarily representative of those at other levels, because the determinants of moving from one level to the next are usually not random. When, for example, only severely ill people are tested and the severity of the infection varies by age, the age distribution of laboratory positive cases is not representative of all individuals with the infection of interest. The relation between different levels of the pyramid may change over time, for example owing to increases of public awareness about the disease influencing healthcare-seeking behaviour or the availability of new diagnostic or typing methods. This may confound the interpretation of surveillance data. There may also be considerable differences between geographic regions or socio-economic groups, for example related to access to healthcare. All of this can result in important biases. There is rarely data available from all levels of the pyramid, so it is up to the epidemiologist to be aware of possible biases and understand their importance.

The lowest level of the pyramid (asymptomatic infection) is usually not observed in any surveillance system, except in serological surveillance (see Chapter 9). For certain pathogens, this level includes healthy carriers of pathogens, as is the case for the pneumococcus and meningococcus. Optimal control of these infections by vaccination requires targeting population subgroups that have the highest prevalence of carriage, which are not necessarily those presenting with the highest incidence of symptomatic disease. For these pathogens, carriage studies in addition to disease surveillance are important to inform vaccine policy.

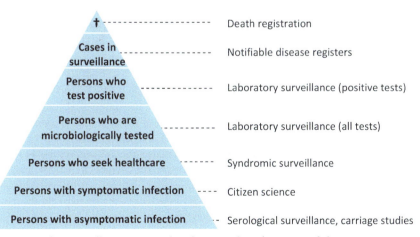

Figure 8.5 The surveillance pyramid with examples of sources of data.
Note: † Fatal cases in surveillance.

In addition to biases in surveillance data owing to selective reporting of cases, data errors can lead to wrong interpretation of results. Errors can be present in the classification of cases (see sensitivity and specificity in Box 8.1) and also in their characteristics. The impact of such errors on the estimation of vaccine effectiveness is discussed in Chapter 13.

8.1.3 Descriptive analyses of vaccine-preventable disease surveillance data

To evaluate the performance of a vaccination programme, descriptive analyses of vaccine-preventable disease data are useful to provide evidence to sustain it (if the programme is doing well) and for hypothesis generation (if it seems to be doing less well). Assessing the impact of a vaccination programme, however, cannot be done by descriptive analyses only, as it requires counterfactual information: what would have happened had the vaccination programme not been introduced? How to handle this is the topic of Chapter 10.

Descriptive analyses involve aggregating the cases by time, place, person and pathogen subtype, and choosing optimal visualisation methods of the results to draw conclusions and generate hypotheses.

The occurrence of cases over time is best presented by a line graph or a histogram of disease counts over time (also called a 'time series'). An example is provided in Box 8.7. In addition to plotting the number of cases over time, it is good practice to also plot the incidence in the target population of the vaccine programme over time, to allow for changes in population size. Regular epidemic cycles in the incidence of a vaccine-preventable disease may indicate inadequate control, allowing endemic circulation of the pathogen in the population, with a regular build-up of susceptibles (see Chapter 4). The time series may become more informative by stratification by age group.

Box 8.7 Descriptive analyses of the incidence of invasive *Haemophilus influenzae* type b infection in the United Kingdom

Following the introduction of *Haemophilus influenzae* type b (Hib) vaccine in the United Kingdom in 1992, a dramatic drop in the incidence of Hib disease was observed in notification-based surveillance data of invasive Hib disease. At that time, it was suggested to stop Hib notification altogether, since the programme was assumed to be highly effective. The importance of continued surveillance was demonstrated by the gradual increase in invasive Hib disease from 1999 onwards. Surveillance was crucial to raise an alarm, which was further investigated by analytic epidemiological studies. The findings of the latter were the basis for the introduction of a Hib booster campaign in 2003 for all children aged between 6 months and 4 years (Figure 8.6) (Trotter, 2003).

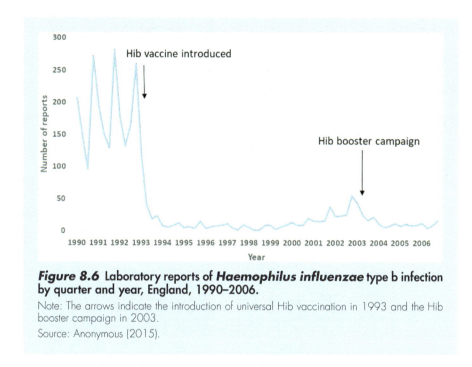

Figure 8.6 Laboratory reports of *Haemophilus influenzae* type b infection by quarter and year, England, 1990–2006.
Note: The arrows indicate the introduction of universal Hib vaccination in 1993 and the Hib booster campaign in 2003.
Source: Anonymous (2015).

When analysing and interpreting time series, reporting delays need to be taken into account for the most recent dates in the series. Nowcasting is a statistical technique to correct for this (see also Box 8.4).

Grouping cases by place is best done by geographical mapping. This can be done as dot maps or as incidence ('chloropleth') maps. These maps can point to areas where the vaccination programme is performing less well, or where other risk factors for the disease may be present (see for example Figure 8.7).

Grouping cases by person means aggregating cases by birth cohort, vaccination status and/or other individual risk factors. An important first step is to categorise cases in three groups: unvaccinated cases who were not eligible for vaccination, cases who were eligible but remained unvaccinated and cases in vaccinated individuals. Considering the distribution of cases across these groups helps to generate hypotheses about why a vaccination programme may be failing to achieve its aims (see also Chapter 11 on outbreaks). It may also provide information on the presence of herd-immunity effects (see Chapters 4, 5 and 10). Changes in the age distribution of cases over time can be due to waning vaccine immunity or inadequate vaccine coverage (see Chapter 5). The assessment of waning immunity is, however, not straightforward and is discussed in Chapter 16.

Grouping the cases by pathogen subtype or genotype can provide insight into the emergence of variants, the presence of serogroup replacement (e.g., for pneumococcal disease) and progress towards elimination (see Section 8.3).

Regional, national and local public health departments usually produce regular reports (often publicly available on the Internet) in which descriptive surveillance data is presented. Disaggregated data is less frequently available. Compliance with the 'FAIR' principles (making sure data is findable, accessible, interoperable and reusable) will help

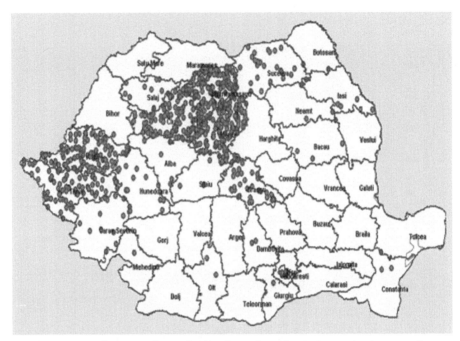

Figure 8.7 Notifications of measles by place of residence, Romania, January–August 2016. Each dot represents one notified case of measles.
Source: Adapted from Romania (2016).

to improve this (Wilkinson et al., 2016). Project Tycho is an example of an initiative based on the FAIR principles (see www.tycho.pitt.edu/).

To interpret descriptive surveillance, it is good practice to compare results from different sources (see Box 8.3) and to interpret these together with data on vaccine coverage. To better understand trends occurring due to other causes (such as changes in disease reporting or surveillance), comparisons with surveillance data of, for example, non-targeted serogroups, or data from other countries, is useful.

8.2 Surveillance of vaccine-preventable pathogens

Pathogen surveillance involves the systematic collection and analysis of data on pathogen subtypes and/or genomic data from pathogens. It is used in the evaluation of vaccination programmes to monitor changes in the ecology of micro-organisms. Such ecological changes can require an adaptation of the vaccination strategy, for example by using a different vaccine that covers more subtypes of the pathogen. Other public health rationales for monitoring pathogen populations include the detection of emerging subtypes that are more virulent, more resistant to antibiotics or more difficult to diagnose. Such evidence can again be used to adapt vaccination programmes. Lastly, pathogen surveillance can aim to generate evidence on the transmission of infection, for example by describing the emergence of a new strain or documenting presence or absence of chains of transmission.

Pathogen surveillance starts with the microbiological characterisation of pathogens obtained from cases of a vaccine-preventable disease. Usually, pathogen surveillance is organised through voluntary submission of identified pathogens (or strains/isolates) by clinical diagnostic laboratories throughout the country to a central (reference) laboratory or public health institute. This can be organised in a sentinel manner, involving only a limited group of laboratories. Box 8.8 provides an example of pathogen surveillance by a single laboratory. For common pathogens, sentinel surveillance may be sufficiently informative, provided sufficient information on the catchment population served by those laboratories is available. Data accompanying the laboratory results usually include basic demographic information such as age and gender, and the date the specimen was taken.

Box 8.8 Surveillance to assess the impact of pneumococcal vaccination in Kenya

Pneumococcal conjugate vaccines (PCVs) protect against invasive pneumococcal disease (IPD) caused by a number of pneumococcal serotypes. Currently licensed PCVs protect against 7, 10 or 13 serotypes and higher-valent PCVs are under development. There are, however, over 80 serotypes against which these vaccines do not protect.

The introduction of universal infant PCV vaccination programmes has resulted in impressive decreases of targeted serotypes in vaccinated children and also in unvaccinated older people due to herd-immunity effects. However, serotypes not targeted have increased in nearly all countries with PCV vaccination programmes. This serotype replacement has substantially decreased the impact of the PCV vaccination programme. Furthermore, the non-vaccine strains may in some instances be more resistant to antibiotics and they may be relatively prone to causing invasive disease. Evidence from pathogen surveillance is needed to assess the impact of vaccination and to justify the use and development of higher-valent vaccines protecting against more serotypes.

In Kenya, 10-valent pneumococcal conjugate vaccine (PCV10) for infants was introduced in January 2011, accompanied by a catch-up campaign in Kilifi County for children less than 5 years of age. To assess the impact of this vaccination programme, pathogen surveillance data from the only hospital in the Kilifi region was linked to data on vaccination status collected in a population-based register. In addition, annual pneumococcal carriage surveys were carried out (Hammitt et al., 2019).

Results show a marked decrease in the incidence of vaccine-type IPD in the age group targeted by the programme (<5-year-olds), and also, through indirect effects, in older age groups (Figure 8.8). The incidence of non-vaccine-type IPD increased in all age groups (albeit not significantly), consistent with the increase of 72% in carriage of non-vaccine-type pneumococci found in children under 5 years of age.

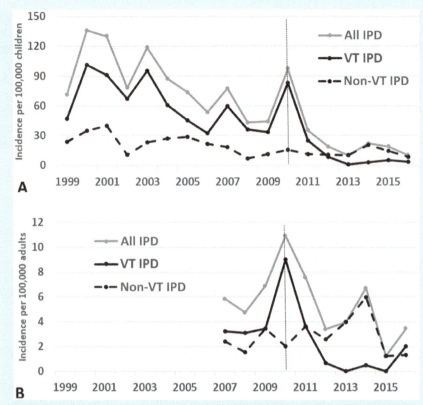

Figure 8.8 Incidence of overall, vaccine-type, and non-vaccine-type invasive pneumococcal disease in the Kilifi Health and Demographic Surveillance System, 1999–2016. (A) In children aged <5 years; (B) in individuals aged ≥15 years. The vertical dotted line indicates PCV10 introduction.

Note: IPD = invasive pneumococcal disease; VT = vaccine serotype.
Source: Adapted from Hammitt et al. (2019).

It is difficult to disentangle whether changes in the pathogen distribution, as for example described in Box 8.8, are truly caused by the vaccination programme, by other factors or are due to secular trends.

WHO has established global networks of subnational, national, regional and global reference laboratories for certain priority diseases such as polio and influenza, with the aim to facilitate high-quality laboratory investigations and surveillance.

Representativeness of results is a key determinant of the validity of conclusions based on pathogen surveillance. For severe diseases such as invasive bacterial meningitis in resource-rich settings, it is likely that the vast majority of strains reach a reference laboratory and are included in nationwide pathogen surveillance. However, these strains may not represent the pathogen population that is mainly present in healthy carriers. For mild diseases, or in resource-poor settings, strains included in pathogen surveillance may only be a very small and biased selection of the pathogen population, which may bias conclusions. It is helpful to consider the surveillance pyramid (see Section 8.1.2) to identify biases and how they might affect inferences drawn from the data. Sentinel surveillance can be a useful tool to obtain a representative sample of strains of pathogens causing a mild disease or in resource-poor settings.

When disease control approaches elimination or eradication, the main aim of pathogen surveillance is to assess whether the case is part of an endemic cluster or the result of an importation from outside the surveillance area. In this way, it can provide evidence to target interventions and certify elimination. This is discussed in the next section.

8.3 Surveillance in the context of elimination and eradication

When a vaccination programme has been successful and the targeted infection is near elimination, the main aim of surveillance is to identify in a timely manner all remaining cases for immediate prevention of transmission and (outbreak) investigation, and to identify remaining pockets of susceptibles in order to target vaccination. An additional aim specific to this context is to provide data to (international) public health authorities who can then verify or certify that elimination or eradication has been achieved (see Chapter 3).

In the context of a very low incidence of the targeted disease, surveillance encounters specific epidemiological challenges, which usually requires enhanced methods. The few remaining true cases of the disease tend to occur among pockets of susceptibles that may be relatively inaccessible. Furthermore, the capacity of clinicians to diagnose cases may have reduced since they are no longer aware of the disease and have lost experience of diagnosing it. This reduces the sensitivity, specificity and timeliness of surveillance. Another complication is that cases which are detected may not be representative of the entire susceptible population, neither in terms of incidence nor characteristics. There may be a gradual build-up of susceptibles due to (even marginally) inadequate vaccine coverage and/or effectiveness, which will only lead to an epidemic when a threshold has been passed and a successful introduction of the pathogen has occurred (see Chapters 4 and 11). This may take years, during which the absence of cases will provide false reassurance. Monitoring vaccine coverage can help, provided it is valid and available at subnational level. In many countries, however, reliable vaccine coverage data is not available, in which case the only way to assess the (hidden) pockets of susceptibles is by serological surveillance (Chapter 9). To what extent susceptible populations remain hidden in disease surveillance data also depends on the transmissibility of the pathogen and visibility of infection by it: measles virus is likely to reveal its susceptibles sooner than, for example, hepatitis B.

When a disease is at or close to the elimination stage, the demand for high-quality surveillance may increase. This is to enable a timely public health response to all cases occurring and to comply with quality criteria from national or international public health authorities. For poliomyelitis, the global eradication goal requires such sensitive surveillance that additional methods have been developed. This includes acute flaccid paralysis (AFP) surveillance (Box 8.9), environmental (sewage) surveillance in high-risk areas (Box 8.11) and laboratory surveillance for enteroviruses. For measles, in an analogy to these enhanced polio surveillance methods, rash/fever surveillance has been proposed but is more challenging primarily because of the much higher incidence of rash and fever compared to AFP. Measles RNA, excreted in urine, has been detected in sewage surveillance, but the added value for measles surveillance has not yet been demonstrated.

> ### Box 8.9 Surveillance for acute flaccid paralysis
>
> The polio eradication objective and its certification require highly sensitive and timely surveillance. Poliomyelitis is characterised by acute flaccid paralysis (AFP), a syndrome that can also be due to other infectious and non-infectious causes. WHO guidelines indicate that polio surveillance should include AFP surveillance in which all cases of AFP are detected and investigated for the presence of poliovirus. Several standards to assess the sensitivity of AFP surveillance have been developed, both from a case detection as well as from a laboratory diagnosis point of view.
>
> The incidence of AFP due to other causes than polio (mainly Guillain-Barré syndrome) is fairly similar across populations. This allows the sensitivity of AFP surveillance to be assessed by a performance criterion: the system should detect at least one non-polio AFP case per 100,000 children under 15 years of age per year.
>
> WHO also set a criterion for the quality of microbiological testing of these AFP cases: from at least 60% of detected AFP cases, at least two adequate specimens should be collected, transported adequately and processed in a WHO-accredited laboratory.
>
> Adequate specimens are defined as having been collected 24–48 hours apart and within 14 days of the onset of paralysis, of adequate volume (approximatively 8–10 g) when arriving in the laboratory, having appropriate documentation (on a laboratory request form) and being in good condition (no leakage or desiccation).
>
> Adequate transport is defined as sealing the specimens in containers that are stored immediately inside a refrigerator or packed between frozen ice packs at 4–8 °C in a cold box. Specimens should arrive at the laboratory within 72 hours of collection. Otherwise they must be frozen (at −20 °C), and then shipped frozen, ideally packed with dry ice or cold packs. There needs to be evidence that the recommended temperature has been maintained (presence of ice or temperature indicator) throughout transport. This procedure is known as the 'reverse cold chain', a variation on the 'cold chain' principle used for vaccines.

When aiming for highly sensitive surveillance, specificity of surveillance may be compromised, leading to a low positive predictive value and a high workload for public health tracing false-positive cases. Adapting the case definition by adding epidemiologic and/or laboratory criteria may help (see Box 8.2). However, when laboratory confirmation is included in the case definition, many mild infections, not normally submitted for laboratory testing, may be missed. To circumvent this, testing rates can be increased by offering less invasive diagnostics free of charge. An example of this is dried blood spot, oral fluid or urine testing for measles and rubella.

SURVEILLANCE 149

In the context of elimination, determining the subtype or genetic sequence of pathogens becomes relevant to detect clusters and to distinguish cases arising from endemic transmission from those due to importation. For vaccine-derived polioviruses, sequencing can provide evidence on the likely period the virus has been circulating, which provides information on the immunity in the population and the quality of surveillance. An example of how surveillance using poliovirus molecular typing data contributed to the elimination of polio in India is provided in Box 8.10. In the pre-elimination phase, constant vigilance is needed to detect all imported cases to prevent and track transmission of infection. International collaboration to share (molecular) case data and coordinate response is becoming more important at this stage.

Box 8.10 The contribution of molecular surveillance to the elimination of poliomyelitis from India

In 2009, surveillance for poliovirus in India included the collection of RNA sequence data from polioviruses isolated from patients and from the environment. This provided evidence that certain areas in Bihar and Uttar Pradesh (Figure 8.9) were endemic reservoirs from which all wild polioviruses (WPV) in India, and in some other countries, originated. This informed a targeted response for improving

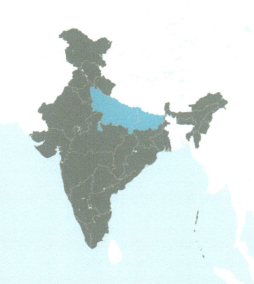

Figure 8.9 Map of India with the states of Uttar Pradesh and Bihar in blue.

routine immunisation coverage and addressing public health issues in underserved populations (Anonymous, 2017).

The last case of poliomyelitis due to WPV in India was detected in January 2011; the WHO South East Asia region was certified polio-free in March 2014. Molecular data provided evidence of elimination of endemic WPV, which contributed to this certification.

For poliovirus, phylogenetic analyses based on assumptions about the 'molecular clock' can provide evidence about how long a virus has been circulating in a population. This can be used to evaluate the sensitivity of disease surveillance and is a direct indicator of the level of control of poliovirus in the country.

Once a disease has been eliminated or eradicated, the main aims of surveillance are to provide evidence that elimination is being maintained and to rapidly detect re-emergence of disease. In the elimination phase, surveillance of outbreaks can provide important additional insights, as discussed in Chapter 10. Re-emergence after eradication can be due, for example, to a deliberate release or to accidents involving viruses handled in laboratories (see Box 8.11). Documenting strains of wild-type viruses targeted for elimination kept in laboratories is a key activity in this phase.

Box 8.11 Wild poliovirus type 2 infection in a laboratory worker after a spill, the Netherlands, 2017

On 3 April 2017, an accidental spill of high-titre monovalent wild poliovirus type 2 (WPV2) occurred at a vaccine manufacturing plant in the Netherlands, 2 years after WPV2 was certified as having been eradicated by the World Health Assembly (WHA). Two fully vaccinated laboratory workers who were possibly exposed to the spill were identified.

The two workers were followed up with throat swabs and stool specimens, which were tested by reverse transcriptase polymerase chain reaction (RT-PCR) and viral culture. Four days after the exposure, a stool sample of one of the workers tested positive in both tests. Sequencing of the viral protein 1 (VP1) gene of the virus demonstrated it was 100% identical to the VP1 region of WPV2. The infected worker was followed up with successive sampling. The last positive sample was taken on 1 May 2017. Sewage monitoring downstream of the infected worker's household was also found to be positive, up to 3 May 2017, inclusive (Duizer, Ruijs, van der Weijden, & Timen, 2017).

Polio vaccination is very effective to protect against disease, but less so against infection. A vaccinated individual who is exposed may therefore still shed viable virus, as occurred in the accident described above.

In addition to the above example, several other laboratory-associated cases of poliomyelitis, and of smallpox, have occurred after these diseases had been eliminated or eradicated, respectively (Anonymous, 1978; Wood, Sutter, & Dowdle, 2000). This highlights the importance of continued surveillance, as well as vigilance, stocktaking and follow-up protocols for laboratory accidents in sites using wild-type viruses that are targeted for elimination or eradication.

Summary

- Surveillance of vaccine-preventable diseases is essential to monitor the impact of vaccination programmes and to identify pockets of susceptibles and changes in the epidemiology of the targeted diseases.
- Methods of vaccine-preventable disease surveillance require adaptation throughout the course of a successful vaccination programme.
- Ideally, surveillance is based on several sources of data, covering the entire population, not just those targeted by the programme. Biases associated with each of the data sources used and errors in the data need to be considered to avoid drawing wrong conclusions.
- Descriptive analysis of surveillance data involves aggregating cases over time, place, person and pathogen (sub)type. It can give an indication of the impact of a vaccination programme and is a basis for generating hypotheses into reasons why programmes may be failing to achieve impact.
- Pathogen surveillance involves the systematic collection and analysis of data on pathogen subtypes or genomic data from pathogens. It is used to monitor the impact of vaccination programmes on the targeted subtypes of pathogens and may also provide evidence on the wider effects of the programme on the ecology of micro-organisms.
- When the targeted infection is near elimination, surveillance with improved sensitivity, specificity and timeliness is required. This necessitates enhanced surveillance.
- After elimination and eradication, continued surveillance and vigilance is needed to detect re-emergence of infections.

References

Anonymous. (1978). Smallpox research after Birmingham. *Lancet*, *2*(8089), 560. Retrieved from www.ncbi.nlm.nih.gov/pubmed/79923.

Anonymous. (2015). *Haemophilus influenzae*: Epidemiological data. Retrieved from www.gov.uk/government/publications/haemophilus-influenzae-epidemiological-data.

Anonymous. (2017). *Report of the 23rd Informal Consultation of the Global Polio Laboratory Network (GPLN)*. Retrieved from http://polioeradication.org/wp-content/uploads/2017/08/GPLN_Meeting_recommendations_2017.pdf.

Chilver, M., Blakeley, D., & Stocks, N. (2016). *Australian Sentinel Practices Research Network, 1 July to 30 September 2016*. Retrieved from www1.health.gov.au/internet/main/publishing.nsf/content/cda-cdi4004-pdf-cnt.htm/$FILE/cdi4004s.pdf.

Chilver, M., Blakeley, D., & Stocks, N. (2017). The Australian Sentinel Practices Research Network, 1 January to 31 March 2017. *Communicable Diseases Intelligence Quarterly Report, 41*(4), E492–E496. Retrieved from www.ncbi.nlm.nih.gov/pubmed/29864394.

Dickson, E. M., Zambon, M., Pebody, R., de Lusignan, S., Elliot, A. J., Ellis, J., ... McMenamin, J. (2020). Do point-of-care tests (POCTs) offer a new paradigm for the management of patients with influenza? *Eurosurveillance, 25*(44). doi:10.2807/1560-7917.ES.2020.25.44.1900420.

Duizer, E., Ruijs, W. L., van der Weijden, C. P., & Timen, A. (2017). Response to a wild poliovirus type 2 (WPV2)-shedding event following accidental exposure to WPV2, the Netherlands, April 2017. *Eurosurveillance, 22*(21). doi:10.2807/1560-7917.ES.2017.22.21.30542.

EuroMOMO. (2020). *EuroMOMO Bulletin, 40*. Retrieved from www.euromomo.eu/bulletins/2020-40.

Guerrisi, C., Turbelin, C., Blanchon, T., Hanslik, T., Bonmarin, I., Levy-Bruhl, D., ... Colizza, V. (2016). Participatory syndromic surveillance of influenza in Europe. *Journal of Infectious Diseases, 214*(Suppl. 4), S386–S392. doi:10.1093/infdis/jiw280.

Guerrisi, C., Turbelin, C., Souty, C., Poletto, C., Blanchon, T., Hanslik, T., ... Colizza, V. (2018). The potential value of crowdsourced surveillance systems in supplementing sentinel influenza networks: The case of France. *Eurosurveillance, 23*(25). doi:10.2807/1560-7917.ES.2018.23.25.1700337.

Hahné, S., Hooiveld, M., Vennema, H., van Ginkel, A., de Melker, H., Wallinga, J., ... Bruijning-Verhagen, P. (2014). Exceptionally low rotavirus incidence in the Netherlands in 2013/14 in the absence of rotavirus vaccination. *Eurosurveillance, 19*(43). Retrieved from www.ncbi.nlm.nih.gov/pubmed/25375899.

Hammitt, L. L., Etyang, A. O., Morpeth, S. C., Ojal, J., Mutuku, A., Mturi, N., ... Scott, J. A. G. (2019). Effect of ten-valent pneumococcal conjugate vaccine on invasive pneumococcal disease and nasopharyngeal carriage in Kenya: A longitudinal surveillance study. *Lancet, 393*(10186), 2146–2154. doi:10.1016/S0140-6736(18)33005-8.

Kyu, H. H., Mumford, J. E., Stanaway, J. D., Barber, R. M., Hancock, J. R., Vos, T., ... Naghavi, M. (2017). Mortality from tetanus between 1990 and 2015: Findings from the global burden of disease study 2015. *BMC Public Health, 17*(1), 179. doi:10.1186/s12889-017-4111-4.

M'ikanatha, N. M., Lynfield, R., van Beneden, C. A., & de Valk, H. (Eds.) (2013). *Infectious disease surveillance* (2nd ed.). Chichester, UK: Wiley-Blackwell.

Romania, M. S. (2016). Epidemie de rujeolă în România. Retrieved from www.facebook.com/permalink.php?story_fbid=327547260933379&id=167611313593642&substory_index=0.

Serfling, R. E. (1963). Methods for current statistical analysis of excess pneumonia-influenza deaths. *Public Health Report, 78*(6), 494–506. Retrieved from www.ncbi.nlm.nih.gov/pubmed/19316455.

Trotter, C. L., Ramsay, M. E., & Slack, M. P. (2003). Rising incidence of *Haemophilus influenzae* type b disease in England and Wales indicates a need for a second catch-up vaccination campaign. *Communicable Disease and Public Health*, 6(1), 55–58.

World Health Organization (WHO). (2016). *The 2016 WHO verbal autopsy instrument*. Retrieved from https://score.tools.who.int/fileadmin/uploads/score/Documents/Count_births__deaths_and_causes_of_death/Verbal_autopsy_instrument/Manual_and_Guidelines_WHO_VA_Tool.pdf.

World Health Organization (WHO). (2018). *Vaccine-preventable diseases surveillance standards*. Retrieved from www.who.int/publications/i/item/surveillance-standards-for-vaccine-preventable-diseases-2nd-edition.

Wilkinson, M. D., Dumontier, M., Aalbersberg, I. J., Appleton, G., Axton, M., Baak, A., ... Mons, B. (2016). The FAIR guiding principles for scientific data management and stewardship. *Scientific Data, 3*, 160018. doi:10.1038/sdata.2016.18.

Wood, D. J., Sutter, R. W., & Dowdle, W. R. (2000). Stopping poliovirus vaccination after eradication: Issues and challenges. *Bulletin of the World Health Organization, 78*(3), 347–357. Retrieved from www.ncbi.nlm.nih.gov/pubmed/10812731.

Chapter 9

Serological surveillance

Serological surveillance refers to the use of biomarker assays to monitor the distribution and determinants of infection or immunity in populations. This information can be used to plan, monitor and, if necessary, adjust vaccination programmes.

Serological surveillance is now fairly common in high-income countries, but is still under-used in low- and middle-income countries owing to limited resources, notably access to high-quality laboratories, sufficient funding and difficulties in conducting representative surveys. However, sampling and laboratory methods used in serological surveys are rapidly evolving and, with expanding field laboratory and epidemiological capacity, the role of serological surveillance is likely to grow. Discussions of serological surveillance methods in contrasting settings may be found in Wilson, Deeks, Hatchette, and Crowcroft (2012) and Cutts and Hanson (2016).

In this chapter we describe some of the uses and methods of serological surveillance of vaccination programmes. Seroprevalence and serological surveys are introduced in Section 9.1. In Section 9.2 we consider how serological surveys may be used to monitor vaccination programmes. Then in Section 9.3 we explore a little further the interpretation of serological data and discuss immunological correlates of protection. Finally, in Section 9.4 we discuss some practical aspects of the design and analysis of serological surveys.

9.1 Seroprevalence and serological surveys

Many vaccine-preventable infections result in the presence of antibodies or other biomarkers of infection in serum or related fluids (such as oral or vaginal fluids). If antibodies are sustained throughout life, their presence indicates that an individual has been infected or vaccinated at some point in the past. Examples of infections inducing such long-lasting antibodies are hepatitis A, rubella and smallpox.

The prevalence of antibodies (or, less commonly, antigens) assessed in such samples from a population is the seroprevalence. For the purpose of estimating antibody seroprevalence, the data are usually dichotomised: individuals are seropositive if (depending on the type of serological test used) antibodies are deemed to be present, or if their concentration lies above a certain threshold, and seronegative if not. Some assays use two thresholds, the values between them defining an equivocal range. The seroprevalence is estimated as the proportion of seropositives in a population. For some other analyses, antibody concentrations or titres may be used directly. Further details are given in Section 9.4.

Seroprevalence is estimated from population-based cross-sectional surveys, called serological surveys. In such a survey, a sample of individuals from the population is selected, blood or other specimens are obtained from them and these specimens are then tested for antibodies or other biomarkers of interest. In Chapter 2, Section 2.8, a variety of serological tests were described. The tests and biomarkers used in serological surveys depend on the infection and the aim of the survey. For example, for rubella and hepatitis A, enzyme-linked immunoassays are commonly used to measure serum concentrations of immunoglobulin G (IgG) antibodies, which provide evidence of past infection or vaccination.

The focus of this chapter is primarily on the serological surveillance of vaccination programmes. However, serological surveys undertaken prior to the introduction of vaccination can play an important role in shaping vaccination policy; an example is provided in Box 9.1. The example helps to illustrate some important aspects of serological surveys and their interpretation, which also apply to serological surveillance of vaccination programmes.

Box 9.1 Hepatitis A seroprevalence in Madagascar

Hepatitis A infection is often asymptomatic in children, the proportion with symptoms increasing with age. Thus, case reports may be inadequate to assess the endemicity of hepatitis A. To this end, a serological survey of hepatitis A was undertaken in Antananarivo, Madagascar (Raharimanga et al., 2008). The survey was conducted in 926 children aged 2 to 24 years, using serum samples collected in 2004. The age-specific seroprevalence profile is shown in Figure 9.1.

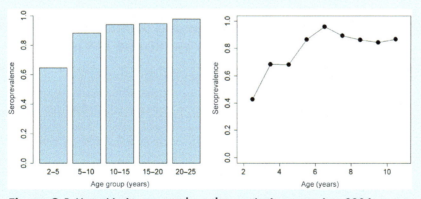

Figure 9.1 Hepatitis A seroprevalence by age in Antananarivo, 2004.

> The bar chart on the left in Figure 9.1 shows that the age-specific seroprevalence increases with age up to age 25 years. The line plot on the right provides more detail for children aged 2–10 years. The seroprevalence is higher at 6 years than at ages 7 to 10 years: this might be due to sampling variation or to changes in incidence over time
>
> These results show that by age 6 years, over 90% of children have antibodies to hepatitis A. Thus, Antananarivo in 2004 was still an area of high endemicity, despite improvements in hygiene and socio-economic conditions. The authors concluded that their findings did not support the introduction of mass vaccination, but that travellers to this area should be immunised.

Some care is needed in interpreting serological survey data, with or without vaccination. This is because infection and vaccination rates generally vary with both age and time, and an age-specific seroprevalence profile reflects this variation. In the absence of vaccination, if the age-specific incidence of infection is broadly constant over time, and provided antibodies are long-lasting, the seroprevalence should increase with age.

These complexities in interpreting serological survey data are compounded by vaccination. In the presence of vaccination, the seroprevalence will reflect the age and time pattern of vaccination and any waning of vaccine-induced antibodies over time, as well as patterns induced by natural infection. Usually, several serological surveys undertaken at different times are needed to disentangle these various effects; several examples will be presented in Section 9.2.

The example in Box 9.1 illustrated a situation in which serological data provide evidence to support the view that mass vaccination is not a priority. In contrast, the example in Box 9.2 illustrates a situation in which serological data provides compelling evidence to support the introduction of mass vaccination and other infection control measures.

> ## Box 9.2 Rubella immunity among women and the burden of congenital rubella syndrome in Cambodia
>
> A nationwide serological survey was conducted in Cambodia in 2012, a year before rubella vaccination was included in the national immunisation programme (Mao et al., 2015). The survey included 2,154 women aged 15–39 years, whose sera were tested for immunity to rubella, polio and measles. Overall, 27% of women of childbearing age were seronegative. Figure 9.2 shows the proportion seronegative for rubella by age group.
>
> Figure 9.2 indicates high susceptibility in all women, particularly those aged 15–19 years and 20–24 years. This is consistent with rubella notification data from Cambodia.

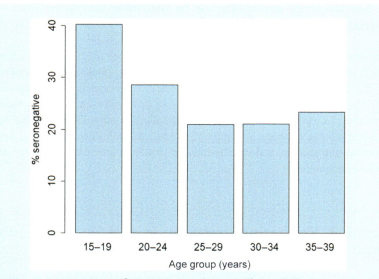

Figure 9.2 Proportion of women seronegative for rubella by age group, Cambodia, 2012.

This pattern of rubella susceptibility is of concern given the risk of congenital rubella syndrome (CRS) when rubella is acquired in pregnancy. Based on these data, it was estimated that about 1 in every 600 children born in Cambodia has CRS.

A nationwide vaccination campaign in children aged 9 months to 14 years with a rubella-containing vaccine was undertaken in 2013, and rubella vaccination has been included in the routine vaccination schedule. However, to close the susceptibility gap in women of childbearing age, catch-up vaccination campaigns in this age group are required. In addition to seroepidemiology, maintaining and enhancing CRS surveillance is essential to guide policy-making.

Serological survey data such as those presented in Box 9.2 are valuable in guiding vaccination policy, and also in providing a baseline against which the impact of the vaccination programme may be assessed.

Serological surveys are particularly useful to describe the epidemiology of infections in which a substantial proportion of cases are subclinical, or when surveillance of clinical cases is likely to be very incomplete or biased, for example owing to age-dependent reporting. They may also be used to undertake other, more advanced analyses to estimate the incidence of infection and its transmission potential. For example, the data in Box 9.2 were used to estimate the burden of CRS in Cambodia. Further examples of such analyses are described briefly at the end of the chapter, but the details lie outside the scope of this book.

9.2 Serological surveillance to monitor vaccination programmes

Unlike other surveillance methods, serological surveillance provides direct information on levels of susceptibility in the population, thus enabling pockets of susceptibles to be identified. Serological data also enables the potential for transmission to be assessed. Thus, serological surveillance is a powerful tool to monitor and improve vaccination programmes. Surveillance of vaccine coverage alone is often inadequate for this purpose, since reliable coverage data may be lacking, the prevalence of natural immunity is not taken into account, and vaccine-induced immunity may wane over time. Box 9.3 provides an example.

Box 9.3 Monitoring immunity to polio in Kano state, Nigeria

In 2015, the World Health Organization (WHO) removed Nigeria from the list of polio-endemic countries after certifying that the transmission of poliovirus had been interrupted. Kano State had been the epicentre of poliovirus transmission in Nigeria, and a series of seroprevalence surveys were undertaken there to guide the eradication effort. These surveys were conducted in children attending the paediatric outpatient department of Murtala Mohammed Specialist Hospital (Kano) in 2001, 2013 and 2014 (Craig et al., 2016). The proportions seropositive in the older age groups studied were high (typically over 85%) for all serotypes. Table 9.1 shows the results for children aged 6–9 months.

As shown in Table 9.1, the seroprevalence in 6–9-month-olds dropped substantially for all three virus types between 2011 and 2013. Provided that the representativeness of the samples did not vary over time, this decline indicated there were problems with the quality of the immunisation activities undertaken in the previous year. Therefore, new strategies were devised to reach young children, especially infants. The seroprevalences for all three virus types recovered in 2014, although they still remained below the 2011 levels.

Table 9.1 Percentage seropositive in children aged 6–9 months by poliovirus type and year, Kano, Nigeria

Year	Type 1 (%)	Type 2 (%)	Type 3 (%)
2011	81	75	73
2013	58	42	52
2014	72	59	64

Serological surveys can also be used to guide adjustments to vaccination programmes, for example to provide evidence on which to base changes to the vaccination schedule, or the inclusion of a booster dose. This is illustrated in Box 9.4.

Box 9.4 Meningococcal serogroup C conjugate vaccination in the United Kingdom

In 1999 the United Kingdom introduced meningococcal serogroup C conjugate (MCC) vaccination into the routine child immunisation schedule at 2, 3 and 4 months of age. In 2000, a catch-up vaccination campaign was also undertaken targeted at young people up to age 18 years, later extended to 24 years. In 2006, the immunisation schedule was adjusted in the light of evidence that direct protection from infant immunisation was short-lived; the revised schedule included vaccinations at 3, 4 and 12 months.

Immunity levels in the population were monitored using a sequence of serological surveys undertaken on sera collected in 1996–1999, 2000–2004 and 2009 (Ishola et al., 2012). Figure 9.3 shows the percentages within each age group with protective levels of serum bactericidal antibody (SBA) in the three surveys.

The pre-vaccination survey (top bar chart in Figure 9.3) shows that proportions protected were low, increasing slightly with age. The two post-vaccination surveys show a marked peak at 6–11 months, resulting from routine infant immunisation. The 2009 survey (bottom bar chart in Figure 9.3) does not suggest that the inclusion of a vaccine dose at 12 months from 2006 onwards had a lasting effect, the proportion protected remaining low in 1–4-year-olds.

The two post-vaccination surveys show marked second peaks corresponding to immunity levels induced by the catch-up vaccination programme, but only for those vaccinated in older childhood. The shift in the location of the second peak from 10–19 years in the 2000–2004 survey (middle bar chart in Figure 9.3) to

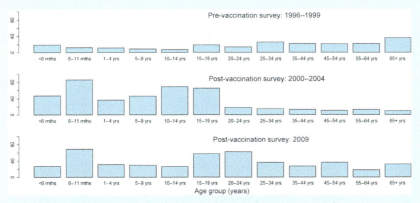

Figure 9.3 Percentages with protective levels of meningococcal group C serum bactericidal antibodies, by age group, in three serological surveys.

15–24 years in the 2009 survey (bottom bar chart) corresponds to ageing of the cohort receiving catch-up vaccines. The similar height of the two peaks suggests that antibodies did not wane substantially in the intervening period.

The authors concluded that these observations indicate that vaccination in early childhood does not confer lasting immunity, but that lasting antibody levels may be achieved by vaccinating at older ages. They suggest that a booster dose administered in older childhood is needed to maintain adequate levels of immunity in the population, and that such a booster is likely to induce longer-lasting protection.

In the light of these and later findings, the vaccination schedule for meningococcal C vaccination in the United Kingdom was altered after 2016 to include two doses: the first dose at 12 months, followed by a booster dose at 13–14 years.

Using the techniques of mathematical modelling, the accrual and ageing of susceptibles identified in serological surveys may be projected forward in time, and the ensuing dynamics of infection may be studied. Even in situations of high vaccination coverage, an outbreak might be triggered if a pool of susceptible individuals reaches an age at which contact rates suddenly rise, for example owing to increased social interactions at school or university. Serological surveys can provide advance warning of such potential problems, allowing time to devise intervention strategies. In this sense, serological surveillance has the potential to guide prevention rather than control. An example is given in Box 9.5.

Box 9.5 The UK measles and rubella vaccination campaign

Measles, mumps and rubella (MMR) vaccination was introduced in the United Kingdom in 1987–1988 for children aged 15 months and soon achieved high coverage, reaching over 90% in the early 1990s. A catch-up campaign aimed at 2–4-year-olds was also implemented at the time the vaccine was introduced. Several serological surveys were undertaken to monitor the vaccination programme. The data for measles susceptibility are given in Figure 9.4.

Figure 9.4 shows that in the pre-MMR serological survey undertaken in 1986–1987, susceptibility to measles declined with age. By 1991, 3 years after the introduction of MMR, it had increased in children aged 7–14 years, reaching 14% in children aged 7–8 years. These children were too old to have been included in the catch-up programme and remained susceptible owing to the drop in incidence of measles virus infection following the introduction of MMR vaccination. Mathematical modelling suggested that the effective reproduction number was likely to increase over time as this pool of susceptibles aged. It was predicted that an epidemic was likely to occur in the mid-1990s (Gay, Hesketh, Morgan-Capner, & Miller, 1995).

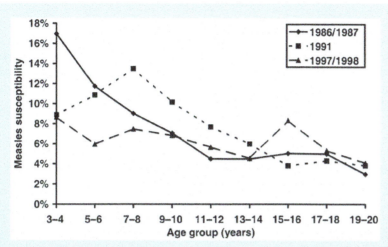

Figure 9.4 Proportion susceptible to measles in England and Wales by age group in three serological surveys.
Source: Reproduced with permission from Vyse et al. (2002).

In consequence, a national measles and rubella (MR) vaccination campaign was undertaken in late 1994, targeting children aged 5 to 16 years (with 92% coverage). In addition, in 1996, a second dose of MMR was introduced for children entering school, in order to maintain low levels of susceptibility among schoolchildren. These measures were monitored with an additional serological survey in 1997–1998. The results, shown in Figure 9.4, show that the susceptible pool in children under the age of 14 years was successfully eliminated. The small peak at ages 15–16 likely corresponds to children aged 5–7 in 1988 who did not receive MMR but remained uninfected, and were among the 8% not reached by the MR campaign.

So far in this chapter, the examples described have involved using serological surveys to monitor the levels of susceptibility in the population, and hence to guide additional interventions or adjustments to the vaccination programme.

To date, for many pathogens it is not possible to distinguish between antibodies elicited by natural infection and those resulting from vaccination. Usually, antibody concentrations are higher when induced by natural infection, but there are exceptions: for example, the level of antibodies induced by meningococcal C vaccination is much higher than that following natural infection. Sometimes, the antibody class can indicate whether natural infection has occurred: for example, IgA (immunoglobulin A) antibodies arise only after natural exposure to polioviruses or to live-attenuated oral poliovirus vaccines (OPV), and hence can be used in populations vaccinated with killed polio vaccine (IPV) to track poliovirus infection. It may also be possible to track pertussis infection in populations vaccinated with acellular pertussis vaccines, by assaying antibodies to antigens not included in the vaccine.

Evaluating vaccine coverage in a population in which natural infection is still occurring may be possible for multi-component or multi-strain vaccines, even if the assay does not distinguish between vaccine-induced and natural immunity. Briefly, seropositivity to all vaccine components over a short time interval after the recommended age of vaccination is suggestive of vaccine-induced rather than naturally induced immunity. The details depend very much on the specific application. An example is described in Box 9.6.

Box 9.6 Human papillomavirus vaccine coverage in the United Kingdom

Vaccination against human papillomavirus (HPV) infection was introduced in the United Kingdom in 2008. The vaccine was offered to girls aged 12–13 years, with a catch-up programme up to 18 years. The vaccine included two strains: HPV16 and HPV18; in 2012 the vaccine was replaced by a quadrivalent one. Some 2,146 serum samples obtained in 2011 from young women aged 15–19 years were analysed (Mesher et al., 2016). The bivalent vaccine was then in use.

HPV vaccination is known to produce close to 100% seroconversion with higher average antibody concentrations than elicited by natural infection. Antibody concentrations (AC) for seropositives were classified as low, moderate and high. Individuals were classified as follows:

- *seronegative*: seronegative to both HPV16 and HPV18;
- *probably infected*: seropositive to one but not both of HPV16 and HPV18;
- *vaccinated or infected*: seropositive to both with low AC for at least one and high AC on neither;
- *probably vaccinated*: seropositive to both with high AC for at least one or moderate AC for both.

Of the 2,146 individuals, 607 were seronegative, 159 probably infected, 60 vaccinated or infected and 1,320 were probably vaccinated. Thus, the vaccine coverage in this sample was estimated to lie between $1,320 / 2,146 = 62\%$ and $(1,320 + 60) / 2,146 = 64\%$. The coverage estimated in this way was found broadly to coincide with the reported coverage, with some age variation, which the authors attributed to under-reporting of vaccination at older ages.

In Box 9.6, antibody concentrations were used to assess vaccine coverage. However, the presence of such antibodies may not necessarily indicate immunity from infection; the interpretation of serological data is the topic of the next section.

9.3 Immunological correlates of protection

The interpretation of antibody levels, and their classification in terms of seropositivity, is highly dependent on the infection, the biomarker studied and the assay used. In this section we discuss the main issues involved.

The usefulness of serological data to monitor vaccination programmes depends on the way vaccine-induced immunity is generated (see Chapter 2). When immunity is mediated mainly through antibodies (or when antibodies are correlated with cell-mediated and/or mucosal immunity), serological data can be used directly to assess population immunity. Examples of such infections include measles, rubella and smallpox.

Serological data are less useful to study immunity against those infections for which immunity arises mainly through cellular or mucosal mechanisms, and for which serum antibodies consequently do not play an important role. Examples include cholera, HPV and typhoid (Cutts & Hanson, 2016). Assays for cellular and mucosal immunity exist, but are at present too complex and insufficiently standardised to be used in assessing population immunity. Serological data are also less useful for infections where the causing pathogen's antigens change over time or immunity may be short-lived. The main example of this is influenza.

The interpretation of serological survey data is greatly simplified if the classification of individuals as seropositive or seronegative can, individually or in groups, be regarded as a proxy measure for presence or absence of immunity. This in turn depends on whether, for any given infection, there is an immunological correlate of protection.

An immunological correlate of protection is a measurement of a (natural or vaccine-induced) immune response that is correlated with protection against infection or disease. An immunological correlate of protection, once properly validated, can thus be used to determine whether individuals are immune. This is important for the evaluation of new vaccines and to assess population immunity. Box 9.7 provides a brief summary of some of the nomenclature and methodological issues that arise in the evaluation of correlates of protection.

Box 9.7 Mechanistic and non-mechanistic correlates of protection

A correlate of protection is an immune marker that is statistically correlated with protection against infection or disease. A correlate of protection may be mechanistic, if it is causally responsible for protection, or non-mechanistic if not.

This nomenclature was suggested by Plotkin and Gilbert (2012), who illustrate the distinction as follows. Immune responses to meningococcal vaccine can be measured by enzyme-linked immunosorbent assay (ELISA) or bactericidal antibodies. Both are correlates of protection. However, only bactericidal antibodies are truly protective. Thus, bactericidal antibodies are a mechanistic correlate of protection, whereas ELISA antibodies are a non-mechanistic correlate of protection. A further example is provided by varicella zoster vaccine. Both antibody and cellular responses have been found to correlate with protection. The cellular

> response, which is more strongly correlated with protection, is a mechanistic correlate of protection, whereas the antibody response is a non-mechanistic correlate of protection. However, the latter is easier to measure, and thus may be more useful in practice.
>
> Some of the methodological issues that arise in assessing correlates of protection are discussed by Qin, Gilbert, Corey, McElrath, and Self (2007). The focus is on the identification of correlates of protection within vaccine trials that fulfil various technical requirements for surrogate end points, developed within the wider statistical literature. The authors also discuss the evidence required to generalise correlates of protection to new situations, using the techniques of meta-analysis.

When a mechanistic serological correlate of protection has been established, stronger inferences may be drawn from serological data. For example, changes in antibody concentrations may be used to document changes in immunity levels. A serological correlate of protection can also help with the interpretation of data on waning vaccine effectiveness over time, a topic further discussed in Chapter 16. Finally, it is worth stressing that for some pathogens the level of the serological correlate of protection may depend on the infectious dose.

9.4 Design and analysis of serological surveys

In this section we discuss two sets of issues relating to the design of serological surveys. First, we discuss sampling strategies to obtain sera for inclusion in serological surveys. Then, we present some statistical considerations relating to the use of assays for seroepidemiology. We do not touch upon laboratory procedures: a basic description is provided in Chapter 2, while detailed descriptions of laboratory methods are outside the scope of this book. Finally, we briefly describe some of the epidemiological analyses that may be undertaken using serological survey data.

9.4.1 Sampling for serological surveys

The purpose of a serological survey is to obtain an unbiased estimate of the seroprevalence within a given population, or within strata of that population (e.g., within age groups). Thus, the sample of individuals from whom sera are collected should be representative (in terms of seropositivity) of the population or strata.

In practice, two approaches are commonly used. The first is to use residual sera, that is, left-over sera originally collected for diagnostic or screening purposes in microbiological or biochemical laboratories. Depending on the study question and the sourcing of the residual samples, such sera may be sufficiently representative. However, seroprevalences may be biased if the infection (or lack of vaccination) is clustered in groups that are under-represented among the residual serum samples available. The use of such a convenience sample raises important ethical issues such as whether sera can be used without consent, how anonymity can be maintained and whether record linkage may be used. An advantage of this approach, however, is that it is straightforward and cheap. A major disadvantage is that information on determinants of infection and other relevant variables, notably vaccination histories, is usually lacking.

The second approach is to sample the population randomly, and explicitly obtain consent to obtain blood specimens from the individuals sampled. A range of standard random sampling methods may be used, including stratified and cluster sampling. A major advantage of this approach is that it allows the collection of detailed personal information on determinants of infections, or linkage with other databases. It is also possible to design the survey so that certain groups of particular interest are over-sampled, by adjusting the sampling fractions. The main disadvantages are the high cost, and the potential for selection bias owing to incomplete participation. To reduce costs, serological surveys can be included in existing population health surveys.

To enhance feasibility and participation, less invasive samples such as oral fluid or dried blood spots rather than serum can be used. Antibody detection in these specimens can approach the results obtained with serum, provided samples are handled appropriately and suitable laboratory assays are used. However, inadequate sensitivity has been reported with dried blood spots and oral fluid (Cutts & Hanson, 2016). Ideally, a venous blood sample is taken from a subsample of the study population to validate results based on less invasive samples. This is especially important in challenging field conditions in developing countries.

Some examples of these different approaches are described in Box 9.8.

Box 9.8 Serological surveys based on residual sera and random sampling

Wilson et al. (2012) describe the national seroepidemiology programmes in Australia, the Netherlands, the United Kingdom and the United States.

Australia and the United Kingdom use convenience samples of residual sera, with only basic demographic information (such as age, sex, location). The UK programme has been in operation since 1986–1987. In Australia, a study was undertaken to compare the results based on convenience and random cluster sampling in children of school age (Kelly, Riddell, Gidding, Nolan, & Gilbert, 2002). The authors found no statistically significant differences in seroprevalence for measles, mumps, hepatitis B or varicella. For rubella, the seroprevalence was slightly higher in the cluster sample.

The Netherlands and the United States, on the other hand, use population-based random sampling. In both these countries, a questionnaire is used to obtain additional demographic and immunisation information. In the Netherlands, municipalities with low immunisation coverage are over-sampled. In the United States, serological data are collected as part of other health surveys.

9.4.2 Statistical considerations relating to the use of assays for serological surveys

The validity (sensitivity and specificity) of the assay used in a serological survey is critical to the interpretation of the survey results. Briefly, the sensitivity of the assay is the proportion of people who test positive among those who are protected by previous infection or vaccination. The specificity is the proportion of people who test negative among those who are not protected by infection or vaccination. High values of both sensitivity and specificity are required. The assays used in serological surveillance are often originally developed for individual diagnostic purposes, whereas seroepidemiology requires a different focus, the aim being to obtain unbiased estimates of seroprevalence in the population. Thus, some validation studies may be required to choose assay thresholds that optimally balance sensitivity and specificity.

Individual sera are often classified as positive, equivocal or negative. A decision must be made about how to treat the equivocal sera; this might involve re-testing them. In some circumstances, it may be appropriate to regard equivocals as low positives, and hence group them with the positives; in others, it may be best to exclude equivocal sera from further analysis.

When serological results are obtained with different assays, or the same assays applied in different laboratories, it may be necessary to standardise assay results. This may be done using a common panel of sera, to translate the results obtained using different assays or in different laboratories into common units. Box 9.9 describes an example.

Box 9.9 Standardisation of hepatitis A assay results

Several Europe-wide seroepidemiology projects have been undertaken to compare immunity levels to a range of infections between countries. These projects have involved a standardisation step, to ensure that data obtained in different countries are comparable. The standardisation methodology has been described by Kafatos, Andrews, and Nardone (2005). The application to hepatitis A described here is in Anastassopoulou et al. (2009).

A panel of 150 sera was distributed to participating laboratories and tested for antibodies to hepatitis A virus (HAV). Antibody concentrations were then compared to those obtained at the reference centre in Greece, and standardisation curves were drawn to translate local results into the scale used at the Greek reference centre. Results for two countries are shown in Figure 9.5.

As shown in Figure 9.5, the assay results from the same sera obtained in laboratories in the Czech Republic and Finland differ. For the purposes of classifying sera as positive or negative, the overriding emphasis is to obtain a well-fitting curve in the region around the positive/negative boundary or in the equivocal range. The standardisation curve and its equation are then used to translate serological survey results into common units.

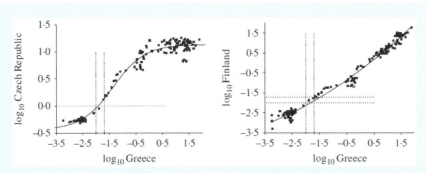

Figure 9.5 Log antibody concentrations and standardisation curves for anti-HAV test results in the Czech Republic (left panel) and Finland (right panel) against the reference results from Greece.

Note: The horizontal dotted lines represent the positive/negative boundary (Czech Republic) or equivocal range (Finland).

Source: Reproduced with permission from Anastassopoulou et al. (2009).

Most often, the assays are applied to sera from individuals, yielding individual test results. In some circumstances, particularly when the prevalence is low, sera may be pooled within strata, thus greatly reducing the number of tests required, and hence the cost of the survey. The assay employed should be sufficiently sensitive to handle the additional dilution involved in pooling sera. The analysis techniques of group testing are then used to retrieve the prevalences (Farrington, 1992).

9.4.3 Descriptive analyses of seroepidemiological data

Most relevant public health questions arising in the monitoring of vaccination programmes may be handled using descriptive statistical methods. Proportions seropositive may be obtained for the population as a whole or for relevant strata, with 95% confidence intervals calculated using standard binomial methods. Thus, if r individuals are seropositive out of n tested and yielding valid test results, the proportion seropositive is $p = r/n$ with approximate 95% confidence limits:

$$p^- = p - 1.96 \times \sqrt{\frac{p \times (1-p)}{n}}, \quad p^+ = p + 1.96 \times \sqrt{\frac{p \times (1-p)}{n}}.$$

If data are sparse, exact methods may be preferable.

Antibody concentrations, or titres, are often expressed on a continuous scale, as for the hepatitis A antibody concentrations in Box 9.9. It is often of interest to quantify the antibody concentrations among seropositives. If the antibody concentrations in the population are right-skew, that is, have a heavy upper tail, it is usual to summarise them using medians or geometric means, rather than arithmetic means, so that large positive values do not distort the average. The geometric mean titre (GMT) of a sample of titres $t_1, t_2, \ldots, t_n$ is most readily calculated by using logarithms:

$$\text{GMT} = \text{antilog}\left\{\sum_{i=1}^{n}\log(t_i)/n\right\}.$$

A practical example of the calculation is given in Box 9.10.

> ### Box 9.10 Obtaining seroprevalence and GMTs
>
> Antibody titres for a given infection were obtained for 20 individuals, and were, in increasing order:
>
> 36, 51, 58, 85, 105, 145, 176, 203, 215, 220, 251, 278, 319, 387, 426, 525, 725, 910, 1317, 2830
>
> Values ≤ 120 are seronegative, values above 120 are seropositive. Thus, in this sample, there are 5 seronegatives and 15 seropositives. The seroprevalence is
>
> $$p = \frac{15}{20} = 0.75$$
>
> or 75%, with 95% confidence limits
>
> $$p^- = 0.75 - 1.96 \times \sqrt{\frac{0.75 \times (1 - 0.75)}{20}} = 0.56,$$
>
> $$p^+ = 0.75 + 1.96 \times \sqrt{\frac{0.75 \times (1 - 0.75)}{20}} = 0.94.$$
>
> To obtain the geometric mean titre of the 15 seropositive titres, first take logs. Any base will do, provided antilogs are then taken in the same base. Using logs to base 10,
>
> $$\text{GMT} = 10^{\{\log_{10}(145) + \log_{10}(176) + \cdots + \log_{10}(2830)\}/15} = 402.1.$$
>
> Thus, the geometric mean titre for the seropositives is 402.1. The median seropositive titre, on the other hand, is 319 (the middle value of the seropositive titres).

9.4.4 Mixture modelling of antibody concentrations

In some circumstances, it may be possible to estimate seroprevalences without classifying individual sera as positive, equivocal or negative according to predetermined cut-off values, by modelling the entire sample as a mixture of seropositives and seronegatives. Such analyses are more complicated from a statistical viewpoint, and are only practical when there are subpopulations with clearly differentiated antibody distributions. An example is described in Box 9.11. Importantly, the designation 'seropositive' in mixture modelling does not necessarily indicate immunological protection. This still depends on the availability of a correlate for protection. Further details on mixture modelling can be found in Held, Hens, O'Neill, and Wallinga (2019).

Box 9.11 Analysis of varicella zoster virus seroprevalence data with mixture models

Del Fava et al. (2016) analysed serological survey data on varicella zoster virus (VZV) in Norway using mixture models. The data and models are in Figure 9.6.

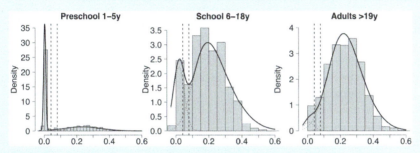

Figure 9.6 Antibody levels to VZV in Norway by age group.
Note: The histograms represent the observed data, the superimposed curves are the mixture models. The two vertical dashed lines indicate the equivocal range.
Source: Reproduced from Del Fava et al. (2016).

The horizontal axes in Figure 9.6 represent the logarithms of the optical densities (plus 1) obtained directly from the serological assay reader. The mixture model comprises two components. The first component, centred close to zero on the horizontal scale, represents the seronegatives. This component is most marked in the preschool group and is still very apparent in the 6–18-year-olds. The second component, centred close to 0.2, represents the seropositives. This component is very flat in the preschool group, increases in importance among 6–18-year-olds and is dominant in adulthood.

Similar results were obtained with this mixture model as with the simpler analysis based on classifying individual sera using a fixed cut-off. One advantage of the mixture model is that no decision needs to be made about how to handle sera in the equivocal range. On the other hand, the mixture model requires additional assumptions relating to the choice of distributions and how their parameters vary with age.

9.4.5 Further analyses of serological survey data

Serological survey data provide opportunities for many other statistical analyses to estimate parameters of interest. These include estimating the force of infection (the rate at which susceptibles become infected), the basic reproduction number and the critical immunisation threshold. If several serological surveys have been undertaken in the same population over time, then variations in the incidence over time may be studied as well as age effects. And if antibodies to several infections are analysed using the same sera, analyses of individual heterogeneities may sometimes be undertaken. Some of these methods, which lie beyond the scope of this book, are described in Farrington, Kanaan, and Gay (2001). Parameter values estimated from serological data may then be used as inputs to mathematical models to chart the epidemiology of the infection and the impact of vaccination programmes into the future, as touched upon in Chapter 4.

Summary

- Serum antibodies, as measured in serological surveys, may be used to estimate the seroprevalence of infections in populations and relevant subgroups, and to plan vaccination programmes.
- Once a vaccination programme has been implemented, serological surveys can be used to monitor levels of susceptibility and identify pools of susceptibles. This information may be used to target supplementary vaccination campaigns, modify vaccination schedules or introduce booster doses.
- The interpretation of serological data is enhanced when serological correlates of protection have been established.
- Different designs have been used for serological surveys, including convenience sampling of residual sera, or random population-based sampling. To allow comparisons between countries, assay results should ideally be standardised.
- When analysing seroepidemiology data for the purpose of monitoring vaccination programmes, descriptive analyses are usually sufficient.
- More advanced statistical analyses include mixture modelling and the estimation of key parameters describing infectious disease dynamics.

References

Anastassopoulou, C. G., Kafatos, G., Nardone, A., Andrews, N., Pebody, R. G., Mossong, J., … Hatzakis, A. (2009). The European Sero-Epidemiology Network 2 (ESEN2): Standardization of assay results for hepatitis A virus (HAV) to enable comparisons of seroprevalence data across 15 countries. *Epidemiology and Infection*, *137*(4), 485–494.

Craig, K. T., Verma, H., Iliyasu, Z., Mkanda, P., Touray, K., Johnson, T., … Vaz, R. G. (2016). Role of serial seroprevalence studies in guiding implementation of the polio eradication initiative in Kano, Nigeria: 2011–2014. *Journal of Infectious Diseases*, *213*(S3), S124–S130.

Cutts, F. T., & Hanson, M. (2016). Seroepidemiology: An underused tool for designing and monitoring vaccination programmes in low- and middle-income countries. *Tropical Medicine and International Health, 21*(9), 1086–1098.

Del Fava, E., Rimseliene, G., Flem, E., de Blasio, B. F., Scalia Tomba, G., & Manfredi, P. (2016). Estimating age-specific immunity and force of infection of varicella zoster virus in Norway using mixture models. *PLoS One, 11*(9), e0163636.

Farrington, C. P. (1992). Estimating prevalence by group testing samples using generalized linear models. *Statistics in Medicine, 11*(12), 1591–1597.

Farrington, C. P., Kanaan, M. N., & Gay, N. J. (2001). Estimation of the basic reproduction number for infectious diseases from age-stratified serological survey data (with discussion). *Applied Statistics, 50*(3), 251–292.

Gay, N. J., Hesketh, L. M., Morgan-Capner, P., & Miller, E. (1995). Interpretation of serological surveillance data for measles using mathematical models: Implications for vaccine strategy. *Epidemiology and Infection, 115*, 139–156.

Held, L., Hens, N., O'Neill, P., & Wallinga, J. (2019). *Handbook of infectious disease data analysis.* Boca Raton, FL: CRC Press.

Ishola, D. A., Borrow, R., Findlow, H., Findlow, J., Trotter, C., & Ramsay, M. E. (2012). Prevalence of serum bactericidal antibody to serogroup C Neisseria meningitidis in England a decade after vaccine introduction. *Clinical and Vaccine Immunology, 19*(8), 1126–1130.

Kafatos, G., Andrews, N., & Nardone, A. (2005). Model selection methodology for interlaboratory standardisation of antibody titres. *Vaccine, 23*(42), 5022–5027.

Kelly, H., Riddell, M. A., Gidding, H. F., Nolan, T., & Gilbert, G. L. (2002). A random cluster survey and a convenience sample give comparable estimates of immunity to vaccine-preventable diseases in children of school age in Victoria, Australia. *Vaccine, 20*(25–26), 3130–3136.

Mao, B., Chheng, K., Wannemuehler, K., Vynnycky, E., Buth, S., Soeung, S. C., ... Gregory, C. J. (2015). Immunity to polio, measles and rubella in women of childbearing age and estimated congenital rubella syndrome incidence, Cambodia, 2012. *Epidemiology and Infection, 143*(9), 1858–1867.

Mesher, D., Stanford, E., White, J., Findlow, J., Warrington, R., Das, S., ... Soldan, K. (2016). HPV serology testing confirms high HPV immunisation coverage in England. *PLoS One, 11*(3), e0150107.

Plotkin, S. A., & Gilbert, P. B. (2012). Nomenclature for immune correlates of protection after vaccination. *Clinical Infectious Diseases, 54*, 1615–1617.

Qin, L., Gilbert, P. B., Corey, L., McElrath, M. J., & Self, S. G. (2007). A framework for assessing immunological correlates of protection in vaccine trials. *Journal of Infectious Diseases, 196*(9), 1304–1312.

Raharimanga, V., Carod, J. -F., Ramarokoto, C. -E., Chrétien, J. -B., Rakotomanana, F., Talarmin, A., & Richard, V. (2008). Age-specific seroprevalence of hepatitis A in Antananarivo (Madagascar). *BMC Infectious Diseases, 8*, 78.

Vyse, A. J., Gay, N. J., White, J. M., Ramsay, M. E., Brown, D. W., Cohen, B. J., ... Miller, E. (2002). Evolution of surveillance of measles, mumps and rubella in England and Wales: Providing the platform for evidence-based vaccination policy. *Epidemiologic Reviews, 24*(2), 125–136.

Wilson, S. E., Deeks, S. L., Hatchette, T. F., & Crowcroft, N. S. (2012). The role of seroepidemiology in the comprehensive surveillance of vaccine-preventable infections. *CMAJ, 184*(1), E70–E76.

Chapter 10

Assessing and monitoring impact

In this chapter we discuss the main methods used for assessing the impact of a vaccination programme. Such assessments should generally be repeated over time since, as seen in Chapter 5, some of the impacts of vaccination programmes may only be apparent long after vaccination has been introduced. We focus on impacts relating to burden of disease and elimination.

We begin in Section 10.1 by contrasting population impacts and effects on individuals and discuss measures of impact. In Section 10.2 we describe methods involving contemporaneous control populations, while in Section 10.3 we describe some informal approaches involving before-and-after comparison methods. In the following two sections we discuss more formal methods: interrupted time-series designs in Section 10.4, and regression discontinuity designs in Section 10.5. Finally, in Section 10.6 we introduce some special methods for monitoring a vaccination programme when elimination has been achieved.

10.1 Population impacts

A vaccination programme is an intervention applied to an entire population. Impacts (there may be several, as described in Chapter 5) are the consequences of the vaccination programme for the population as a whole. Typically, impacts relating to the burden of disease are measured by comparing an indicator (such as a risk or rate of disease) in the population in which the vaccination programme has been introduced, to that same indicator in a comparator (or counterfactual) population in which the vaccination programme has not been introduced.

While impacts relate to the population as a whole, the direct and indirect effects of vaccination are experienced by individuals within that population. In the presence of a mass vaccination programme, indirect effects will most likely vary between individuals and subgroups within the population, owing to heterogeneity in vaccine coverage. The impact of vaccination on the burden of disease is the aggregate result of its direct and indirect effects in individuals.

DOI: 10.4324/9781315166414-11
This Chapter has been made available under a CC-BY-NC-ND license.

ASSESSING AND MONITORING IMPACT   173

Population impact, effects in individuals and how to evaluate them in principle are discussed further in Box 10.1 in the context of vaccination programmes.

Box 10.1 Individual effects and population impact of mass vaccination programmes

Individuals within a population in which a vaccination programme has been introduced experience direct and indirect effects of vaccination. Vaccination directly protects vaccinated individuals by inducing immunity in these individuals: this is the *direct effect* of vaccination; it benefits only vaccinated individuals. Vaccination may also indirectly protect people by herd immunity: these are the *indirect effects* of vaccination; they benefit all individuals within the population, whether vaccinated or not.

Most vaccination programmes will induce indirect effects. Exceptions are when the targeted pathogen is predominantly acquired from a non-human reservoir (such as tetanus), when the targeted disease results from a reactivation of a chronic infection (such as herpes zoster), or when the vaccine protects against disease but not infection.

Impacts are the consequences of a vaccination programme for the population as a whole, such as an overall reduction in disease burden. Impact results from the totality of the individual effects experienced by people within the population, and

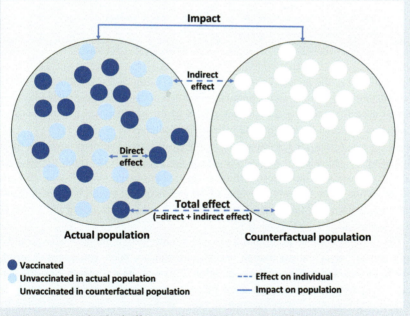

Figure 10.1 Individual effects and population impact of vaccination.

is dependent on the implementation of the vaccination programme, in particular on the vaccine coverage achieved.

Individual effects and population impact are represented in Figure 10.1.

The large circle on the left of Figure 10.1 represents the actual population in which the vaccination programme has been implemented; the individuals within this population are represented by dots: the darker ones are vaccinated, the lighter ones are unvaccinated. The large circle on the right represents the same population (with the same individuals) in which the vaccination programme has not been introduced: this is the counterfactual population.

- The *direct effect* of vaccination is assessed (in principle) by comparing infection rates in vaccinated individuals to those in unvaccinated individuals within the actual population in which the vaccination programme has been introduced. This and other effects are indicated by the arrows in Figure 10.1.
- The *indirect effect* of vaccination is assessed by comparing unvaccinated individuals within the actual population to individuals within the counterfactual population in which this vaccination programme has not been introduced.
- The *total effect* of vaccination on an individual is assessed by comparing vaccinated individuals in the actual population to individuals in the counterfactual unvaccinated population.
- The *impact* of the vaccination programme on the population as a whole is assessed by comparing global indicators of disease burden in the actual and counterfactual populations.

In practice, the counterfactual population is not observed, so some other comparable but unvaccinated population is used.

The main aim of the present chapter is to describe methods for assessing the impact of a vaccination programme on the population burden of disease. These methods can often also be used for assessing the indirect effects of the programme on individuals in the population in which the programme is being implemented.

As set out in Box 10.1, evaluating the impact of a vaccination programme involves comparing an indicator of disease burden in the population in which the vaccination programme has been introduced (which is the *actual population* in Figure 10.1), to its counterfactual value, namely the value of the indicator that would have been measured in this population, had the vaccination programme not been introduced (this is the *counterfactual population* in Figure 10.1).

The difficulty is that we do not know the counterfactual: namely what would have happened in our actual population had vaccination not been introduced. Instead, we have to use a comparable control population. This may be a contemporaneous population, in which no intervention has taken place. Or a comparison might be made between the pre-vaccination and post-vaccination eras. In either case, the comparability of the control population with the actual population (and hence its validity for representing the counterfactual) is a major issue. In particular, before-and-after comparisons are confounded by time: an observed difference may be due, at least in principle, to a temporal effect unrelated to vaccination but coinciding with it, such as seasonality or epidemic cycles.

Occasionally, a natural experiment may occur in which the vaccination programme is altered or suspended in such a way as to allow inferences on impact to be made. The example of whooping cough vaccination in the United Kingdom described in Chapter 5 is one such instance. Vaccination against pertussis was introduced in the 1950s and was accompanied by a steep decline in whooping cough notifications. However, it could be objected that the decline had begun several years earlier (see Chapter 5) and thus could be due to more general improvements in health provision rather than the impact of the vaccine. However, the upsurge in whooping cough notifications in England and Wales in the mid-1970s, which occurred when vaccine coverage dropped from over 80% to less than 40% (this variation constituting the natural experiment in this case), provides powerful evidence that the decline in the burden of whooping cough observed in the 1950s was not wholly due to improvements in public health unrelated to pertussis vaccination.

In most cases, however, such opportunities for demonstrating impact are unavailable, and assessing impact relies on strong assumptions. Some study types for assessing impact are reviewed by Lopez Bernal, Andrews, and Amirthalingam (2019).

A variety of different measures of impact on burden of disease may be used, depending on the context. Absolute measures include the number of cases prevented by vaccination, and the difference in incidence (incidence of infection or disease before minus incidence after the introduction of the vaccination programme), also called vaccine-preventable disease incidence or VPDI (Gessner & Feikin, 2014):

$$DIFF = IR_{pre\text{-}vaccine} - IR_{post\text{-}vaccine}.$$

Here, $IR_{pre\text{-}vaccine}$ and $IR_{post\text{-}vaccine}$ denote the incidence rate before and after the introduction of the vaccination programme, respectively. Relative measures of impact, such as the relative difference in incidence, are also commonly used:

$$RDIFF = \frac{IR_{pre\text{-}vaccine} - IR_{post\text{-}vaccine}}{IR_{pre\text{-}vaccine}} = 1 - IRR,$$

where IRR is the incidence rate ratio. These and other impact measures, and how they relate to measures such as vaccine effectiveness (the topic of Chapter 12), are discussed by Hanquet, Valenciano, Simondon, and Moren (2013). Our emphasis in the present chapter is, for the most part, on measures of impact that reflect the full effect of a vaccination programme as a whole.

All impact measures are highly context-dependent, and their values relate very specifically to the population and the conditions under which the vaccine has been introduced. Often, a graphical representation may convey more effectively the impact of a vaccination programme over time than a single numerical summary. Indeed, impact is likely to evolve: owing to the non-linear processes at play, and the possibility of threshold effects, impacts cannot be extrapolated but instead need to be monitored over time.

10.2 Contemporaneous comparisons

One situation in which it is possible to evaluate impact through comparison with a contemporaneous unvaccinated control population is when the vaccination programme is introduced in one location, but not in another. It is then possible to evaluate the impact of the programme by comparing the two locations, provided the two locations are comparable. Situations where this is possible are relatively uncommon. One example is described in Box 10.2.

Box 10.2 Impact of cholera vaccination in South Sudan

In December 2013, violence erupted in South Sudan leading to the displacement of one in five persons within the country. A preventive cholera vaccination programme was targeted at six settlements of internally displaced persons, but not at persons in the host community (Azman et al., 2016). The risk of cholera (per 10,000 persons) was compared in different locations, using suspected cholera cases (persons with clinician-diagnosed acute watery diarrhoea). Two-dose vaccine coverage of the eligible populations was assessed.

In one comparison, the risk of cholera was contrasted in two camps, one unvaccinated and one with 92.2% coverage. The risk was 38.8 per 10,000 in the vaccinated camp and 236.4 per 10,000 in the unvaccinated camp. Provided that the determinants of transmission (such as contact rates and frequencies of importations) are comparable in the two camps, this suggests that vaccination may have reduced the risk of cholera by about 84% through its direct and indirect effects within the camp setting.

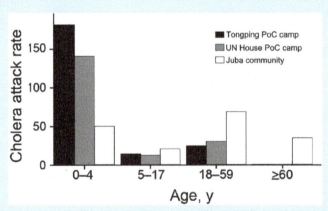

Figure 10.2 Estimated risk of cholera (per 10,000) by age in three locations in South Sudan: Tongping PoC camp (93% vaccine coverage); UN House PoC camp (95% vaccine coverage); Juba community (unvaccinated).
Source: Reproduced from Azman et al. (2016).

A second comparison was made between two camps (with vaccine coverage 93% and 95% respectively) in the region of Juba and the non-camp population of Juba without access to improved sanitation. In this case, the camps and the community settings are not truly comparable as the determinants of transmission will most likely differ. Thus, overall risks, which were only slightly higher in the community than in the camps, are not comparable.

However, the age distribution of cases was markedly different, with a much higher incidence of cases in children under 5 years old in the camps, as shown in Figure 10.2.

The authors note that the difference in age distributions does not appear to be the result of differences in population structure, age-specific vaccine coverage or presence of other diarrhoeal pathogens in the camps. This suggests that the vaccine may be less effective in younger children in the special conditions prevailing at these camps.

Another situation where impact may be assessed contemporaneously is when a vaccination programme is introduced in different areas at different times. This is the idea behind the stepped-wedge design, which will be described in Chapter 12 on vaccine effectiveness. It also applies when a vaccination programme is piloted in some areas prior to being rolled out more generally. An example is described in Box 10.3.

Box 10.3 Impact of vaccinating school-age children against influenza in England

The phased introduction of childhood vaccination with the live-attenuated influenza vaccine in the United Kingdom began in 2013 (Pebody et al., 2015). During the 2014–2015 influenza season, all children aged 2–3 years were offered the vaccine. Vaccination of children aged 4–11 years (and some of age 11–13 years) was piloted in selected areas in England. The pilot areas and non-pilot areas were county-wide and geographically distinct. The dominant strains of influenza A and B found to be circulating during the 2014–2015 influenza season did not match the relevant components of the vaccine.

We focus on the impact of vaccinating children aged 4–11 years. This was assessed by comparing indicators of influenza virus infection and disease in pilot areas and non-pilot areas in various age groups.

The impact in the targeted age group (children of primary school age, 57% coverage) was large and statistically significant: consultations rates for influenza-like illness (ILI) were reduced by 94%, confirmed influenza hospital admissions were reduced by 93%. There were also large yet not statistically significant impacts (owing to small numbers of cases) in younger children: ILI consultations were 92% lower and confirmed hospitalisations 61% lower in children of preschool age. Impacts were also observed for some older age groups. On the other hand, the impacts were less pronounced in all age groups for more severe end points including excess mortality.

However, the authors point out that caution is required in interpreting these results, owing to differences between pilot and non-pilot areas in past incidence of influenza and in the vaccination coverage in 2–4-year-olds. An impact as large as that observed would perhaps not be expected, since vaccine strains differed from circulating strains.

As illustrated in Box 10.3, a major difficulty confronting contemporaneous comparisons between populations lies in ensuring that the populations are comparable. The validity of the comparison may be investigated when data are available for the period preceding the introduction of the vaccination programme, through before-and-after comparisons. As will be seen in the next section, before-and-after comparisons are also used to assess impact directly.

10.3 Before-and-after comparisons

Before-and-after comparisons involve comparing some quantitative measure of infection or disease, using measurements made both before and after the introduction of vaccination in the population. They are the most commonly used method of assessing impact. Comparisons of this sort have already been described in Chapter 9 on serological surveillance, which involved comparing age-specific seroprevalences before and after vaccination was introduced.

Before-and-after comparisons are often based on numbers of case reports or on risks or incidences of infection or disease, and can provide estimates of the difference or relative difference in incidence before and after introduction of the vaccination programme. More generally, if the vaccination programme has had an impact, this should be reflected in the observed patterns of infection before and after the introduction of vaccination. An example of this approach is described in Box 10.4.

Box 10.4 Impact of *Haemophilus influenzae* type b vaccination in the Gambia

Prior to the introduction of vaccination against *Haemophilus influenzae* type b (Hib) in the Gambia, the incidence was high with a case fatality rate of 30% for Hib meningitis. Following a successful trial of the vaccine in 1993–1995, routine vaccination was introduced in 1997, with three doses of a conjugate vaccine administered with diphtheria, tetanus and pertussis (DTP) vaccine.

A study of the impact of the vaccination programme was undertaken in the western region of the Gambia (Adegbola et al., 2005). Possible cases of Hib

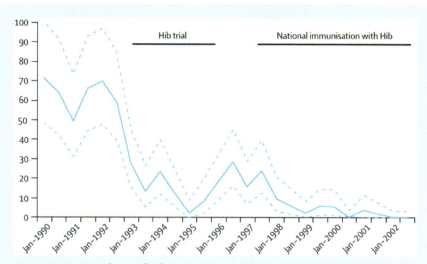

Figure 10.3 Incidence of Hib meningitis in children younger than 5 years: rates per 100,000 per year and 90% confidence intervals.
Source: Reproduced with permission from Adegbola et al. (2005).

disease in children under 6 years of age were enrolled and investigated for Hib infection. Accurate denominators were obtained by interpolating from census data and cluster sampling data. Figure 10.3 shows the incidence of Hib meningitis over time in children aged less than 5 years; the trend in children under 1 year is similar.

Figure 10.3 shows a sharp decline in the incidence of Hib disease coinciding with the Hib trial in 1993–1995, followed by a resurgence after the end of the trial. The introduction of routine immunisation in 1997 is accompanied by a further drop. The annual incidence dropped from 60 cases per 100,000 before any use of Hib to 0 cases in the last year of the study. This impact was achieved with vaccine coverage of 94% for dose 1, 84% for dose 2 and 68% for dose 3, though vaccine supply was erratic.

Two main sets of issues need to be taken into consideration when interpreting a trend such as that presented in Figure 10.3. The first is whether the case ascertainment procedures were adequate and whether changes in these procedures, perhaps related to the introduction of vaccination, might explain the observed effects. The second is whether these effects might be explained by naturally occurring changes in the incidence of disease, which are unrelated to vaccination but that happen to coincide with its introduction.

In the case of the example in Box 10.4, both alternative explanations are unlikely. Surveillance of Hib in the study area was instituted in 1990 and maintained with the same methods; if anything, surveillance is likely to have been reinforced after the introduction of the vaccine. Thus, changes in surveillance procedures are unlikely to account for the observed trend. Furthermore, the resurgence of Hib disease after the end of the trial and before the beginning of routine vaccination suggests (but does not definitively prove) that the observed pattern is caused by the vaccine.

More generally, it is important to keep in mind that observing a difference in incidence before and after introduction of a vaccination programme does not imply that this difference is caused by the programme. The strength of the evidence for impact is greatly enhanced if other effects, notably secular trends in incidence, caused by changes in surveillance procedures or natural variation in incidence, can be discounted or taken into account in the analysis.

One way to achieve a degree of control is to use another infection as a contemporaneous control. Such a control infection should ideally fulfil three criteria:

- it should not be affected by the vaccination programme or by other changes in prevention measures;
- it should be documented using similar surveillance procedures as those applied for the infection of interest; and
- it should be transmitted by the same route as the infection of interest.

The first condition ensures that the vaccination programme will have no effect, direct or indirect, on the incidence of the control infection within the control cohorts; this also applies to other changes in prevention measures, including any directed at the control infection. The other conditions ensure that changes in surveillance methods or changes in contact rates in the population should be reflected in any trends observed for the control infection. This type of control is called a negative control and is discussed more formally by Lipsitch, Tchetgen Tchetgen, and Cohen (2010).

Observed difference in secular trends between the infection of interest and the control infection can then reasonably be attributed to the vaccination programme, rather than to changes in surveillance or contact rates. However, other confounding factors can never completely be ruled out. For example, the epidemic or seasonal cycles observed for some infections may complicate the interpretation; these can be handled by the modelling techniques described in Section 10.4.

An example of an impact assessment reinforced by the consideration of a control infection is described in Box 10.5.

Box 10.5 Impact of human papillomavirus vaccination on anogenital warts in Québec

In Québec, Canada, a human papillomavirus (HPV) vaccination programme in schools was introduced in 2008 with the quadrivalent vaccine, aimed at girls and young women aged 9–17 years. To assess the early impact of the vaccination programme, a study was undertaken to compare the incidence of anogenital warts in the pre-vaccination period (2004–2007) and the post-vaccination period (2009–2012), by age group and sex (Steben, Ouhoummane, Rodier, Sinyavskaya, & Brassard, 2018).

Sex- and age-specific annual rates of anogenital warts per 100,000 were calculated using data obtained from an administrative health database. For women aged 15–19 years, the average annual incidence of anogenital warts per 100,000 was 65.43 in 2004–2007 and 36.47 in 2009–2012. Thus, the difference in incidence is

$$DIFF = 65.43 - 36.47 = 28.96$$

and the relative difference is

$$RDIFF = \frac{65.43 - 36.47}{65.43} = 0.443,$$

an incidence reduction of 44%. For women aged 20–24 years the decline was 19%, and for women aged 25–29 years it was 11%. The relative difference is greatest for women aged 15–19 years and for women aged 20–24 years; these age groups include women targeted by the vaccination programme.

Rates were also calculated for chlamydia, another sexually transmitted infection, using the same data source as for anogenital warts, and over the same period. In the present context, chlamydia may be regarded as a control infection: unaffected by the HPV vaccine or changes in other control measures, ascertained using similar methods as the anogenital warts data and sexually transmitted as for HPV infection.

The age-specific rates in women for both infections over the period 2004–2012 are shown in Figure 10.4.

The left panel of Figure 10.4 shows the decline in the incidence of anogenital warts in women between the pre-vaccination (2004–2007) and post-vaccination (2009–2012) periods, in all three age groups. The right panel of Figure 10.4 shows that the incidence of chlamydia in women increased steadily in the same age groups over the same period. The contrast in the trends for anogenital warts and for chlamydia suggests that the drop in incidence of anogenital warts is unlikely to be due to reporting artefacts or to secular trends in sexually transmitted infections caused by behavioural changes.

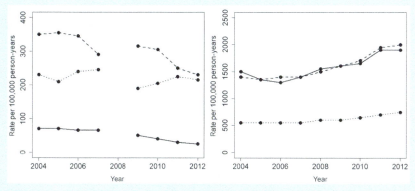

Figure 10.4 Incidence of anogenital warts (left) and chlamydia (right) in women, by age group, 2004–2012. Full lines: 15–19 years; dashed lines: 20–24 years; dotted lines: 25–29 years.

In the HPV example in Box 10.5, chlamydia was used as a control infection. The use of control infections provides a method to validate inferences drawn about the impact of vaccination, when the trend observed for the infection of interest, which is targeted by vaccination, differs markedly from that observed for the control infection.

Before-and-after methods can also be used to provide evidence of impact of a vaccination programme through the indirect effects of vaccination. Typically, such effects are evaluated by estimating the impact of the vaccination programme on groups that remain unvaccinated. The approach is illustrated in Box 10.6 for the examples previously discussed in this section.

Box 10.6 Obtaining evidence of indirect effects of vaccination

In Box 10.4 it was shown that the introduction of routine vaccination in the Gambia had a big impact on Hib disease incidence. Evidence for the indirect effects of vaccination may be obtained from the impact on the incidence of infection in children too young to be directly protected by vaccination. The median age of cases prior to the introduction of vaccination was 7 months; and the average age at vaccination with the second dose was 6.5 months (this is the dose that provides most protection). These being roughly equal, it follows that a large proportion of cases could not be protected directly by vaccination. Since the vaccination programme achieved big reductions in incidence in all age groups, the vaccination programme is likely to have had a substantial impact in reducing the incidence of Hib disease in very young children, which in turn suggests that indirect effects due to herd immunity were important.

For the HPV data of Box 10.5, it was possible to evaluate impacts due to the indirect effects of vaccination. A 21% reduction in incidence of anogenital warts was observed in young men aged 15–19 years after the introduction of HPV vaccination in girls and young women. The incidence of chlamydia in young men aged 15–19 years increased over time (as it did for young women). Thus, the drop in the rate of anogenital warts in young men aged 15–19 years is an impact attributable to the indirect effects of vaccination, though a contribution from direct effects resulting from vaccinations obtained outside the public sector cannot be excluded.

In this section we have focused on descriptive methods to assess the impact of vaccination programmes, typically involving graphical presentations as well as numerical summaries based on average incidences before and after the introduction of vaccination. In the next section, we discuss some more advanced methods that allow for trends and cycles in the data.

10.4 Interrupted time-series methods

An interrupted time series, in the present context, is a regular sequence of disease counts observed before and after the introduction of a vaccination programme. The data discussed in Boxes 10.4 and 10.5 are interrupted time series.

When patterns are present in the pre-vaccination era, for example epidemic or seasonal cycles or secular trends, more advanced statistical modelling approaches for before-and-after data are needed than those described in Section 10.3. These techniques involve explicitly modelling the counterfactual, that is, the state of nature that would have occurred had the vaccination programme not been introduced.

This approach involves fitting a trend function to data on the incidence of infection or disease before the introduction of vaccination, and then extrapolating that trend over the periods during and after which the vaccination programme is introduced. This extrapolation seeks to capture the counterfactual, by representing the course of the infection that would have been observed had the vaccination programme not been introduced.

Provided the extrapolation is valid, the difference between the numbers of cases observed after the vaccination programme has been introduced, and the numbers expected under the extrapolated counterfactual, aggregated since the beginning of the vaccination programme, provides an estimate of the numbers of cases averted by the vaccination programme. An example is described in Box 10.7.

Box 10.7 Impact of vaccination on diphtheria and poliomyelitis in the Netherlands

In this study, data on numbers of notifications of several infectious diseases were used to calculate the impact of vaccination programmes in the Netherlands, expressed in terms of the the total number of notifications prevented (van Wijhe et al., 2018). Data predating the introduction of vaccination were used to model the underlying trends, taking into account the effects of seasonality, epidemic cycles, secular trends and correlations between successive monthly counts, using a Poisson regression model. These trends were then extrapolated.

The data for diphtheria and poliomyelitis, and the extropolated values derived for the vaccination era, are shown in Figure 10.5.

The authors estimate that between the introduction of the diphtheria vaccination programme in January 1953 and December 1965, the number of notified cases of diphtheria averted was 18,900 with 95% confidence interval (CI) from 12,000 to 28,600. For poliomyelitis, the number of notified cases averted between the introduction of the polio vaccination programme in July 1957 and June 1970 was 5,000, with 95% CI from 2,200 to 13,500.

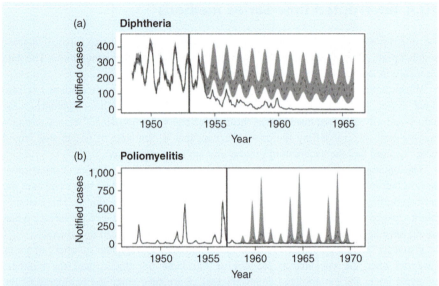

Figure 10.5 Notified cases of diphtheria and polio in the Netherlands by year. The full lines represent the observed monthly counts of notified cases.

Note: The vertical lines denote the introduction of vaccination. The shaded grey areas represent ranges of likely counterfactual values, with median values indicated by dashed lines.

Source: Reproduced with permission from van Wijhe et al. (2018).

Some applications of interrupted time series in epidemiology involve fitting a separate model to the post-vaccination time series, and contrasting the pre- and post-vaccination models (Lopez Bernal, Cummins, & Gasparrini, 2017). In the case of vaccine-preventable infectious diseases, accurate modelling of long time series post-vaccination is likely to be challenging in view of the range of possible impacts. Thus, we recommend using the observed post-vaccination data minus expected values (i.e., values extrapolated from the pre-vaccination model) to quantify the total cases averted as in Box 10.7.

This modelling approach relies on three requirements. The first is the availability of reliable historical data on the pre-vaccination era. Such data are often not available in mid- and low-income countries. Efforts such as project Tycho (www.tycho.pitt.edu/) aim to address this gap. The second is the application of suitable statistical modelling techniques to represent the pre-vaccination data. Some of the statistical issues are discussed in Mealing, Hayen, and Newall (2016). A wide range of statistical techniques may be used, which lie outside the scope of this book. The third requirement is that the extrapolation should validly represent the counterfactual.

For single data series, such as those presented in Box 10.7, the validity of the extrapolated counterfactual is unknowable even once obvious sources of bias have been ruled out, these including, for example, the accuracy of the data, the specificity of the case definitions used and changes in diagnostic procedures over time. Some reassurance that the modelling strategy adopted has good predictive performance may be obtained by splitting the historical data into training and test sets to verify that observed pre-vaccination trends can be reproduced in this way. However, this would require substantial amounts of historical data.

In some circumstances, inferences may be strengthened using negative control data, as described in Section 10.3. The control data are incorporated in the analysis so as to provide a benchmark against which changes in the time series of primary interest are assessed. So, for example, if the primary time series and the control series experience the same relative changes before and after the introduction of the vaccination programme, the net impact is nil. An example is given in Box 10.8.

Box 10.8 Impact of rotavirus vaccination in Kenya

Monovalent rotavirus vaccination was introduced in Kenya in 2014, with two doses at 6 and 10 weeks; there was no catch-up campaign. An interrupted time-series study was undertaken in two surveillance sites to evaluate the impact of the vaccination programme on rotavirus-associated hospitalisations and on all-cause diarrhoea (Otieno et al., 2019).

Monthly data on hospitalisations of children under the age of 5 years for the period 2010–2017 were used. Rotavirus-negative diarrhoea hospitalisations acted as the control series for the analysis of rotavirus-associated hospitalisations; non-diarrhoea hospitalisations acted as controls for the analysis of all-cause diarrhoea. Since vaccine coverage varied after the introduction of vaccination in July 2014, separate relative impact estimates were obtained for the first, second and third year post-introduction. A log-linear model was used, with the control data as offset (this provides the required benchmark), and relevant covariates including month of the year.

Similar impacts were observed in the two centres studied. In the Kilifi centre, the percentage reduction in rotavirus-associated hospitalisations was 57% in year 1, 80% in year 2 and 76% in year 3. For all-cause diarrhoea, the percentage reductions were 41% in year 1, 48% in year 2 and 46% in year 3. The confidence intervals indicated that these declines were highly statistically significant.

The authors calculate that an 80% relative impact equates to 8,000 rotavirus-related hospitalisations prevented per year in Kenyan children under 5 years of age.

An important assumption in controlled interrupted time-series analyses, including that of Box 10.8, is that the control series reflects the counterfactual trend in the primary series that would have been observed had the vaccination programme not been introduced. Thus, the method relies strongly on an appropriate choice of control series.

For targeted vaccination programmes, control may be achieved with the same infection in groups not targeted by the vaccination programme, provided indirect effects can be discounted (since otherwise the full impact of the vaccine will not be measured). An example of such a controlled interrupted time-series analysis is described in Box 10.9.

Box 10.9 Impact of herpes zoster vaccination in the United Kingdom

Vaccination against herpes zoster (shingles) was introduced in the United Kingdom in 2013, targeted at individuals aged 70 years, along with a catch-up programme aimed at some older individuals. A study was undertaken to evaluate the impact of the first 3 years (2014–2016) of the vaccination programme in England (Amirthalingam et al., 2018).

The data comprise cohorts of individuals aged 60 to 89 years, stratified by age on 1 September 2013, observed between 2005 and 2016. The cohorts that become eligible for vaccination at some point are interrupted time series; the cohorts that were never eligible for vaccination act as control cohorts.

The data were obtained from sentinel GP practices. The denominator data consisted of monthly numbers of registered patients stratified by age, time, gender and GP; the numerators were aggregate numbers of consultations for herpes zoster and postherpetic neuralgia, classified according to the same strata. Poisson modelling was used to analyse the data. The impact analysis was based on more than 3.35 million person-years of data.

It was estimated that the vaccination programme reduced herpes zoster incidence by 35% in persons eligible for routine vaccination, and postherpetic neuralgia by 50%. This translates to 17,000 fewer episodes of herpes zoster and 3,300 fewer episodes of postherpetic neuralgia among the 5.5 million people targeted by the vaccination programme in its first 3 years. These impacts were achieved with vaccination coverage in the range 46%–70% within the eligible cohorts.

The example in Box 10.9 is unusual in that vaccination against varicella zoster does not induce indirect effects. Thus, the control infection can be the same as the infection of interest, but restricted to cohorts not eligible for vaccination. The conditions for a control infection set out in Section 10.3 are still satisfied. Therefore, in this case the impact of the programme may still be estimated. Had there been indirect effects, a separation of vaccinated and unvaccinated populations (or the use of different controls) would have been required to assess impact.

In the example described in Box 10.9, the interrupted time-series analysis is well controlled and provides powerful evidence of impact. Further information on the use of controlled interrupted time series in epidemiology may be found in Lopez Bernal, Cummins, and Gasparrini (2018).

10.5 Regression discontinuity designs

Regression discontinuity designs (RDDs) are quasi-experimental designs that may be applicable to evaluate limited aspects of the impact of vaccination programmes involving an eligibility cut-off measured on a variable called the assignment variable. Such a cut-off may be defined in terms of age or time and may arise when the vaccination programme is introduced. Thus, the cut-off may be used to define two groups of individuals on either side of it, one comprising individuals eligible for vaccination and the other comprising individuals who are not eligible for vaccination. The RDD design estimates the impact of the vaccination programme in eligible individuals at the cut-off. It thus depends on vaccine coverage within the eligible cohort.

For example, consider a vaccination programme targeted at children under 14 years of age (this example is based on that of Box 10.11). The incidences in non-eligible 14-year-olds and in eligible 13-year-olds are used to estimate the difference between the two groups when the vaccine is first introduced.

Provided the choice of cut-off on the assignment variable is arbitrary in terms of disease transmission (so, for example, it does not coincide with a sudden change in transmission rates), then allocation to the eligible or non-eligible groups is uninformative about the probability of infection. The RDD design thus, in principle, replicates this feature of random allocation.

The difference in disease incidences at the cut-off provides an unbiased estimate of the impact of the vaccination programme in individuals eligible for vaccination (irrespective of whether they have actually been vaccinated) compared to those who are ineligible within the same population. However, this is just the impact at one point in time: at this point, all individuals experience the same indirect effects of vaccination, should any exist. Thus, the comparison can only provide information on impact resulting from the direct effects of vaccination, and only does so at one point in time. The method is not appropriate for estimating the full impact of vaccination over longer time periods.

Box 10.10 provides a little more detail about the technicalities of the method.

Box 10.10 The RDD for estimating impact at cut-off

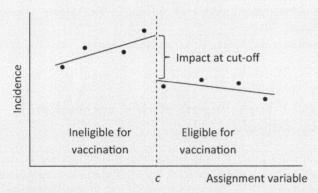

Figure 10.6 RDD design.

Note: The value c is the cut-off value on the assignment variable. The dots represent observed incidences close to the cut-off for the two groups (eligible and ineligible for vaccination), with regression lines. The effect measured is the level change between the two lines at the cut-off.

Figure 10.6 shows a schematic representation of the RDD as applied to vaccination.

As illustrated in Figure 10.6, interest focuses exclusively on the change in level at the cut-off; the regression lines (or curves) fitted to the data on either side of the cut-off aim simply to improve the estimation of this change in level. The regression or linear predictor is typically of the form:

$$E(y) = \beta_0 + \beta_1(x-c) + \beta_2 I(x>c) + \beta_3(x-c)I(x>c)$$

where x is the assignment variable and $I(x>c)$ takes the value 1 when $x>c$ and 0 otherwise. The parameter β_2 then represents the change in level at the cut-off.

The key assumption for the RDD method is that the incidence of infection is continuous at the cut-off, which must therefore not coincide with a sudden change in factors associated with infection transmission or disease. The effect estimated is the difference in incidences (absolute or relative). This measures the impact of the vaccination programme in persons eligible for vaccination, whether or not they have been vaccinated.

Under stronger assumptions, the direct effect of vaccination in vaccinees (as opposed to impact in eligible individuals) may also obtained. This is achieved by scaling the difference in incidences at the cut-off by the difference in vaccine uptake at the cut-off.

A key feature of the RDD, which distinguishes it from an interrupted time series, is that the impact of the vaccination programme is estimated at the cut-off exclusively. The time series on either side of the cut-off are used solely to improve the estimation at the cut-off; typically, only a narrow data window is used. The impact measure estimated in a RDD will therefore typically be a difference in incidence, or a relative difference in incidence, rather than a number of cases averted. Further details of the method, its assumptions and statistical aspects may be found in Bor, Moscoe, Mutevedzi, Newell, and Barnighausen (2014).

An application of the RDD to HPV vaccine in Canada is described in Box 10.11.

Box 10.11 Early impact of HPV vaccination in Ontario, Canada

The Province of Ontario, Canada, began offering HPV vaccination free of charge to all grade 8 girls in September 2007. An RDD was used to estimate the impact of this vaccination programme on the incidence of cervical dysplasia (Smith et al., 2015).

The data for the study were extracted from administrative databases. Two cohorts were defined: girls eligible for HPV vaccine, who were in grade 8 in 2007/2008 and 2008/2009; and girls not eligible for HPV vaccine, who were in grade 8 in 2005/2006 and 2006/2007. As school grade was not available, date of birth was used as a proxy. Thus, in this RDD, date of birth is the assignment variable, with cut-off date at midnight on 31 December 1993. Incident cases of cervical dysplasia in these two cohorts was ascertained at grades 10–12.

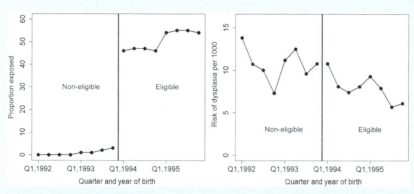

Figure 10.7 Proportions fully vaccinated by quarter and year of birth and the risks of cervical dysplasia.

Note: Left: proportions having received three doses of HPV vaccine, by quarter and year of birth. Right: risks of cervical dysplasia per 1,000, by quarter and year of birth. The vertical lines mark the eligibility cut-off.

The proportions fully vaccinated by quarter and year of birth and the risks of cervical dysplasia, on either side of the cut-off, are shown in Figure 10.7.

The panel on the left on Figure 10.7 shows that very few non-eligible women were vaccinated. In the eligible cohort the vaccine coverage was around 50%. The change in level for the risk of dysplasia (shown in the right panel of Figure 10.7) at the cut-off was estimated using a regression model with an adjustment for birth quarter. The impact of the vaccination programme on cervical dysplasia was estimated to be a risk reduction of −2.32 per 1,000, with 95% CI (−4.61, −0.61) and therefore statistically significant; the corresponding relative risk reduction was 21%.

The authors also estimated the direct effect of vaccination in vaccinees, by scaling the risk reduction by the difference in vaccine uptake at the cut-off. The risk reduction was then −5.70 per 1,000, with 95% CI (−9.91, −1.50), which translates to a relative risk reduction of 44%.

It is particularly important when reporting RDD analyses to provide graphical presentations of the data at the cut-off, as in Figure 10.7 of Box 10.11. Note also that the RDD design is not immune from bias resulting from factors that may differentially affect eligible and ineligible groups. Other applications of RDD to vaccination programmes are discussed in Basta and Halloran (2019).

10.6 Monitoring elimination

All the methods so far described for evaluating the impact of a vaccination programme have been based on calculations of incidences. When the infection has been eliminated in a given population, there is no sustained transmission of infection. Infections do still occur, resulting from limited spread from imported cases, but the incidence of infection may be of little help in monitoring the vaccination programme. Instead, more detailed analyses of the pattern of infections are needed, in order to monitor any changes and ensure that the elimination state is maintained.

The elimination state is characterised by the fact that the effective reproduction number of the infection, R, in the presence of the vaccination programme, is less than 1. Thus, the introduction of a single infectious individual in this population will lead to direct spread to R secondary cases on average, R^2 cases on average at the next generation, then R^3 and so on. Summing this geometric series $1 + R + R^2 + R^3 + \cdots = (1-R)^{-1}$ gives the total number of cases generated by a single infectious imported case. Thus, the proportion of imported cases P is related to R by the equation $R = 1 - P$, and so R may be estimated as one minus the proportion of imported cases.

This method requires intensive investigation of cases so as to identify their origin. Alternatively, more sophisticated statistical methods can be used to estimate R based on the size or duration of outbreaks, and also to evaluate the probability that $R > 1$ (this latter analysis being undertaken in a Bayesian statistical setting). These outbreak surveillance methods are described in De Serres, Gay, and Farrington (2000), with statistical details in Farrington, Kanaan, and Gay (2003). An example is described in Box 10.12.

Box 10.12 Measles surveillance post-elimination in the United States in the 1990s

In the mid-1990s, the annual numbers of cases of measles in the United States had dropped to a few hundred, suggesting that the elimination state had been achieved. If so, how far below 1 was the effective reproduction number?

In 1995–1997, there were 318 cases of measles reported in the United States, of which 16.5% were imported (De Serres et al., 2000). The corresponding estimate of the effective reproduction number is

$$R = 1 - 0.165 = 0.835.$$

Single cases without any secondary spread are likely to be unreported. However, the methods can be adapted to handle data on outbreaks of minimum size or generations of spread. In 1997–1999 there were 41 outbreaks in the United States comprising at least 2 cases, each originating from a single case, with a total 207 cases (Farrington et al., 2003). The distribution of outbreak sizes is in Figure 10.8.

The largest of these outbreaks had 33 cases. Based on these data, the effective reproduction is estimated to be $R = 0.66$ with 95% CI (0.55, 0.78).

Also available were data on the duration of the outbreaks, which ranged from 9 to 100 days; data on outbreak durations may be less sensitive to unreported cases. Using a serial interval distribution with mean 11 days (the time interval between cases in successive generations), the effective reproduction number was estimated to be $R = 0.53$ with 95% CI (0.40, 0.68).

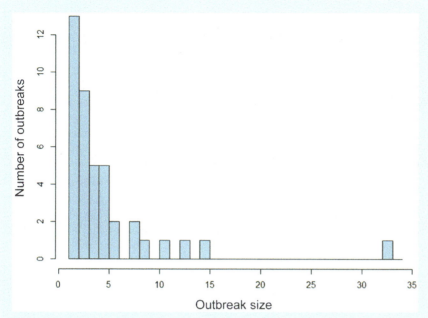

Figure 10.8 Distribution of outbreak sizes of 41 outbreaks with at least two cases.

Further analyses in a Bayesian statistical setting showed that, for analyses based on outbreak size or duration, the probability that $R > 1$ was negligible. Calculations such as this are particularly useful for monitoring whether the elimination state is being maintained. For example, additional measures might be indicated if the probability $P(R > 1)$ were to exceed a certain threshold.

These analyses suggest that measles was well controlled at this time in the United States, the effective reproduction number being well below 1, thus ensuring that elimination was maintained.

The methods described in Box 10.12 are based on surveillance of outbreaks and rely on information on the proportion of imported cases, the distribution of outbreak sizes or the distribution of outbreak durations. Such information can be obtained using traditional surveillance methods.

More recently, as described in Section 8.3, whole-genome sequencing of infective organisms has been introduced and has proved invaluable to identify circulating strains, establish epidemiological links between cases and assess the potential for sustained transmission. Genomic surveillance data has played a key role in determining which countries have achieved World Health Organization (WHO) elimination status, as illustrated in Box 10.13.

Box 10.13 WHO measles elimination status in the United Kingdom

The WHO defines measles elimination as the absence of circulating measles, in the presence of high vaccine coverage, with good surveillance systems to identify cases of the disease. The United Kingdom first achieved WHO measles elimination status in 2017, based on data from 2014–2016.

However, in 2018 there was a substantial increase in the numbers of confirmed measles cases: 991 confirmed cases in England and Wales compared with 284 cases in 2017. Measles, mumps and rubella (MMR) vaccine coverage at 5 years of age was 95.1% for the first dose but only 87.4% for the second dose, below the WHO target of 95%.

The same strain of measles, called B3 Dublin, was detected by gene sequencing for more than 12 months in the United Kingdom across 2017 and 2018. In consequence, on 19 August 2019, WHO concluded that measles transmission had been re-established, and that measles could no longer be considered to have been eliminated in the United Kingdom.

Following the loss of the UK elimination status, renewed emphasis was placed on increasing vaccination coverage above the recommended 95% level. Evidence suggested that improving access to local health services was the key to maintaining high vaccination coverage.

Summary

- The impact of a vaccination programme on a population results from the totality of its direct and indirect effects, as compared to the counterfactual population without the programme.
- Impact on disease burden may be assessed by the number of cases prevented or the reduction in the incidence. Graphical representations of impact are particularly informative.
- Impact may be assessed using contemporaneous comparisons (in different locations) or in before-and-after studies. In the latter, control infections may be used to strengthen inferences.
- Statistical techniques for assessing impact include interrupted time series and RDDs. The latter can only be used to evaluate the impact of a vaccination programme resulting from direct effects of vaccination.
- Special methods may be used to monitor vaccination programmes that have achieved local elimination of the infection, based on proportions of imported cases, outbreak sizes or durations. Genomic analysis of circulating strains is an invaluable tool in this regard.

References

Adegbola, R. A., Secka, O., Lahai, G., Lloyd-Evans, N., Nije, A., Usen, S., ... Milligan, P. J. (2005). Elimination of *Haemophilus influenzae* type b (Hib) disease from the Gambia after the introduction of routine immunisation with a Hib conjugate vaccine: A prospective study. *Lancet, 366*, 144–150.

Amirthalingam, G., Andrews, N., Keel, P., Mullett, D., Correa, A., de Lusignan, S., & Ramsay, M. (2018). Evaluation of the effect of the herpes zoster vaccination programme 3 years after its introduction in England: A population-based study. *Lancet Public Health, 3*, e82–e90.

Azman, A. S., Rumunu, J., Abubakar, A., West, H., Ciglenecki, I., Helderman, T., ... Luquero, F. J. (2016). Population-level effect of cholera vaccine on displaced populations, South Sudan, 2014. *Emerging Infectious Diseases, 22*(6), 1067–1070.

Basta, N. E., & Halloran, M. E. (2019). Evaluating the effectiveness of vaccines by regression discontinuity design. *American Journal of Epidemiology, 188*(6), 987–990.

Bor, J., Moscoe, E., Mutevedzi, P., Newell, M. -L., & Barnighausen, T. (2014). Regression discontinuity designs in epidemiology. *Epidemiology, 25*(5), 729–737.

De Serres, G., Gay, N. J., & Farrington, C. P. (2000). Epidemiology of transmissible diseases after elimination. *American Journal of Epidemiology, 151*(11), 1039–1048.

Farrington, C. P., Kanaan, M. N., & Gay, N. J. (2003). Branching process models for surveillance of infectious diseases controlled by mass vaccination. *Biostatistics, 4*(2), 279–295.

Gessner, B. D., & Feikin, D. R. (2014). Vaccine-preventable disease incidence as a complement to vaccine efficacy for setting vaccine policy. *Vaccine, 26*, 3133–3138.

Hanquet, G., Valenciano, M., Simondon, F., & Moren, A. (2013). Vaccine effects and impact of vaccination programmes in post-licensure studies. *Vaccine, 31*, 5634–5642.

Lipsitch, M., Tchetgen Tchetgen, E., & Cohen, T. (2010). Negative controls: A tool for detecting confounding bias in observational studies. *Epidemiology, 21*(3), 383–388.

Lopez Bernal, J. A., Andrews, N., & Amirthalingam, G. (2019). The use of quasi-experimental designs for vaccine evaluation. *Clinical Infectious Diseases, 68*(10), 1769–1776.

Lopez Bernal, J., Cummins, S., & Gasparrini, A. (2017). Interrupted time series regression for the evaluation of public health interventions: A tutorial. *International Journal of Epidemiology, 46*(1), 348–355.

Lopez Bernal, J., Cummins, S., & Gasparrini, A. (2018). The use of controls in interrupted time series of public health interventions. *International Journal of Epidemiology, 47*(6), 2082–2093.

Mealing, N., Hayen, A., & Newall, A. T. (2016). Assessing the impact of vaccination programmes on burden of disease: Underlying complexities and statistical methods. *Vaccine, 34*(27), 3022–3029.

Otieno, G. P., Bottomley, C., Khagayi, S., Adetifa, I., Ngama, M., Omore, R., ... Nokes, D. J. (2019). Impact of the introduction of rotavirus vaccine on hospital admissions for diarrhoea among children in Kenya: A controlled interrupted time series analysis. *Clinical Infectious Diseases, 70*(1), 2306–2313.

Pebody, R. G., Green, H. K., Andrews, N., Boddington, N. L., Zhao, H., Yonova, I., ... Zambon, M. (2015). Uptake and impact of vaccinating school age children against influenza during a season with circulation of drifted influenza A and B strains, England, 2014/15. *Eurosurveillance, 20*(39). https://doi.org/10.2807/1560-7917.es.2015.20.39.30029.

Smith, L. M., Strumpf, E. C., Kaufman, J. S., Lofters, A., Schwandt, M., & Levesque, L. E. (2015). The early benefits of human papillomavirus vaccination on cervical dysplasia and anogenital warts. *Pediatrics, 135*(5), e1131–e1140.

Steben, M., Ouhoummane, N., Rodier, C., Sinyavskaya, L., & Brassard, P. (2018). The early impact of human papillomavirus vaccination on anogenital warts in Quebec, Canada. *Journal of Medical Virology, 90*, 592–598.

van Wijhe, M., Tulen, A. D., Korthals Altes, H., McDonald, S. A., de Melker, H. E., Postma, M. J., & Wallinga, J. (2018). Quantifying the impact of mass vaccination programmes on notified cases in the Netherlands. *Epidemiology and Infection, 146*, 716–722.

Chapter 11

Outbreak investigation of vaccine-preventable diseases

From the perspective of monitoring vaccination programmes, outbreaks of vaccine-preventable diseases targeted by such a programme are usually worth investigating, since they point towards potential failures or weaknesses of the programme, and the investigation can provide valuable evidence on how to address these. In addition, outbreaks may allow more fundamental study of the effects of vaccination, immunity, the pathogen, its transmission and the epidemiological and microbiological characteristics of the infection.

In this chapter we discuss the aims and methods of vaccine-preventable disease outbreak investigations, with a focus on obtaining evidence relevant for the evaluation and improvement of vaccination programmes. This excludes investigations where the evidence is primarily needed for non-vaccine interventions, for example to identify contaminated food products in hepatitis A outbreaks.

Sometimes, a distinction is made between the terms 'outbreak' and 'epidemic' (Porta, 2014). In this book we use these terms interchangeably, indicating a situation where the occurrence of cases of a disease is in excess of normal expectation. This definition implies that to declare an outbreak, one needs to have (some) information on the background incidence of the disease.

We start by outlining the main three causes of vaccine-preventable disease outbreaks in the context of a universal vaccination programme. We then describe the aims of vaccine-preventable disease outbreak investigations. Lastly, we go through the '10 steps of an outbreak investigation', a systematic approach for epidemiological outbreak investigations. We discuss each step with a focus on those aspects particularly relevant for vaccine-preventable disease outbreaks. Microbiological and environmental aspects are touched upon, but a detailed description falls outside the scope of this book. General methods for epidemiological outbreak investigation can be found in Giesecke (2017).

To make sure the results of outbreak investigations can contribute to vaccine policy, investigators need to be aware of previous and past vaccine policy, and how vaccine

DOI: 10.4324/9781315166414-12
This Chapter has been made available under a CC-BY-NC-ND license.

policy is set. This differs between countries and sometimes even between districts within a country. A brief and general overview of this can be found in Chapter 3. At the end of the current chapter, we address outbreak reports and recommendations based on outbreak investigations.

11.1 The three principal causes of vaccine-preventable disease outbreaks

Outbreaks of infections targeted by a universal vaccination programme have three principal causes: inadequate uptake of the vaccine in individuals eligible for vaccination (also referred to as failure to vaccinate), inadequate effectiveness of the vaccine (also referred to as vaccine failure) and susceptibility among individuals not targeted by the programme who have hitherto missed out on natural infection (Figure 11.1).

In most outbreaks all three causes are likely to be present to a certain extent. It is important to study which of them contributed most to the outbreak, since this will guide further investigations, control and prevention of future outbreaks and vaccine policy. In the context of one or more of these causes being present, the outbreak will only start when the infectious pathogen reaches the susceptible population. The actual timing of this is a chance event. In what follows we will discuss the three principal causes of outbreaks of vaccine-preventable diseases in the context of mass vaccination programmes.

11.2 Outbreaks due to failure to vaccinate

Failure to vaccinate indicates a situation where an individual has been targeted for vaccination but did not receive the vaccine. This can be due to three main issues: (1) a lack of availability of the vaccine, (2) problems with the health system infrastructure

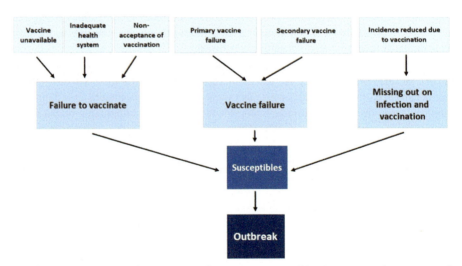

Figure 11.1 Causes of outbreaks of vaccine-preventable diseases in the context of a vaccination programme.

to deliver it or (3) a lack of acceptance of the vaccine by the target population. The first two issues can be due to lack of resources, mismanagement or to inequity in the health system. The third issue, non-acceptance of vaccination, can be related to a many different causes including social, political or cultural factors, religious and philosophical objections and concerns about vaccine safety (see Chapter 6).

Failure to vaccinate can result in an outbreak when the proportion of the population that is immune has fallen below a certain threshold. The risk of outbreaks due to failure to vaccinate increases with the degree of socio-geographic clustering of unvaccinated individuals, and with the frequency and intensity of contacts between them (see Chapter 4).

In weak health systems, routine vaccination programmes are often inadequately implemented and/or disrupted due to a range of problems including ineffective (preventive) healthcare management, lack of funding and lack of staff. Vaccination being a low priority among parents may compound the effects of this. This results in inadequate vaccine coverage in the target population, which is then prone to outbreaks. An example of an outbreak related to these factors is provided in Box 11.1.

Box 11.1 A large measles outbreak in Pakistan

Pakistan introduced measles vaccination in 1974 with a single dose at the age of 9 months. In 2009 a second dose of measles vaccine at age 15 months was included in the routine vaccination schedule. Despite supplementary immunisation activities (SIAs), measles vaccine coverage remains low with wide variation

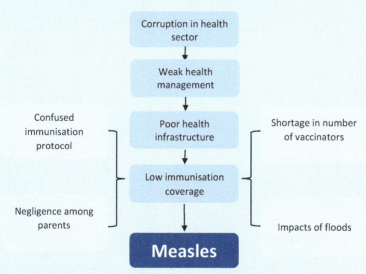

Figure 11.2 Schematic representation of causes of measles outbreaks.
Source: Adapted from Khan (2014).

between districts. In 2012, the reported coverage was 65% for the first dose and 32% for the second dose. This inadequate coverage in combination with extensive flooding and population movements resulted in a large measles outbreak in 2012–2014, with nearly 41,000 cases reported in 2013 (Mere et al., 2019). Khan (2014) summarised causes of the low vaccination coverage in Pakistan contributing to the outbreak (Figure 11.2). In 2017–2018, another outbreak occurred, with over 33,000 cases in 2018 (Mere et al., 2019).

Unfortunately, outbreaks due to the factors as described in Box 11.1 are common in many low- and middle-income countries. Measles is one of the first pathogens to cause outbreaks when routine vaccination coverage is inadequate, since due to its high transmissibility the coverage needed to control it is high (see Chapter 4). Box 11.2 includes an example of an outbreak of another vaccine-preventable disease caused by failure to vaccinate.

Box 11.2 Diphtheria outbreaks in newly independent states of the former Soviet Union in the 1990s

Diphtheria is caused by toxigenic strains of *Corynebacterium diphtheriae* or *Corynebacterium ulcerans*. It is an acute infectious disease of the upper respiratory tract and sometimes the skin. Diphtheria toxin can lead to paralysis and cardiac failure.

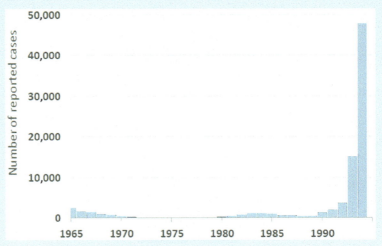

Figure 11.3 Number of reported diphtheria cases by year, (former) Soviet Union, 1965–1995.
Source: Adapted from Hardy et al. (1996).

Since the late 1950s, universal infant diphtheria vaccination programmes successfully controlled diphtheria in the former Soviet Union for several decades, as in most Western countries. This was possible since in populations with high diphtheria vaccine coverage, toxigenic strains of the bacteria causing diphtheria lose their selective advantage and disappear.

Since 1990, the number of cases of diphtheria increased exponentially in the Soviet Union (Figure 11.3), coinciding with the process of its dissolution. The outbreak included nearly 50,000 reported cases by 1995, with observed case fatality ranging from 3% to 28% between states, mainly depending on the sensitivity of the surveillance system to include all cases. The majority of reported cases (70%) were in adults.

Factors contributing to the outbreak included reduced childhood vaccination coverage (due to disruptions of vaccine supply), mass population movement, socio-economic instability, a deteriorating health infrastructure and lack of mass vaccination to control the outbreak. All of these were directly related to the political and social instability of the country during its transition into newly independent states (Hardy, Dittmann, & Sutter, 1996).

Even though the relative importance of these determinants may differ, they continue to lead to diphtheria outbreaks more recently, for example in Venezuela and in refugee populations such as the Rohingya in Bangladesh (Finger et al., 2019; Paniz-Mondolfi et al., 2019).

Outbreaks due to failure to vaccinate that are related to non-acceptance of the vaccine among the target population can be related to a wide variety of factors. An example of an outbreak where religion was a key factor is provided in Box 11.3.

Box 11.3 A rubella outbreak due to failure to vaccinate

In the Netherlands, about 40% of the members of the Dutch Orthodox Reformed Church (a minority religion in the Netherlands) refrain from vaccination based on their religious beliefs. These communities are socially and geographically clustered in the so-called bible belt (most of the dark shaded areas in Figure 11.4a). In 2004–2005, a large outbreak of rubella occurred in this population (Figure 11.4b). Of 398 reported cases, 98% were unvaccinated. The outbreak resulted in 14 infants born with congenital rubella virus infection. The rubella outbreak spread to a similar community in Canada with historic ties to the Dutch Orthodox Reformed communities, resulting in 309 reported cases of which 99% were unvaccinated in Canada (Hahné et al., 2009). Since even a single dose of rubella vaccine has long-lasting effectiveness, rubella outbreaks are generally due to failure to vaccinate rather than vaccine failure.

200 MONITORING VACCINATION PROGRAMMES

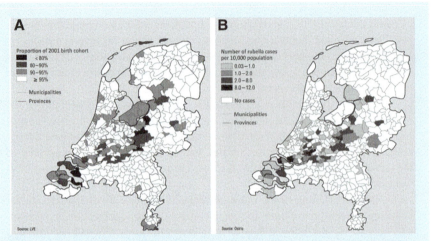

Figure 11.4 (A) Proportion of the 2001 birth cohort who received MMR-1, by municipality, the Netherlands, January 2004; (B) number of notified rubella cases per 100,000 population, by municipality, the Netherlands, 1 September 2004–31 July 2005.
Source: Adapted from Hahné et al. (2009).

An important public health aim of epidemiological investigations of outbreaks due to failure to vaccinate is to document the burden of disease and death. When the failure to vaccinate is related to complex political and health system factors (such as the examples in Boxes 11.1 and 11.2), health service and socio-political investigations may be used to disentangle its root causes. In humanitarian emergencies, a first step is to perform a risk assessment to inform prioritisation of vaccination (WHO, 2017).

When the failure to vaccinate is due to resistance by the target population, it is important to disentangle whether there is genuine resistance to vaccination or whether health system-related factors such as limited access, inadequate health infrastructure (including lack of training of healthcare workers) or political factors play a role. Box 11.4 presents an example of an outbreak caused by a range of socio-political factors (see also Chapter 6). When there is evidence of vaccine refusal by the target population, further research into concerns and fears about vaccination and determinants of uptake is important, to inform interventions to improve uptake (see Chapter 7 on vaccine coverage).

Box 11.4 A poliomyelitis outbreak in Nigeria caused by a boycott of the vaccine

In 2003, religious and political leaders of three northern Nigerian states (Kano, Zamfara and Kaduna) stated that polio vaccine was contaminated with anti-fertility agents, HIV and agents causing cancer. They decided polio vaccination should be stopped. This led to low coverage and an outbreak of several hundreds of polio cases, with spread of the outbreak to at least seven other countries (Pincock, 2004). After an 11-month boycott, polio vaccination was resumed, after it was declared safe based on tests performed by an Indonesian company.

While some dismissed the boycott as 'religious opposition to vaccination', its context was more complex and multifactorial: increasing polarisation between Muslims and other religions, general limited use of health services in the area, population distrust due to government-led fertility regulation programmes in the 1980s and a general distrust of free vaccination being actively provided in a context where all other healthcare has to be paid for (Jegede, 2007).

Epidemiological studies in this context can contribute by documenting evidence on the extent of the outbreak and its associated burden of disease and death, and by establishing the key factors leading to refusal of the vaccine.

11.3 Outbreaks due to vaccine failure

Outbreaks due to vaccine failure can be due to primary or secondary vaccine failure, or a combination of both. Primary vaccine failure is defined as the occurrence of infection in a person who never responded to the receipt of a dose of vaccine targeted against that infection. Secondary vaccine failure is the occurrence of infection in a person who responded to a vaccine but in whom immunity waned over time (see Chapter 2).

Outbreaks due to vaccine failure are much less common than outbreaks due to failure to vaccinate. When they do occur, both primary and secondary vaccine failure may play a role. It is important to distinguish which of these was the outbreak's main cause, since it determines the public health interventions required to prevent future outbreaks. Outbreaks due to primary vaccine failure may require a different vaccine to be used in the programme, or improving the quality of vaccine storage and delivery. Evidence that the outbreak was mainly due to secondary vaccine failure can also be used to choose a different vaccine for the programme (when available), but mainly to guide changes to the vaccine schedule (timing and number of doses).

An example of an outbreak likely due to an inadequate cold chain causing primary vaccine failure is provided in Box 11.5.

Box 11.5 A measles outbreak in Polynesia due to cold chain problems

In June 2014, a measles outbreak started in Pohnpei State, one of the four states of the Federated States of Micronesia (FSM). This was surprising, as it followed a measles, mumps and rubella (MMR) supplementary immunisation activity (SIA) in 2011 targeting children aged 1–6 years with 96% coverage.

The outbreak included 251 cases with a median age of 24 years, of whom 71% had received one dose of measles containing vaccine (MCV) and 54%

had received at least two doses. In a household study, vaccine effectiveness was estimated separately for MCV doses given prior to and as part of the 2011 SIA. Vaccine effectiveness for pre-SIA doses was estimated in different time periods.

The adjusted vaccine effectiveness for 1 and 2 pre-SIA doses was 23% and 63%, respectively, which is lower than expected. The vaccine effectiveness was much lower for doses administered before 2010 compared to that of doses administered after 2010. This observation could be explained by primary or secondary vaccine failure, but the absence of a decreasing trend in vaccine effectiveness by time since vaccination pointed towards primary vaccine failure as an important determinant of the outbreak (although secondary vaccine failure may have contributed). This was consistent with evidence of suboptimal storage and handling of the vaccine, which was improved in the mid-2000s (Hales et al., 2016).

Box 11.6 provides an example of an outbreak mainly due to secondary vaccine failure.

Box 11.6 A mumps outbreak among vaccinated students in Norway, 2015 to 2016

In Autumn 2015, a cluster of mumps cases was notified among university students in Trondheim, Norway. The outbreak spread to Bergen, with a second peak in the number of infections in early 2016. The median age of cases was

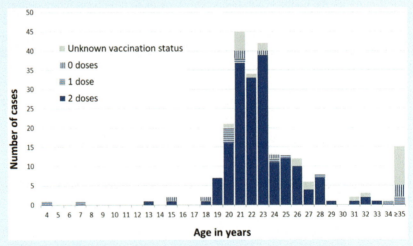

Figure 11.5 Mumps cases by age and MMR vaccination status, Norway, September 2015–May 2016 (n = 231*).

* One person aged 25 years who was vaccinated three times is excluded from the graph.
Source: Adapted with permission from Veneti et al. (2018).

23 years, with the vast majority of cases (185 cases (89%)) having received at least two doses of MMR vaccine prior to the outbreak (see Figure 11.5) (Veneti et al., 2018).

Mumps outbreaks among students have occurred in many countries with long-standing universal mumps vaccination programmes. Waning immunity (in combination with intense social contact) is considered their main cause, based on the large proportion of cases that was vaccinated, serological findings in vaccinated cases and epidemiological studies of vaccine effectiveness over time since vaccination (see Chapter 16). Several studies have found that among cases of mumps, those vaccinated have a lower risk of severe mumps disease and complications than those unvaccinated, a finding that is also consistent with waning immunity playing an important role.

11.4 Outbreaks in birth cohorts having missed infection and vaccination

After implementation of a vaccination programme with reasonable coverage, transmission of infection is reduced. As a result, individuals within birth cohorts not targeted by the programme are likely to escape infection and thus remain susceptible for longer than would otherwise be the case. These susceptible individuals can contribute to outbreaks when they reach an age at which contacts with infectious individuals are more frequent. This type of vaccine-preventable disease outbreak is referred to as a post-honeymoon outbreak (McLean & Anderson, 1988), indicating the occurrence of an outbreak after several years of low incidence (this is the 'honeymoon') subsequent to implementation of a vaccination programme (see Box 11.7, and also Chapter 5). A higher than expected average age of infection suggests this phenomenon may be present. It can be avoided by combining the introduction of routine infant vaccination with a catch-up programme for older birth cohorts.

Box 11.7 Post-honeymoon outbreaks

Figure 11.6 displays schematically the number of cases of a highly transmissible vaccine-preventable disease over time before and after the implementation of a vaccination programme. The time series is characterised by regular epidemics prior to the implementation of the programme, resulting from the accumulation of susceptibles in the population due to births (once maternal antibodies have waned) or immigration. When the proportion of susceptibles exceeds a certain threshold, introduction of the pathogen may start an epidemic (see Chapter 4).

Infant vaccination programmes reduce the rate at which susceptibles enter the population. However, they may also result in pools of susceptible individuals among older, unvaccinated individuals missing out on acquiring natural immunity due to reduction in incidence post-introduction of vaccination. This can arise even

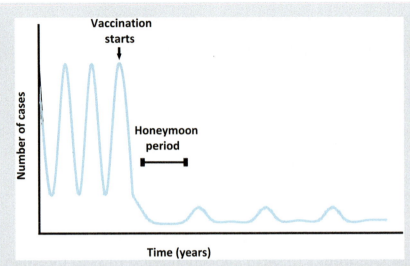

Figure 11.6 Number of cases of a hypothetical vaccine-preventable disease over time, with regular epidemic cycles pre-introduction of a vaccination programme, a 'honeymoon period' and three 'post-honeymoon' epidemics.
Source: Adapted from Chen (1993).

when vaccine coverage is high among the targeted population, and with high vaccine effectiveness. Modelling studies have suggested that this (as well as low coverage or low vaccine effectiveness) can result in the reoccurrence of outbreaks as displayed in Figure 11.6 (Anderson, Crombie, & Grenfell, 1987).

The post-honeymoon period is characterised by smaller epidemics separated by longer inter-epidemic periods and a higher average age of infection compared to the pre-vaccine era. The latter can have implications for the severity and burden of disease (see Chapter 5).

Methods for investigating post-honeymoon outbreaks include descriptive epidemiology to assess changes in the age of cases and analytical epidemiology to assess vaccine effectiveness and the presence of waning immunity (see Chapters 12–16).

11.5 Aims of vaccine-preventable disease outbreak investigations

The primary aim of an outbreak investigation of a vaccine-preventable disease is to understand why the outbreak happened in order to provide evidence to control it and prevent future reoccurrence. Outbreak investigations can help to identify subgroups of the population in which vaccine coverage is low, for example due to socio-economic or cultural reasons (see Box 11.8). Investigations can also reveal loss of potency of the vaccine due to problems with the cold chain or other aspects of the vaccine delivery system (see Box 11.5). Evidence documented by outbreak investigations can hence help to improve programme implementation.

Box 11.8 A measles outbreak in northern Pakistan

The investigation of a measles outbreak in a northern Pakistani village included an assessment of the vaccine coverage among children up to the age of 14 years. This revealed a particularly low coverage (5%) among the Sunni minority living in the village. The first measles cases in the outbreak occurred in this community, and they had an increased risk of measles, even when adjusting for vaccination status. This was likely due to relatively high contact rates between Sunni children. The low vaccine coverage turned out to be related to the limited use of the available health service in the village by the Sunni minority (Murray & Rasmussen, 2000).

Outbreak investigations may also provide evidence to support or improve vaccine policy. Changes to vaccine policy include changing the vaccination schedule (in terms of number and timing of doses), introducing a booster and/or catch-up vaccination for older age groups and recommending efforts to increase uptake or to vaccinate additional target groups (see Chapter 3). Of course, non-vaccine interventions may also be necessary to control vaccine-preventable disease outbreaks, such as recalling hepatitis A contaminated food from shops.

Investigation of outbreaks occurring in the context of high vaccination coverage in the affected population are particularly important, since these outbreaks are likely to reduce trust in the programme. The aim of such investigations is to distinguish which of the three predominant causes of the recurrence of disease prevailed, in order to inform the public and guide outbreak control. Trust in the vaccination programme is especially at stake when a high proportion of cases is vaccinated and, intuitively, vaccine failure seems a likely cause. In this situation it is important to study vaccine effectiveness, which may be adequate if the vaccine coverage in the population is high (see Section 11.6). A rapid evaluation method, called the screening method, is available for this purpose; it is described in Chapter 15.

In addition to these programme-specific aims, it is also usually important to document the burden of disease and death due to the outbreak, since this provides an argument to policy makers to act and aids prioritisation of interventions. Lastly, outbreaks of vaccine-preventable diseases can be considered an opportunity to study the infection, immunity and vaccine effects.

11.6 Steps in the investigation of outbreaks of vaccine-preventable diseases

To achieve its aims rapidly and reliably, an outbreak investigation should take a systematic approach following the steps set out in Box 11.9. Not all of these are always needed: for example, a descriptive analysis of cases is often sufficient to provide evidence to inform vaccine policy. Also, it is important to implement interventions as soon as evidence becomes available to justify them, rather than waiting until all the steps have been executed. Further note that the steps listed in Box 11.9 only include actions relevant to the epidemiological investigation of outbreaks. Steps relevant for outbreak management (such as establishing an outbreak control team) are not included.

> **Box 11.9 The 10 steps of an outbreak investigation**
>
> 1. Establish the presence of an outbreak.
> 2. Identify the pathogen causing the outbreak.
> 3. Agree upon a case definition.
> 4. Find and investigate cases.
> 5. Undertake a descriptive analysis of the cases' characteristics.
> 6. Establish questions that need to be studied and generate hypotheses.
> 7. Perform analytical epidemiological studies to test hypotheses.
> 8. Draw conclusions.
> 9. Prepare an outbreak report.
> 10. Communicate recommendations for interventions to those who need to know.
>
> (Adapted from FEMWiki, not dated)

11.6.1 Step 1: Establish the existence of an outbreak

An outbreak is defined as the occurrence of more cases than expected in a certain population and time period. To determine whether a reported number of cases of a certain disease constitutes an outbreak therefore requires a comparison with baseline surveillance data. According to this definition, a single case of paralytic polio constitutes an outbreak in an area where polio has been eliminated. When establishing the presence of an outbreak, it may already be clear which vaccine-preventable disease is involved. If not, this is established in step 2.

Even though one of the aims of surveillance is to detect outbreaks, in practice many first alerts about outbreaks come from astute health professionals. Prior to declaring an outbreak, alternative explanations for the observed increase in cases need to be ruled out. These might include false-positivity due to contamination, the availability of a new diagnostic method, raised awareness and errors or delays in data management or reporting.

11.6.2 Step 2: Identify the pathogen causing the outbreak

This involves collecting clinical data from some patients involved in the outbreak and testing some of them with microbiological or serological assays. In larger clusters it is sufficient to test a representative sample of cases, since patients with similar symptoms who are epidemiologically linked to a confirmed case are likely to be caused by the same pathogen. Confirmation of the pathogen causing the outbreak is a crucial step, although some of the subsequent steps in the outbreak investigation can proceed without this.

However, outbreak control by a vaccination campaign will require the identification of the pathogen, and delays in this will result in missed opportunities for prevention. This is a major problem especially in low- and middle-income countries, due to a range of factors including limited laboratory capacity. The confirmation of cholera in the outbreak of watery diarrhoea in South Sudan described in Box 11.10 took over a month, in which valuable time for outbreak control through a vaccination campaign was lost. In 2010, severe delays in laboratory testing of stool samples from cases of acute flaccid paralysis led to late confirmation of polio and hence less effective outbreak control in the Republic of Congo (see Box 11.16).

Box 11.10 Delays in laboratory diagnosis of cholera hampering outbreak control

In June 2015, cholera broke out in Juba, the capital of South Sudan, in a context of a civil war and large population movements. Among several types of delay that occurred until outbreak control vaccination started, the culture confirmation of cholera and subsequent declaration of an outbreak was the longest: 34 days (Figure 11.7) (Parker et al., 2017).

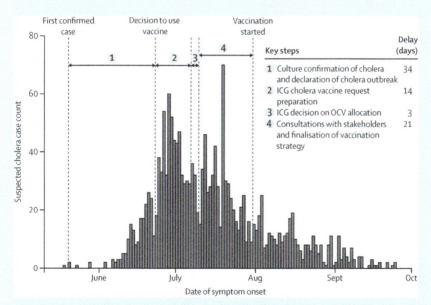

Figure 11.7 Epidemic curve and key time delays in vaccination in Juba, South Sudan, 2015.
Note: Bars represent numbers of suspected cases, defined as all individuals with acute watery diarrhoea regardless of dehydration. ICG: International Coordination Group. OCV: oral cholera vaccine.
Source: Adapted from Parker et al. (2017).

Delays also occur in high-income countries, for example by attributing clinical symptoms to the wrong infection. In these settings, where the incidence of most vaccine-preventable diseases has become low, clinicians are no longer experienced in their diagnosis. This is especially problematic for infections such as rubella that generally cause mild symptoms, which do not warrant diagnostic testing. Furthermore, diagnosing vaccine-preventable diseases in vaccinated individuals can be difficult as clinical symptoms may differ from those in unvaccinated cases. Diagnostic tests to identify infections in vaccinated individuals require appropriate interpretation and may need adaptation. For example, for measles and mumps, the IgM response usually indicating acute infection may be absent in infected individuals who have been vaccinated (see Chapter 2).

Based on the results from steps 1 and 2, the existence of an outbreak can be declared. This is an important trigger for a range of public health actions, including further epidemiological investigations.

11.6.3 Step 3: Agree upon a case definition

Standard case definitions for surveillance of vaccine-preventable diseases may be available in each country (see Chapter 8). These definitions usually have a time, place, person, clinical and microbiological component. For the purpose of an outbreak investigation, they usually need to be adapted to represent the characteristics of outbreak cases (see Box 11.11). This can be difficult, since at the start of the investigation, the scale and characteristics of the outbreak may be unclear. The case definition is usually based on the first individuals presenting with the outbreak disease. As for surveillance purposes, it is often useful to classify cases as confirmed, probable and possible, and vary the subset of cases included in subsequent analyses.

Box 11.11 Examples of case definitions used in vaccine-preventable disease outbreak investigations

Below we provide some example case definitions:

- *Mumps outbreak among students, the Netherlands, 2010* (Greenland et al., 2012): a case was defined as a student with self-reported mumps (swelling of one or both cheeks with symptoms lasting at least 2 days) who was a member of one of four student associations, in Delft, Leiden or Utrecht, with symptom onset after 1 September 2009.
- *Meningococcal W outbreak among Hajj pilgrims in several European countries, 2000* (Aguilera, Perrocheau, Meffre, Hahné, & W135 Working Group, 2002): a confirmed case was defined as invasive disease caused by *Neisseria meningitidis* of serogroup W135 2a P1.2, 5 or belonging to the ET-37 complex. A probable case was defined as illness in a pilgrim or a pilgrim contact, with either invasive disease due to *N. meningitidis* serogroup W135 of unknown serotype or with a clinical diagnosis of invasive meningococcal infection without microbiologic confirmation. Cases included were those

with dates of hospital admission from 18 March 2000, until 31 July 2000 and occurring in Europe.

- *Measles outbreak in a northern Pakistani village, 1990* (Murray & Rasmussen, 2000): a case was a person who had an illness with a generalised rash of 3 or more days' duration, fever and at least one of the following: cough, coryza or conjunctivitis having occurred in the month prior to the survey in the village of Hassis, Pakistan.

11.6.4 Step 4: Find and investigate cases

Case finding can be based on existing surveillance systems, which are usually in place for vaccine-preventable diseases included in a national vaccination programme. Often, however, existing surveillance needs to be enhanced for the purposes of an outbreak investigation. An example of this is the outbreak of meningococcal C disease in men who have sex with men (MSM) in Western countries (Box 11.12). Since MSM were not previously known to be at increased risk of meningococcal disease, the notification form needed to be adapted to document sexual behaviour of cases to allow the identification of cases linked to the outbreak.

Box 11.12 Outbreak of meningococcal serogroup C disease in MSM

In 2001, a rise in incidence of invasive meningococcal disease was detected in Toronto, Canada. Six cases were found to be caused by a unique strain, and all of these were in MSM (Tsang et al., 2003). Since data on sexual preference and practice were not routinely collected during public health investigations of meningococcal disease, the epidemiology of meningococcal disease among MSM, including estimates of baseline incidence, was largely unknown prior to this outbreak. Modification of surveillance and outbreak investigation forms to include information on sexual behaviour of cases allowed the detection of multiple outbreaks of meningococcal serogroup C disease in various cities, including Berlin, Paris and New York.

Especially for relatively mild infections, surveillance systems usually underestimate the true number of cases. Completeness of case finding can be enhanced by actively searching cases among cases' contacts (a procedure known as contact tracing). When the outbreak is confined to a defined population, such as a village or a school, enhanced case finding may be undertaken by administering a questionnaire ascertaining exposures and symptoms to all individuals (or their parents).

To avoid bias in outbreak investigations, case finding needs to result in a set of cases that is representative of all cases in the outbreak. For vaccine-preventable diseases, it is especially important that the likelihood of including cases in the investigation is independent from their vaccination status. This is further discussed in Chapter 13.

Subsequent to finding cases, they need to be investigated. Epidemiological case investigation involves documenting information to characterise cases and their (potential) exposures. This includes demographics, information on vaccination status and clinical information including date of onset and criteria included in the case definition. It is also useful to collect information on severity of disease. Vaccination status information ideally consists of which vaccines were received, the dates of vaccination and lot numbers. The most reliable source of vaccination status information is a vaccine register completed at the time of vaccination. In practice, this is very seldom available, and information must be obtained from patient-held vaccination booklets or recall by patients or parents. Booklets can be biased in that vaccination records may be missing. Recall is the least reliable. It can be biased in many ways, for example towards giving socially desirable answers (such as 'completed vaccination schedule'). Misclassification of vaccination status is a major source of bias in outbreak investigations of vaccine-preventable diseases (see Chapter 13).

There are several ways in which laboratory tests can support the outbreak investigation. Serological testing of cases can help to distinguish primary and secondary vaccine failure (see Chapter 2). Furthermore, it is sometimes possible to validate vaccination status of cases by serological testing, for example for tetanus (as antibodies against tetanus can only be induced by vaccination), for pertussis, for polio (when cases have immunity against all types of poliovirus present in the vaccine, this suggests they are vaccinated) or, similarly, for combined vaccines such as MMR (in a setting where these diseases are rare, immunity against all three infections suggests an MMR vaccination history).

In addition to serology, analyses of the pathogen's genome in vaccine-preventable disease cases can be a powerful tool to characterise the outbreak and its causes. For cases of poliovirus infection, RNA sequence analysis is essential to distinguish whether they are due to wild or vaccine-derived virus (see Chapter 8). Phylogenetic analyses combined with assumptions about the speed at which the genome changes ('the molecular clock'), can provide insight into how long the virus has been circulating in a particular population.

11.6.5 Step 5: Undertake a descriptive analysis of cases

Methods for descriptive epidemiologic analyses in an outbreak investigation are similar to descriptive analyses of surveillance data. They involve grouping cases in time, place, person and pathogen (subtype) (see Chapter 8). Descriptive analyses of the age and the vaccination status of cases provides important clues as to which of the three main causes of vaccine-preventable disease outbreaks prevailed (failure to vaccinate, vaccine failure or susceptibility among older individuals having missed out on infection and vaccination (see Section 11.1)). To assess the presence of the latter cause, cases can be grouped into those eligible and not eligible for vaccination, according to their year of birth.

To assess the presence of failure to vaccinate or vaccine failure, information on the proportion of cases vaccinated needs to be interpreted in the context of information on the vaccine coverage in the population the cases arose from. A high proportion of cases vaccinated can be consistent with adequate vaccine effectiveness when the outbreak is in a highly vaccinated population. When the proportion of cases vaccinated is lower than the vaccine coverage in the population, failure to vaccinate is likely to be an important cause of the outbreak. In contrast, when the proportion of cases vaccinated is similar (or higher) than the vaccine coverage in the population, vaccine failure is a likely cause.

Clustering of cases of vaccine failure by residence or healthcare provider may indicate primary vaccine failure (see Chapter 2) due to errors in vaccine handling, storage or administration in certain localised settings. Clustering of vaccine failures at family level may indicate primary vaccine failure due to a genetic risk factor. The age distribution of cases of vaccine failure may point towards secondary vaccine failure (waning immunity). However, to assess whether secondary vaccine failure contributed or caused an outbreak raises some complex methodological challenges, which are discussed in Chapter 16. Besides epidemiological analyses, laboratory investigations can help to disentangle the presence of primary and secondary vaccine failure (see Chapter 2).

In many instances, descriptive epidemiology is sufficient to provide evidence for vaccine policy, without the need for analytical epidemiologic studies (see Boxes 11.13 and 11.14).

Box 11.13 Descriptive epidemiology of a meningococcal disease outbreak investigation

In 2000 and 2001 a meningococcal serogroup W disease outbreak occurred in several European countries among pilgrims to the Hajj in Mecca. Based on descriptive epidemiology of cases in England and Wales (Figure 11.8), it was clear that the population at risk included mostly pilgrims and contacts of pilgrims, and that there was very limited spread of the outbreak strain in the general population. This provided sufficient evidence that a recommendation for targeted meningococcal serogroup W vaccination of pilgrims would likely be a sufficient intervention to prevent future outbreaks.

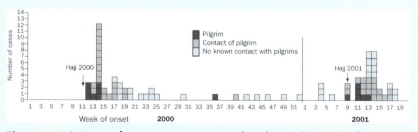

Figure 11.8 Cases of invasive meningococcal W disease by week of onset and pilgrim status, England and Wales, 2000 and 2001 (up to week 19).
Source: Adapted from Hahné, Gray et al. (2002).

Inadequate vaccine coverage among pilgrims to the Hajj in 2001 led to the occurrence of another outbreak (Figure 11.8). Subsequently, quadrivalent meningococcal vaccination (against serogroups A, C, W and Y) was made a Hajj visa requirement, which prevented future meningococcal outbreaks due to these serogroups in this population (Hahné, Gray et al., 2002).

Box 11.14 An outbreak investigation assessing risk factors for failure to vaccinate

During a large measles outbreak in Germany in 2006, 80% of cases were unvaccinated. A questionnaire study among parents of cases collected information on reasons for this (see Table 11.1) (Wichmann et al., 2009).

The most frequently reported reason for non-vaccination was that parents had forgotten to get the child vaccinated, suggesting that reminders, recall and an

Table 11.1 Reasons for not being vaccinated, measles patients (n = 272), Duisburg, Germany, 2006

Reasons for not being vaccinated[a]	Number	%
Parents forgot about the vacination	115	36.4
Parents rejected the vaccination	88	27.8
Afraid of side effects	41	
Generally against vaccinations	38	
Believed measles were not harmful	9	
Family doctor or paediatrician recommended against vaccination	53	16.8
Underlying diseases of the child[b]	19	
Held opinion that 'it is not necessary'	15	
Concerns about side effects	4	
No reasons given	15	
Child was too young for vaccination (<12 months)	41	13.0
Vaccination was not offered by family paediatrician	19	6.0

Source: Adapted from Wichmann et al. (2009).

[a] More than one reason was given by 44. Patients with missing data (n = 33) or who answered 'don't know' (n = 68) were excluded.
[b] In 18 of these 19 cases, the reasons provided were not considered true contraindications by the outbreak investigation team (e.g., eczema, 'often sick'). In one child an immunodefect was considered a true contraindication.

outreach system might improve vaccination coverage. Surprisingly, in a considerable proportion (17%) of cases, parents claimed that a health professional advised against vaccination; a much higher proportion than expected based on true medical contraindications. This suggests education of health professionals may also be required to improve vaccine uptake.

11.6.6 Step 6: Establish detailed questions to be investigated and develop hypotheses

Hypotheses as to why the outbreak occurred in the presence of a vaccination programme are first informed by the descriptive analyses of cases (see step 5 above). In addition, the investigator needs to do background research to obtain historical information about the vaccination programme (including time since implementation, schedules, vaccines used, time series of coverage). Studying the literature on the specific pathogen and vaccine is part of the background research. It is also important to be aware of the procedures for outbreak control and for vaccine policy-making in the setting of the outbreak, so that the investigation is more likely to result in policy-relevant and actionable evidence and it is clear to whom the evidence needs to be presented.

Many different study questions may need answering to inform outbreak control and vaccination policy. Examples relevant to vaccination programmes include assessing the determinants of vaccine uptake (when the outbreak is due to a failure to vaccinate), the type of vaccine failure (when there are indications the vaccine effectiveness is lower than expected), risk factors for vaccine failure and the assessment of vaccine effectiveness (see Chapters 12–16).

In addition to study questions directly related to vaccine policy, the outbreak investigation can also aim to assess parameters relevant to understanding the dynamics of transmission and the severity of the outbreak. Lastly, an outbreak can also provide an opportunity to assess the validity of new diagnostic methods or answer more fundamental questions about, for example, the natural history of disease and sequelae of infection.

From a vaccination programme perspective, the prioritisation of these questions requires a careful assessment of feasibility of obtaining the evidence and its potential to contribute to vaccine policy-making or implementation (see Box 11.15).

This process may eventually lead to the specification of precise hypotheses to be investigated or tested in analytic epidemiological studies.

Box 11.15 Relevant study questions during the meningococcal W outbreak investigation among Hajj pilgrims

The example described in Box 11.13 posed a public health emergency: it was an outbreak of a severe disease against which a safe and effective vaccine was available.

Questions relevant to vaccine policy included:

- *To determine who was at risk of this infection: was transmission occurring in an identifiable risk group or was it spreading in the general population?* This question could be answered by descriptive epidemiology (Hahné, Gray et al., 2002): there were very few outbreak cases in people who did not go to the Hajj and did not have contact with pilgrims. This suggested the outbreak did not spread into the general population, and that targeted vaccination might be effective to control it.
- *To assess the burden of morbidity and mortality: was this outbreak serious enough to warrant changing vaccine policy?* This question could also be answered by descriptive epidemiology (Hahné, Gray et al., 2002). The burden of morbidity and mortality was considerable. Given that a change in vaccine policy was relatively easy from a public health perspective (changing visa vaccination requirements), this burden warranted a change in policy.
- *How to best control the outbreak and prevent it from occurring again in the future?*
  - *Would it be effective to give antibiotics to all returning pilgrims (as was done in France but not the United Kingdom)?* The progression of the outbreak was compared between the United Kingdom and France, but this did not allow drawing any conclusions on the effectiveness of providing antibiotics to all returning pilgrims (Aguilera et al., 2002).
  - *Will the available polysaccharide vaccine provide protection against meningococcal W carriage so that vaccinating pilgrims is sufficient to also protect their contacts back home?* Descriptive epidemiology suggested the vaccine had some effect on carriage: the vaccine coverage among pilgrims who were likely sources for infections in their contacts was much lower (6%) than the estimated coverage in the entire pilgrim population (50%) (Hahné, Handford, & Ramsay, 2002). Large and expensive cohort studies assessing carriage would provide more robust evidence on this.
- *Is there something special about the outbreak strain, or is the relatively high case fatality rate related to host determinants such as age?* This required an analytical study (see step 7). The null hypothesis (that the case fatality rate of the outbreak strain was the same as that of other meningococcal infections) could not be rejected, possibly due to low power of the analyses (Aguilera et al., 2002).

11.6.7 Step 7: Perform analytical epidemiologic studies to test hypotheses

To answer study questions regarding, for example, the contribution of risk factors to the outbreak, and to assess vaccine effectiveness, analytical epidemiological studies are needed. The essential difference with descriptive epidemiology is that usually information from non-cases is required. A range of different methods may be available. The epidemiologic study designs and methods available for analytical outbreak investigations do not differ from any other analytical epidemiological study, and include cohort, case-control, cross-sectional and ecological designs. For this reason, they are not discussed in detail in this book. Further information can be found in Giesecke (2017). Chapters 12–16 provide more detail on analytical studies to assess vaccine effectiveness. An example of an analytical outbreak investigation is provided in Box 11.16.

Box 11.16 A polio outbreak investigation assessing risk factors for dying

A large wild poliomyelitis virus type 1 outbreak occurred in the Republic of Congo in the second half of 2010, with 445 cases reported between September 2010 and January 2011. A high proportion of cases was in adults, consistent with the gaps in population immunity caused by disruptions in vaccination programmes during periods in the past when there was little or no wild-virus circulation. There was a delay of more than 2 months in recognising the outbreak, resulting in late implementation of studies and mass vaccination campaigns (Patriarca, 2012). The case fatality was unusually high (47%) in one particular region (Pointe Noire), even when taking into account the adult age of cases (polio, as some other viral infections, is more severe in adults than in children).

An analytical epidemiological study (a cohort study) was performed to understand determinants of dying from polio (Gregory et al., 2012). A questionnaire was administered to a cohort of 369 polio cases (or, when deceased, someone who could represent them) resulting in 96 cases for whom an interview was available. The major risk factor identified was age greater than 15 years. The authors comment that a delay in eradication of polio is likely to result in more outbreaks of polio in older age groups who are not routinely targeted by polio vaccination campaigns, and in whom the case fatality rate is likely to be high.

11.6.8 Step 8: Interpret the findings and draw conclusions

When interpreting results of epidemiologic investigations, it is important to consider whether chance, bias and/or confounding, or any errors by the investigators, could have contributed to the findings. Depending on the completeness of data collection, additional statistical analyses may be used to assess confounding. When information from a reference population is available, the presence of selection bias may be assessed. The presence of information bias requires an evaluation of the quality of, for example, a questionnaire used. It cannot usually be assessed quantitatively. The interpretation of epidemiological investigation of vaccine-preventable disease outbreaks does not fundamentally differ from other epidemiological studies. Further information may be found in Giesecke (2017) and Rothman, Greenland, and Lash (2020).

To draw conclusions, all epidemiological, microbiological and, where relevant, environmental evidence resulting from investigations of the outbreak is combined with prior knowledge (assembled during the background research described in step 6). These conclusions can be about the cause of the outbreak, limitations of the vaccine or vaccination programme, or non-vaccination-related causes of the outbreak.

11.6.9 Step 9: Prepare an outbreak report

In order to inform outbreak control and/or vaccine policy-making, methods and results of the outbreak investigation need to be documented in an outbreak report. Communication about the outbreak report can be delivered orally or in written form, aiming to reach those who need to know of the results. Prior to starting the report, it is important to consider the main target audience so that the format of the report is tailored to their needs.

In general, vaccine policy and outbreak control are the responsibility of public health authorities. In nationwide outbreaks, or outbreaks spanning several districts, this is usually the Ministry of Health, while in more localised outbreaks it is a local health authority. These authorities sometimes work with advisory bodies collecting evidence on the needs, risks and benefits of outbreak control, including vaccination. If so, outbreak reports should be addressed to these advisory bodies rather than directly to, for example, the Ministry of Health. It is important to liaise with public health authorities and their advisory bodies prior to starting an outbreak investigation report, to understand when, where and how the report can be delivered.

The outbreak investigation report usually includes the following sections: introduction, background, methods, results, discussion and recommendations. It is most efficient to start writing it during the investigation.

In addition to the outbreak investigation report aimed at decision makers as described above, it is often useful to report the findings in a scientific journal to reach a wider audience.

11.6.10 Step 10: Communicate recommendations to those who need to know

People who may be able to benefit from evidence obtained during outbreak investigations include the following groups:

- the general population;
- persons involved in the outbreak;
- population subgroups at increased risk;
- health professionals;
- vaccine policy makers;

- those involved in prioritising public expenditures;
- vaccine manufacturers;
- regulatory authorities;
- scientists;
- students of field epidemiology.

The recommendations need to be couched in a format and communicated in such a way as to maximise the chance that the group they are targeted at will take notice and implement them (see Box 11.17 for an example).

Box 11.17 Public health campaign during mumps outbreak in Canada

In 2007–2008, mumps emerged in Canada among post-secondary students. Alberta Health Services implemented an MMR vaccination programme to provide a second dose of MMR vaccine to at risk students. To aid implementation, sex-specific mumps ads previously employed in Nova Scotia were used. These posters aimed to directly engage students to take responsibility for their own health, by focusing on the social implications of mumps (Stark, 2017).

Summary

- Outbreaks of vaccine-preventable diseases are usually worth investigating, since they may point towards failures or weaknesses within the programme. The investigation can provide evidence how to address them.
- Outbreaks of infections targeted by a universal vaccination programme can have three principal causes: inadequate uptake of the vaccine (failure to vaccinate), problems with the effectiveness of the vaccine (vaccine failure) and susceptibility among those not targeted by the programme who also missed out on infection. Most outbreaks are mainly due to failure to vaccinate, although the other two causes may also be present to some extent.
- The overall aim of a vaccine-preventable disease outbreak investigation is to understand the main cause of the outbreak to provide evidence to control it, prevent reoccurrence and inform vaccine policy and its implementation. Documenting the burden of disease and death is usually important to provide a rationale for action and aid prioritisation.
- Outbreaks may also provide an opportunity for studying more fundamental research questions about the diagnosis, pathogenesis and sequelae of the disease, and about natural immunity.
- The 'ten-steps of an outbreak investigation' describe a systematic approach to outbreak investigation that helps to achieve its aims rapidly and reliably.

References

Aguilera, J. F., Perrocheau, A., Meffre, C., Hahné, S., & W135 Working Group. (2002). Outbreak of serogroup W135 meningococcal disease after the Hajj pilgrimage, Europe, 2000. *Emerging Infectious Diseases*, 8(8), 761–767. doi:10.3201/eid0805.010422.

Anderson, R. M., Crombie, J. A., & Grenfell, B. T. (1987). The epidemiology of mumps in the UK: A preliminary study of virus transmission, herd immunity and the potential impact of immunization. *Epidemiology and Infection*, 99(1), 65–84. Retrieved from www.ncbi.nlm.nih.gov/pubmed/3609175.

Chen, R. M., B. (1993). *A measles outbreak in a highly vaccinated population: Health sector Muyinga, Burundi 1988–1989*. Atlanta, GA: CDC.

FEMWiki. (not dated). *Outbreak investigations: 10 steps, 10 pitfalls*. Retrieved from https://wiki.ecdc.europa.eu/fem/w/wiki/outbreak-investigations-10-steps-10-pitfalls.

Finger, F., Funk, S., White, K., Siddiqui, M. R., Edmunds, W. J., & Kucharski, A. J. (2019). Real-time analysis of the diphtheria outbreak in forcibly displaced Myanmar nationals in Bangladesh. *BMC Medicine*, 17(1), 58. doi:10.1186/s12916-019-1288-7.

Giesecke, J. (2017). *Modern infectious disease epidemiology*. Boca Raton, FL: CRC Press.

Greenland, K., Whelan, J., Fanoy, E., Borgert, M., Hulshof, K., Yap, K. B., ... Hahné, S. (2012). Mumps outbreak among vaccinated university students associated with a large party, the Netherlands, 2010. *Vaccine*, 30(31), 4676–4680. doi:10.1016/j.vaccine.2012.04.083.

Gregory, C. J., Ndiaye, S., Patel, M., Hakizamana, E., Wannemuehler, K., Ndinga, E., ... Kretsinger, K. (2012). Investigation of elevated case-fatality rate in poliomyelitis outbreak in Pointe Noire, Republic of Congo, 2010. *Clinical Infectious Diseases*, 55(10), 1299–1306. doi:10.1093/cid/cis715.

Hahné, S., Gray, S. J., Jean, F., Aguilera, Crowcroft, N. S., Nichols, T., ... Ramsay, M. E. (2002). W135 meningococcal disease in England and Wales associated with Hajj 2000 and 2001. *Lancet*, 359(9306), 582–583. Retrieved from www.ncbi.nlm.nih.gov/pubmed/11867116.

Hahné, S., Handford, S., & Ramsay, M. (2002). W135 meningococcal carriage in Hajj pilgrims. *Lancet*, 360(9350), 2089–2090. doi:10.1016/s0140-6736(02)11991-x.

Hahné, S., Macey, J., van Binnendijk, R., Kohl, R., Dolman, S., van der Veen, Y., ... de Melker, H. (2009). Rubella outbreak in the Netherlands, 2004–2005: High burden of congenital infection and spread to Canada. *Pediatric Infectious Diseases Journal*, 28(9), 795–800. doi:10.1097/INF.0b013e3181a3e2d5.

Hales, C. M., Johnson, E., Helgenberger, L., Papania, M. J., Larzelere, M., Gopalani, S. V., ... Marin, M. (2016). Measles outbreak associated with low vaccine effectiveness among adults in Pohnpei state, federated states of Micronesia, 2014. *Open Forum Infectious Diseases*, 3(2), ofw064. doi:10.1093/ofid/ofw064.

Hardy, I. R., Dittmann, S., & Sutter, R. W. (1996). Current situation and control strategies for resurgence of diphtheria in newly independent states of the former Soviet Union. *Lancet*, 347(9017), 1739–1744. Retrieved from www.ncbi.nlm.nih.gov/pubmed/8656909.

Jegede, A. S. (2007). What led to the Nigerian boycott of the polio vaccination campaign? *PLoS Med*, 4(3), e73. doi:10.1371/journal.pmed.0040073.

Khan, T. Q., J. (2014). Measles outbreaks in Pakistan: Causes of the tragedy and future implications. *Epidemiology Reports*, 2(1). doi:10.7243/2054-9911-2-1.

McLean, A. R., & Anderson, R. M. (1988). Measles in developing countries. Part II. The predicted impact of mass vaccination. *Epidemiology and Infection*, 100(3), 419–442. Retrieved from www.ncbi.nlm.nih.gov/pubmed/3378585.

Mere, M. O., Goodson, J. L., Chandio, A. K., Rana, M. S., Hasan, Q., Teleb, N., & Alexander, J. P. Jr. (2019). Progress toward measles elimination: Pakistan, 2000–2018. *Morbidity and Mortality Weekly Report, 68*(22), 505–510. doi:10.15585/mmwr.mm6822a4.

Murray, M., & Rasmussen, Z. (2000). Measles outbreak in a northern Pakistani village: Epidemiology and vaccine effectiveness. *American Journal of Epidemiology, 151*(8), 811–819. Retrieved from www.ncbi.nlm.nih.gov/pubmed/10965978.

Paniz-Mondolfi, A. E., Tami, A., Grillet, M. E., Marquez, M., Hernandez-Villena, J., Escalona-Rodriguez, M. A., ... Oletta, J. (2019). Resurgence of vaccine-preventable diseases in Venezuela as a regional public health threat in the Americas. *Emerging Infectious Diseases, 25*(4), 625–632. doi:10.3201/eid2504.181305.

Parker, L. A., Rumunu, J., Jamet, C., Kenyi, Y., Lino, R. L., Wamala, J. F., ... Cabrol, J. C. (2017). Adapting to the global shortage of cholera vaccines: Targeted single-dose cholera vaccine in response to an outbreak in South Sudan. *Lancet Infect Dis, 17*(4), e123–e127. doi:10.1016/S1473-3099(16)30472-8.

Patriarca, P. A. (2012). Research and development and the polio eradication initiative: too much, too soon ... too little, too late? *Clinical Infectious Diseases, 55*(10), 1307–1311. doi:10.1093/cid/cis720.

Pincock, S. (2004). Poliovirus spreads beyond Nigeria after vaccine uptake drops. *BMJ, 328*(7435), 310. doi:10.1136/bmj.328.7435.310-c.

Porta, M. (2014). *A dictionary of epidemiology*. New York: Oxford University Press.

Rothman, K. J., Greenland, S., & Lash, T. (2020). *Modern epidemiology* (4th ed.). Philadelphia, PA: Lippincott Williams &Wilkins.

Stark, R. (2017). Mumps in the post-secondary environment: Targeted advertising in the 2007–2008 Alberta mumps vaccination campaign. *Arcadia, 4*. Retrieved from www.environmentandsociety.org/arcadia/mumps-post-secondary-environment-targeted-advertising-2007-2008-alberta-mumps-vaccination.

Tsang, R. S., Kiefer, L., Law, D. K., Stoltz, J., Shahin, R., Brown, S., & Jamieson, F. (2003). Outbreak of serogroup C meningococcal disease caused by a variant of Neisseria meningitidis serotype 2a ET-15 in a community of men who have sex with men. *Journal of Clinical Microbiology, 41*(9), 4411–4414. Retrieved from www.ncbi.nlm.nih.gov/pubmed/12958279.

Veneti, L., Borgen, K., Borge, K. S., Danis, K., Greve-Isdahl, M., Konsmo, K., ... Riise, O. R. (2018). Large outbreak of mumps virus genotype G among vaccinated students in Norway, 2015 to 2016. *Eurosurveillance, 23*(38). doi:10.2807/1560-7917.ES.2018.23.38.1700642.

Wichmann, O., Siedler, A., Sagebiel, D., Hellenbrand, W., Santibanez, S., Mankertz, A., ... Krause, G. (2009). Further efforts needed to achieve measles elimination in Germany: Results of an outbreak investigation. *Bulletin of the World Health Organization, 87*(2), 108–115. Retrieved from www.ncbi.nlm.nih.gov/pubmed/19274362.

World Health Organization (WHO). (2017). *Vaccination in acute humanitarian emergencies: A framework for decision making*. Geneva, Switzerland: World Health Organization.

Part III

Vaccine effectiveness

Chapter 12

Vaccine effectiveness

The effectiveness of a vaccine is the degree to which it prevents infection, disease or infectiousness, through its action on individuals. It depends on how well the vaccine-induced immune response blocks the replication of the pathogen (or neutralises its toxin), the intensity of exposure to the pathogen and on the time since vaccination.

Assessing and monitoring vaccine effectiveness is a key aspect of the epidemiological assessment of vaccination programmes. Vaccine effectiveness is an important surveillance indicator and can be the focus of dedicated studies when there is an increase in cases or an outbreak of a disease targeted by vaccination. In this situation it is important as a first step to generate hypotheses about the causes of the increase. This is done by considering descriptive epidemiological characteristics (mainly vaccination status and age) of a subset of cases that are thought to be representative of all cases and reviewing existing evidence about vaccine coverage and effectiveness. The public health questions that require priority will depend on the context. If, for example, in a measles outbreak the vast majority of cases are unvaccinated, it may be more important from a public health perspective to assess reasons for non-vaccination rather than vaccine effectiveness (see Chapter 11). Nevertheless, outbreaks provide opportunities to study many aspects of vaccines and vaccination programmes, including vaccine effectiveness.

When considering vaccine effectiveness, the primary emphasis is on individuals, rather than on populations: this is what distinguishes measures of effectiveness from measures of impact. For example, an effective vaccine that is only administered to a small proportion of individuals within a given population is likely to have a low impact. Nevertheless, effectiveness in individuals and impact in populations are related, and it is important to clarify the relationship between them. Furthermore, effectiveness is sometimes evaluated by comparing different subpopulations, and may therefore encompass indirect as well as direct effects.

A question often asked is 'How effective should a vaccine be?' There is no simple answer to this question: it depends entirely on context, in particular on the infection and the severity of infection-related disease, on the aims of the vaccination programme and on the availability of other means and therapeutics.

DOI: 10.4324/9781315166414-13
This Chapter has been made available under a CC-BY-NC-ND license.

In this chapter we focus on concepts of effectiveness, whereas Chapters 13 to 16 describe the methods for estimating vaccine effectiveness in the field and the methodological issues involved. Since most field studies focus on protective effectiveness (the degree of protection that the vaccine imparts directly to an individual, by reducing that individual's risk of infection or disease) this is where we begin, in Section 12.1.

In line with the book's focus on public health epidemiology, we concentrate on the effectiveness of licensed vaccines used in the field, rather than on the process of demonstrating a vaccine's efficacy for scientific or licensure purposes. The distinction between field effectiveness and experimental efficacy is discussed in Section 12.2.

In Section 12.3, we discuss different concepts of protective vaccine effectiveness according to which outcome is studied: disease, infection or progression of disease (severity). Since from a disease control perspective the effectiveness of vaccination in reducing infectiousness is of key importance, we have dedicated Section 12.4 to this. This brings us to the final Section 12.5, in which we combine different measures of vaccine effectiveness into a single one, the vaccine effectiveness against transmission, and discuss how this relates to the indirect effects of vaccination and reproduction numbers. Further information may be found in Halloran, Longini, and Struchiner (2010).

12.1 Protective vaccine effectiveness

Protective vaccine effectiveness is the proportionate reduction in the risk of infection or infection-related disease in vaccinated individuals, compared to the risk in unvaccinated individuals. Protective vaccine effectiveness is usually just called vaccine effectiveness, and denoted VE. Thus:

$$VE = \frac{R_u - R_v}{R_u},$$

where R_u is the risk of infection or disease in unvaccinated individuals and R_v is the risk in vaccinated individuals. The risk is the probability of infection or disease over a given period; rates may also be used to calculate vaccine effectiveness. Risks and rates are often used interchangeably in epidemiology: in fact, they are different quantities, and may yield different results, a point we shall return to in Chapter 13, but that we will gloss over until then. The measure VE of vaccine effectiveness is also known as the preventive fraction. Often, VE is expressed as a percentage:

$$VE = \frac{R_u - R_v}{R_u} \times 100.$$

It can also be written in terms of the relative risk $RR = R_v / R_u$, as follows:

$$VE = 1 - \frac{R_v}{R_u} = 1 - RR.$$

Box 12.1 explains the calculation and interpretation of vaccine effectiveness using these two formulas.

Box 12.1 Calculating vaccine effectiveness

This measure of effectiveness was proposed by Greenwood and Yule (1915), who called it efficiency. For example, if in a given setting the infection risk in unvaccinated individuals is 0.25 and 0.05 in vaccinated individuals, the vaccine effectiveness is

$$VE = \frac{0.25 - 0.05}{0.25} = 0.8$$

or equivalently as a percentage, 80%. Alternatively, the relative risk is $RR = \frac{0.05}{0.25} = 0.2$, so

$$VE = 1 - 0.2 = 0.8.$$

A vaccine effectiveness of zero means that vaccination does not affect the infection risk. In this case, $R_v = R_u$ (and the relative risk is 1). A positive effectiveness means that the vaccine is associated with a reduction in the risk. The maximum effectiveness is 1 (or 100%), which occurs when $R_v = 0$ and $R_u > 0$. On the other hand, if $R_v > R_u$, then the vaccine effectiveness is negative. This implies that the infection risk is higher in vaccinated than in unvaccinated persons.

It is usual to quote an estimate of vaccine effectiveness with an indication of its uncertainty. This uncertainty may be represented by a 95% confidence interval (CI), as described in Box 12.2.

Box 12.2 Confidence intervals for VE

In practice, VE is estimated using relative risks obtained from epidemiological studies, which are described in Chapters 14 and 15. The estimated relative risk RR is usually associated with a 95% CI (RR^-, RR^+) that quantifies its statistical uncertainty. The estimated vaccine effectiveness is then

$$VE = 1 - RR$$

and its 95% confidence limits are

$$VE^- = 1 - RR^+, \quad VE^+ = 1 - RR^-.$$

For example, if the relative risk is estimated to be 0.20 with 95% CI (0.08, 0.32), the estimated vaccine effectiveness is 0.80 with 95% CI (0.68, 0.92). Alternatively, using percentages, the vaccine effectiveness is 80% with 95% CI (68%, 92%). This is written $VE = 80\%$, 95% CI (68%, 92%).

If the lower 95% confidence limit for VE is negative, so that the confidence interval includes 0, there is little evidence that the vaccine provides any protection.

A confidence interval quantifies the uncertainty associated with an estimate of VE within one study. At least as important is the variability of VE estimates between studies. This variability arises because the effectiveness of a vaccine generally depends on the characteristics of the population in which it is evaluated (an example will be described in Box 12.8). VE may also vary according to environmental determinants such as the setting and the intensity of contacts involved, and because of differences in study design. As in any epidemiological study, bias and confounding can distort VE estimates, the extent of which usually varies between different studies. Some of these issues will be addressed in more detail in Chapter 13. Between-study variability is illustrated in Box 12.3.

Box 12.3 Influenza vaccine effectiveness in the community and in households

This example contrasts the results of two vaccine effectiveness studies of the seasonal influenza vaccine undertaken during the 2010–2011 influenza season in the United States. The vaccine strains included in the vaccine were antigenically similar to the circulating virus strains during this influenza season.

The first study was undertaken in the community, with confirmed influenza cases ascertained from a range of medical facilities (Treanor et al., 2012). The overall vaccine effectiveness in this setting was found to be 60%, 95% CI 53% to 66%. The conclusion from this study was that the vaccine was moderately effective in preventing medically attended influenza.

A second study was undertaken during the same influenza epidemic, based on confirmed symptomatic influenza cases. This study evaluated vaccine effectiveness both within the community and within households (Ohmit et al., 2013). The overall vaccine effectiveness within the community was estimated to be 31%, 95% CI −7% to 55%. Furthermore, there was no evidence of any protective efficacy against acquisition of influenza within households: the vaccine effectiveness was −51%, 95% CI −254% to 36%.

The estimates of VE for community-acquired influenza differ substantially between the two studies. Furthermore, the second study suggests that, once influenza enters a household, the vaccine does not provide any protection against transmission within that household.

The example in Box 12.3 illustrates a commonly encountered conundrum in studies of vaccine effectiveness: different studies can yield very different results. Making sense of such variation requires detailed understanding of vaccine effectiveness and the methods to estimate it, key aspects of which are discussed in this book.

12.2 Vaccine efficacy and vaccine effectiveness

Vaccine efficacy is calculated in exactly the same way as vaccine effectiveness, as described in Section 12.1. The difference between the terms 'vaccine efficacy' and 'vaccine effectiveness' arises from the context in which they are assessed. The term 'vaccine efficacy' is used more restrictively to denote an effect measure obtained under strict experimental conditions in a double-blind, randomised controlled trial. In contrast, 'vaccine effectiveness' is an effect measure relating to the vaccine when used in the field, usually as part of a vaccination programme, and evaluated using non-randomised observational studies. Thus, efficacy is obtained under ideal experimental conditions, whereas effectiveness is pragmatic. In this book, we will not cover experimental vaccine trials in any detail; a very brief outline is provided in Chapter 1.

Our focus is very much on the evaluation of licensed vaccines used in vaccination programmes, that is, on pragmatic vaccine effectiveness. The evaluation of vaccine effectiveness in this context is based on observational epidemiological studies, often using data available through pre-existing surveillance systems. This is because, once a vaccination programme is implemented, vaccine efficacy trials in which a part of the study population no longer receive the vaccine are usually considered unethical. Unlike vaccine efficacy trials, observational studies can be as large, and involve as much follow-up time, as the data allow. However, because they are not randomised, field evaluations of vaccine effectiveness are subject to the same biases as any other observational epidemiological study.

When vaccines are administered under conditions of routine use, rather than under the strict protocol of a trial, procedures to administer the vaccine may depart from those recommended under the vaccination programme. This may result in reduced vaccine effectiveness. Examples of such programmatic errors are discussed in Box 12.4.

Box 12.4 The potential impact of programmatic errors

Programmatic errors are significant departures from the recommended procedures governing a vaccination programme. These errors may relate, for example, to the timing of vaccinations, the composition or combination of vaccines used, dosage, storage and handling issues, including problems with the cold chain, or use of incorrect vaccination sites.

Examples of programmatic errors are: lack of appropriate training of persons administering vaccines; mixing different vaccines that should have been administered separately; storing vaccines in a domestic fridge with no temperature monitoring; and vaccines stored at temperatures lower than the recommended range, for example at the back of the fridge where they tend to freeze (Craig et al., 2011).

Programmatic errors may reduce the effectiveness of the vaccine. In their report, Craig et al. (2011) discuss the steps taken to mitigate the impact of the programmatic errors identified, notably the risk of adverse reactions upon revaccination, and the ethical issues involved. They emphasise that, since programmatic errors inevitably occur, robust monitoring systems are required so that poor practice can be identified and corrected.

The distinction between vaccine efficacy and vaccine effectiveness can be overstated as, essentially, they measure the same quantity. The difference between them lies in the rigour of the administration of the vaccine and the study design and other methods used to evaluate it.

The distinction between efficacy and effectiveness may be blurred in randomised introductions of a vaccine – in which the vaccine is introduced for immediate public health purposes using a randomised study design. Such studies combine aspects of the methodological rigour of randomised clinical trials, but are carried out in the context of a vaccination programme. One example is given in Box 12.5. This is a cluster randomised trial, which introduced what has become known as the 'stepped-wedge design'.

Box 12.5 The stepped-wedge design: hepatitis B vaccination in the Gambia

The stepped-wedge design is a phased introduction of mass vaccination. The vaccine is introduced sequentially in different areas, the order of introduction being decided at random. The idea behind the design is illustrated in Figure 12.1 in a simplified scenario involving just three areas.

Baseline incidences in the three areas are established during period 1. The vaccine is introduced in area A during period 2, in area B during period 3 and in area C during period 4. The incidences in different areas within each period are then compared: for example, during period 2, vaccinees in area A are compared with unvaccinated individuals in areas B and C, after adjustment for differences

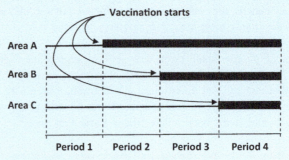

Figure 12.1 The stepped-wedge design with three areas.

between areas. In period 3, vaccinees in areas A and B are compared to unvaccinated persons in area C.

The Gambia hepatitis intervention study was launched in 1987 to assess the long-term efficacy of hepatitis B vaccination in preventing liver cancer and other long-term sequelae (Hall et al., 1987). It introduced the stepped-wedge design, in this instance with 17 areas. The hepatitis B vaccine was administered within the existing Expanded Programme of Immunisation (EPI) framework, along with other EPI vaccines (see Chapter 3). The vaccine effectiveness against HBsAg carriage in 15-year-olds was found to be 95% with 95% CI (91%, 100%) (Viviani et al., 2008).

As with other study designs comparing different populations, the vaccine effectiveness obtained from a stepped-wedge design may encompass indirect as well as direct protection. The hepatitis B vaccine study described in Box 12.5 was planned for several decades of follow-up and involved an implementation period of several years. Very different circumstances prevailed for the Ebola vaccine trial described in Box 12.6. Here, the randomised introduction of the vaccine was precipitated by an outbreak of Ebola. The design also involved cluster randomisation, but used ring vaccination (see Chapter 3).

Box 12.6 The Guinea Ebola ring vaccination trial

This trial was undertaken in Guinea during the 2014–2016 outbreak of Ebola virus in West Africa. The candidate vaccine had at this stage not been evaluated in phase III trials. The trial design involved enumerating contacts, and contacts of contacts, of new Ebola cases. These were grouped in clusters, which were then randomly assigned to immediate vaccination, or vaccination delayed by 21 days. Attack rates were obtained over 21 days after randomisation (post-vaccination if vaccination was immediate, pre-vaccination if it was delayed), and compared between clusters. An interim analysis suggested high efficacy, at which point the delayed vaccination arm was discontinued.

In the final analysis, there were no cases meeting the case definition in the 51 clusters assigned to immediate vaccination, and 16 cases in 7 of the 47 clusters assigned to delayed vaccination. The resulting vaccine efficacy was 100% with 95% CI (69%, 100%). When data from 19 non-randomised clusters were included, the vaccine effectiveness was 100%, 95% CI (79%, 100%) (Henao-Restrepo et al., 2017).

The interventions described in Boxes 12.5 and 12.6 both used innovative designs to achieve important public health objectives (namely, introducing vaccination while at the same time evaluating its effectiveness) in challenging conditions, while remaining within the methodological framework of randomised controlled trials. Whether they result in a measure of (experimental) efficacy or (pragmatic) effectiveness is perhaps a moot point. More importantly, such intervention trials can be used as an opportunity to build capacity, as described by the investigators of another Ebola vaccine trial conducted during the 2014–2016 epidemic (Carter et al., 2018).

Both vaccine efficacy and vaccine effectiveness involve an interplay with the population in which the vaccine is being evaluated. Thus, context plays a key role both in randomised efficacy trials and in observational effectiveness studies. Box 12.7 provides an illustration.

Box 12.7 Efficacy and effectiveness of rotavirus vaccines vary by population studied

Several randomised controlled trials and observational studies have been carried out in different countries to evaluate the efficacy and effectiveness of rotavirus vaccines. Here, we consider studies using the pentavalent rotavirus vaccine.

This rotavirus vaccine was evaluated in several large multi-centre randomised controlled trials. One was undertaken in several mainly high- or middle-income countries, and found an efficacy of 95%, with 95% CI (91%, 97%) against hospitalisations due to rotavirus gastroenteritis (Vesikari et al., 2006). In contrast, studies from low- and lower-middle-income countries found much lower efficacy: a randomised trial in Ghana, Kenya and Mali found an efficacy of 39%, 95% CI (19%, 55%) against severe rotavirus gastroenteritis (Armah et al., 2010), while another in Bangladesh and Vietnam found the efficacy to be 48%, 95% CI (22%, 66%) (Zaman et al., 2010).

Observational studies have obtained vaccine effectiveness estimates against hospitalisation for rotavirus gastroenteritis that were comparable to trial results in each setting. In the United States, the effectiveness was found to be 92%, 95% CI (75%–97%) (Cortese et al., 2013). In contrast, a study in Nicaragua obtained an effectiveness of 45%, 95% CI (25%–59%) (Patel et al., 2016); another in Rwanda an effectiveness of 75%, 95% CI (31%–91%) (Tate et al., 2016).

As illustrated in Box 12.7, a vaccine can have very different efficacy or effectiveness in different settings. In this example, the efficacy and effectiveness of the pentavalent rotavirus vaccine were found to be very high in high- and middle-income countries, and much lower (but still significantly protective, and highly beneficial) in low-income countries. Results from trials and from observational studies in similar settings were comparable. Both vaccine efficacy and vaccine effectiveness may depend on the populations, environment and circumstances in which the vaccine is used. When summarising data from different studies, for example in systematic reviews and meta-analyses, it is essential to acknowledge such variability, and seek to understand it.

12.3 Protection against infection, disease and disease progression

An important decision to make in vaccine effectiveness studies is against which clinical entity one wants to study the protection afforded by the vaccine. The main options available include protection against infection (or colonisation), protection against clinical disease and protection against progression to severe disease. In this section we consider these three options and discuss the relationships between them. Which option to choose depends on the aims set by the vaccination programme, the biological mechanism by which the vaccine confers protection, the microbiological characteristics of the pathogen, the feasibility of obtaining data about the end points and the question one wants to answer.

Investigating vaccine protection against infection is particularly relevant when the causative micro-organisms can infect and then colonise their host without causing symptoms (such as Hib or pneumococcal disease). It is also relevant when there are substantial numbers of mild or subclinical cases, which may contribute to transmission, but do not present with significant symptoms. Vaccine effectiveness against infection is then important for understanding and quantifying how vaccination affects the transmission of infection. Vaccine effectiveness against infection is calculated using the expression:

$$VE_{Infection} = 1 - \frac{\text{risk of infection in vaccinated}}{\text{risk of infection in unvaccinated}}.$$

Box 12.8 gives an example relating to Hib colonisation.

Box 12.8 Effectiveness of Hib conjugate vaccination against colonisation

Haemophilus influenzae type b (Hib) bacteria can colonise a person's nose and throat, rarely (but more often so in children) leading to severe invasive disease. Several studies have reported that vaccination against Hib with the conjugate vaccine reduces Hib carriage. This suggests that vaccination may reduce Hib transmission, thus giving rise to herd immunity.

The Hib vaccination programme in the United Kingdom was phased in at different times in different areas, as in a stepped-wedge design (see Box 12.5). A study was undertaken to compare proportions of infants with Hib carriage in Oxfordshire, where the vaccine was introduced, and in neighbouring Buckinghamshire, where it was not. The relative risk of carriage in vaccinated relative to unvaccinated infants between the ages of 6 and 12 months was $RR = 0.23$, with 95% CI (0.056, 0.91). Thus, the vaccine effectiveness against carriage was

$$VE = 1 - RR = 1 - 0.23 = 0.77,$$

or 77%, with 95% CI (9% to 94%) (Barbour, Mayon-White, Coles, Crook, & Moxon, 1995). The wide confidence interval indicates substantial uncertainty in this estimate. When the comparison was restricted to infants whose family members carried Hib, the same *VE* was observed: the carriage rates were 8.7% in vaccinated and 38.5% in unvaccinated infants, though the numbers were small.

In 1999, a resurgence of Hib disease was observed, which was attributed to low protective effectiveness of the vaccine against Hib disease in infants (see Chapter 5). Further studies suggested that this was due to low antibodies, associated with inadequate protection against invasive disease. There was, however, no increase in Hib transmission: the prevalence of carriage remained close to zero in infants (McVernon, Howard, Slack, & Ramsay, 2004). This suggests vaccine effectiveness against colonisation was adequate.

When direct health benefits are of primary interest, it is logical to use disease, specified using a suitable case definition, as the end point of the study. The risks to be compared are then the risk of disease in vaccinated and unvaccinated individuals; most studies of vaccine effectiveness are of this type. Vaccine effectiveness is then

$$VE_{Disease} = 1 - \frac{\text{risk of disease in vaccinated}}{\text{risk of disease in unvaccinated}}.$$

For example, the primary purpose of vaccination programmes against influenza is to prevent influenza-related disease, particularly among the elderly. It is appropriate to reflect this purpose when evaluating influenza vaccine effectiveness, and thus to use a suitable indicator of disease as the end point. An example is given in Box 12.9.

Box 12.9 Effectiveness of influenza vaccines against hospitalisation in Canada

When evaluating the effectiveness of influenza vaccines, there is particular interest in assessing its potential to prevent disease in the elderly. This was the aim of a multi-centre study undertaken during the 2011–2012 influenza season in persons aged 65 years or more in Canada (Andrew et al., 2017).

The vaccine was the seasonal trivalent inactivated influenza vaccine. The outcome of interest was hospitalisation due to laboratory confirmed influenza, by any strain. The overall vaccine effectiveness was *VE* = 58% with 95% CI (34%, 73%). The effectiveness was similar against influenza A (*VE* = 63%) and influenza B (*VE* = 58%). It declined with increasing frailty of the patients, as measured by a validated frailty index.

Some vaccines offer no protection against infection, but do protect against infection-related disease. Consequently, the vaccine cannot be expected to have any impact on transmission of the infection, or induce any herd immunity, but can protect individuals from becoming ill. For such vaccines, vaccine effectiveness against disease is clearly of primary interest. An example is described in Box 12.10.

> **Box 12.10 Effectiveness of pneumococcal polysaccharide vaccines against bacteraemia**
>
> Pneumococcal polysaccharide vaccines do not induce mucosal immunity, and consequently do not affect carriage or transmission, and have limited effect on pneumococcal respiratory tract infections (Pletz, Maus, Krug, Welte, & Lode, 2008). However, these vaccines can prevent pneumococcal bacteraemia (presence of bacteria in the blood), as shown in a large study in the United States (Jackson et al., 2003).
>
> This study, which was conducted in persons aged 65 years or older, found that receipt of the 23-valent pneumococcal polysaccharide vaccine was associated with a reduction in the risk of pneumococcal bacteraemia, but was not associated with any difference in community-acquired pneumonia.
>
> The rates of pneumococcal bacteraemia (per 1,000 person-years) were 0.68 for unvaccinated persons, and 0.38 for vaccinated persons. The relative risk for pneumococcal bacteraemia was $RR = 0.56$, 95% CI (0.33, 0.93). This gives a vaccine effectiveness against pneumococcal bacteraemia of 44%, 95% CI (7%, 67%).

For infections with an appreciable proportion of subclinical cases, such as mumps, it may not be realistic to seek to estimate vaccine effectiveness against infection per se. This is because cases are usually identified using clinical signs, the pathogen involved then being confirmed by laboratory methods. In fact, this is true more generally: it can be difficult to disentangle vaccine effectiveness against infection from vaccine effectiveness against disease, because methodological issues relating to the sensitivity and specificity of the case definitions, to be described in Chapter 13, are likely to intrude.

Some vaccines may modify the clinical manifestation of infection-related disease. There are two different approaches to studying this. First, one can choose severe disease as the end point in the vaccine effectiveness study, for example by choosing a particular disease manifestation or by including hospitalised or deceased cases only. Effectiveness against severe disease is defined in exactly the same way as the protective effectiveness against disease was defined previously:

$$VE_{Severe} = 1 - \frac{risk\ of\ severe\ disease\ in\ vaccinated}{risk\ of\ severe\ disease\ in\ unvaccinated},$$

where the risks of severe disease in vaccinated and unvaccinated individuals are determined using an appropriate case definition. The example in Box 12.10 was of this nature.

Alternatively, the effectiveness of the vaccine in preventing progression to severe disease, denoted VP, can be studied. This is a different indicator from the VE against severe disease described above. The estimation of VP involves comparing the severity of disease between vaccinated and unvaccinated persons with the disease. The advantage of estimating VP rather than VE against severe disease is that it requires samples of vaccinated and unvaccinated cases only: population denominators, or samples of non-cases, are not needed.

To calculate VP, the risks of a case being severe (defined using some objective criterion) in vaccinated and in unvaccinated cases of disease are compared. Suppose that the risk of a severe case among vaccinated cases is S_v, and that the risk of a severe case among unvaccinated cases is S_u. If 'severe' means death, then these risks are also called case fatality rates (or risks). The vaccine effectiveness against progression (to severe disease) is then

$$VP = 1 - \frac{S_v}{S_u}.$$

Like the protective vaccine effectiveness VE, this measure is also of the form $VP = 1 - RR$, where RR is a relative risk, but now the relative risk relates to the ratio of probabilities of a case being severe. This measure of effectiveness against disease progression was proposed by Halloran, Longini, and Struchiner (1999). It measures the relative severity of cases in vaccinated and unvaccinated persons, not whether vaccination affects the case load. A vaccine that has a low protective vaccine effectiveness, but a moderate or high vaccine effectiveness against severe disease, or a high vaccine effectiveness against progression to severe disease, can still be of considerable public health benefit. However, it is important to bear in mind that medical treatment of cases may interfere with studies of the effects of vaccines on severity or progression of disease.

An example of these different measures relating to pertussis vaccine is presented in Box 12.11.

Box 12.11 The effectiveness of pertussis vaccination against progression to severe disease

This study was undertaken in Niakhar, Senegal, during 1993, an epidemic year for pertussis (Préziosi & Halloran, 2003). The study area was the site of an active surveillance programme for pertussis. Potential cases were children with a cough lasting over a week. Cases of pertussis were confirmed by culture or serology. The clinical severity of each case was assessed on an ordinal scale, by a physician blinded to the vaccination status of the case. In the following analysis, only completely vaccinated (three doses of pertussis vaccine) or unvaccinated cases are included.

A total 834 cases of pertussis in children aged 6 months to 8 years were recorded. Cases were classified as severe if they scored above the median severity score. The vaccine effectiveness for all confirmed cases, irrespective of clinical severity, was $VE = 29\%$ with 95% CI (19%, 39%). The vaccine effectiveness for severe cases was $VE = 64\%$ with 95% CI (55%, 71%).

Some 32% of vaccinated cases and 61% of unvaccinated cases were deemed to be severe. Thus, the vaccine effectiveness against progression to severe disease is:

$$VP = 1 - \frac{0.32}{0.61} = 0.48$$

or 48%, with 95% CI (39%, 55%). Thus, vaccinated cases are about half as likely as unvaccinated cases to be classified as severe.

In Box 12.11, disease modification resulting from pertussis vaccination is captured in two ways: by the contrasting VE values according to severity (29% for all cases, 64% for severe cases); and by the progression measure $VP = 48\%$. Generally, it is advisable to obtain vaccine effectiveness across a severity range of disease manifestations, in order to capture both changes in caseload and in disease severity.

Vaccine effectiveness against severe disease VE_{Severe}, vaccine effectiveness against infection $VE_{Infection}$ and the vaccine effectiveness against progression (from infection to severe disease) VP, all expressed as numbers less than 1 (rather than percentages), are related as follows:

$$VE_{Severe} = 1 - (1 - VP) \times (1 - VE_{Infection}).$$

This relationship is based on the assumption that protection against infection and progression to severe disease are independent. If they are not independent, for example because both quantities vary with age, then the relationship applies within strata (such as age groups).

For the data of Box 12.11, one can tentatively take $VE_{Infection} \approx 0.29$, the vaccine effectiveness against all confirmed cases irrespective of severity, and $VP = 0.48$, giving $VE_{Severe} \approx 0.63$, close to the value 0.64 observed.

So far, all end points considered have been directly related to the infection targeted by the vaccine. However, it may also be relevant to consider vaccine effectiveness against a syndrome: influenza-like illness (ILI), say, rather than influenza. From a vaccinology point of view, the effectiveness of the vaccine against a specific infection is usually the first study priority, whereas from a public health perspective, the level of protection against a syndrome may be more relevant. This measure of syndromic vaccine effectiveness is thus:

$$VE_{Syndromic} = 1 - \frac{Syndromic\ risk\ in\ vaccinated}{Syndromic\ risk\ in\ unvaccinated}.$$

Box 12.12 provides an example.

Box 12.12 Influenza vaccine effectiveness against influenza-like illness in pilgrims to the Hajj

This study of influenza vaccine effectiveness was undertaken among Pakistani pilgrims attending the Hajj in 1999 (Qureshi et al., 2000). Pilgrims travel in groups; five groups were recruited prior to attending the Hajj, and were offered influenza vaccine. Among those followed up, 1,120 had chosen to be vaccinated and 950 had chosen not to be; 11% of the vaccinated and 5.7% of the unvaccinated had a history of cardiorespiratory illness.

The main end point of the study was influenza-like illness (ILI), defined as sore throat in combination with cough or fever of at least 38ºC. The risks of ILI were 62% in unvaccinated pilgrims and 36% in vaccinated pilgrims. The risks varied between the five pilgrim groups, so the analyses were stratified by group. The vaccine effectiveness was 38%, with 95% CI (29% to 45%); the risk difference was 22%, with 95% CI (16% to 27%).

The interpretation of these results is that 38% of cases of ILI could be prevented by vaccinating pilgrims attending the Hajj, corresponding to an absolute risk reduction of 22%. The effectiveness of the influenza vaccine in protecting against influenza (as distinct from ILI) was not estimated.

Typically, the syndrome of interest will also include disease not caused by the infection targeted, and so syndromic vaccine effectiveness will tend to be lower than the vaccine effectiveness against infection-related disease. However, the absolute reduction in the risk of the syndrome may be higher than the absolute reduction in the estimated risk of the disease specifically caused by the targeted infection, since case definitions for infection-related disease may not be 100% sensitive.

Using a clinical syndrome as the end point in a vaccine effectiveness study may also help to uncover the burden of disease preventable by vaccination. This approach has been described as using the vaccine as a probe (Feikin, Scott, & Gessner, 2014). An example is given in Box 12.13.

Box 12.13 Using the cholera vaccine as a probe in Bangladesh

The sensitivity of *Vibrio cholera* O1 diagnoses based on microbiological culture of stool samples from patients with acute watery diarrhoea (AWD) has been questioned. If such cultures were found to be insensitive, the global burden of cholera could be seriously underestimated. To investigate this issue, a vaccine probe study with a killed whole-cell oral cholera vaccine of proven effectiveness was undertaken in culture-negative samples obtained in a previous vaccine study (Im et al., 2019).

> The study sought to estimate the effectiveness of two vaccine doses against first episodes of culture-negative (for cholera) AWD in children. The rationale was that, if some cholera patients had culture-negative samples, then the cholera vaccine effectiveness should be positive, since the vaccine had previously been shown to be effective in preventing cholera.
>
> The overall vaccine effectiveness was $VE = -1.7\%$ with 95% CI (−23%, 16%) for cholera-negative AWD. In contrast, the effectiveness for cholera-positive AWD was 52%, 95% CI (40%, 61%). Thus, the study did not demonstrate any effectiveness against cholera-negative AWD. This finding does not support the hypothesis that culture is insensitive for cholera diagnosis and that the global burden of cholera is underestimated.

12.4 Vaccine effectiveness against infectiousness

So far, we have focused on the protective effectiveness of a vaccine, namely the proportionate reduction of the infection or disease rate in vaccinated compared to unvaccinated persons, and on the effectiveness of the vaccine in modifying disease severity. These are undoubtedly important measures of vaccine effectiveness, as they quantify the direct benefits of vaccination to individuals. However, vaccination can produce other benefits, perhaps not for the person vaccinated, but for those around them.

Thus, a vaccine that does not protect an individual from acquiring infection (or infection-related disease) may nevertheless reduce the infectiousness of that individual if they became infected. This could occur in different ways. For example, the infectious period may be shorter for a vaccinated infected person than for an unvaccinated infected person. Alternatively, the probability of transmission of the infection, when contact is made with a susceptible person, may be lower. The precise mechanisms are usually infection-specific; an important example involving nasopharyngeal carriage of bacterial infections is discussed in Box 12.14.

> **Box 12.14 Conjugate vaccines and nasopharyngeal carriage of bacterial infections**
>
> Bacteria such as *Neisseria meningitidis* and *Streptococcus pneumoniae* may cause serious invasive disease (such as meningitis and sepsis), and have been successfully prevented by vaccination. While invasive disease caused by these bacteria is rare, nasopharyngeal carriage is common, and plays a key role in the transmission of these infections. Conjugate vaccines have been shown to protect against invasive disease, and to reduce carriage of the serotypes included in the vaccine.
>
> Recent research has focused on the determinants of carriage density of bacterial infections, as distinct from carriage frequency (or carriage rates). Carriage density

is likely to be associated with infectiousness (Thors et al., 2016). A key question is whether vaccination impacts upon carriage density as well as carriage frequency, and thus on the infectiousness of carriers.

Protection against infectiousness provides a contribution to herd immunity over and above that resulting from protection against infection. On the other hand, if a vaccine only protects against disease, and does not reduce the risk of infection or reduce infectiousness, it does not contribute to herd immunity.

The effectiveness of a vaccine against infectiousness will be denoted VI. It is defined as the proportionate reduction in a susceptible individual's risk of infection when exposed to a vaccinated infectious person compared to when exposed to an unvaccinated infectious person. Thus:

$$VI = \frac{R_{ui} - R_{vi}}{R_{ui}},$$

where R_{ui} is the risk of infection from an unvaccinated infectious person and R_{vi} is the risk of infection from a vaccinated infectious person. VI may be expressed as a percentage by multiplying by 100:

$$VI = \frac{R_{ui} - R_{vi}}{R_{ui}} \times 100$$

or it may be written in the relative risk form:

$$VI = 1 - \frac{R_{vi}}{R_{ui}}.$$

Note that the quantities R_{ui} and R_{vi} are risks, usually calculated over the duration of exposure, or the duration of the infectious period if this is brief. For infections with long infectious periods (such as some sexually transmitted infections) the period of exposure relates to a contact during which transmission may take place (such as a sexual contact).

Because the definition of VI requires knowledge of exposure, its estimation (discussed in Chapter 14) is less straightforward than protective effectiveness, and is likely only to be practicable in secondary attack rate studies within households. Box 12.15 provides an example.

Box 12.15 Effectiveness against infectiousness: mumps vaccine in the Netherlands

A large mumps outbreak occurred in 2007 in areas of the Netherlands with low vaccine coverage. A study was undertaken in primary school children and their household contacts (Snijders et al., 2012). Within the household, the protective vaccine effectiveness was $VE = 67\%$, 95% CI 65% to 95%.

> Laboratory investigations found that viral titres were significantly lower, and mumps virus RNA was less likely to be found in throat swabs and urine samples, for vaccinated cases than for unvaccinated cases (Fanoy et al., 2011). These laboratory results suggest that vaccinated mumps cases may be less infectious than unvaccinated cases.
>
> Accordingly, the vaccine effectiveness against infectiousness was also estimated, and found to be $VI = 11\%$, 95% CI (–4%, 88%). The wide confidence interval, which includes zero, suggests low power.

The study reported in Box 12.15 found only a moderate mumps vaccine effectiveness against infectiousness. However, the laboratory investigations summarised there suggest that this effect, though it may be small, is likely to be genuine.

The wider implications of vaccine effectiveness against infection and infectiousness are explored in the next section.

12.5 Effectiveness against transmission and population impact on transmission

Both vaccine protective effectiveness (against infection, VE) and vaccine effectiveness against infectiousness (VI) are individual measures of effect: they describe how the vaccine, administered to an individual, affects that individual's potential for acquiring infection, and for infecting others, respectively. Thus, both relate to how an individual may transmit infection. In this section, we consider how vaccination affects transmission of infection within the wider population. The discussion is primarily conceptual: while there are some explicit expressions, their validity is usually subject to assumptions.

As a first step, the two measures VE and VI may be combined into an overall measure of the individual vaccine effectiveness against transmission, which is denoted VT. With some independence assumptions discussed in Farrington (2003), VT may be expressed in terms of VE and VI (both expressed as numbers less than 1, not as percentages) as follows:

$$VT = 1 - (1 - VE) \times (1 - VI).$$

The key conceptual aspect of this expression is that it emphasises the equivalent roles of protective vaccine effectiveness against infection VE, and vaccine effectiveness against infectiousness VI, as far as transmission is concerned. In particular, if the vaccine provides 100% protective effectiveness against infection, then $VE = 1$ and so $VT = 1$: vaccination completely interrupts transmission by vaccinated individuals. Exactly the same result is obtained if the vaccine provides 100% effectiveness against infectiousness, so that $VI = 1$: in this case also, $VT = 1$ and vaccination completely interrupts transmission by vaccinated individuals. Box 12.16 provides a practical example.

Box 12.16 Impact of mumps vaccination on household transmission in the Netherlands

This example is based on the study described in Box 12.15. Within households, the protective effectiveness conferred by mumps vaccination was $VE = 0.67$. This was against clinical mumps in conditions of household exposure; we shall assume the same value applies for protective effectiveness against infection. The vaccine effectiveness against infectiousness was $VI = 0.11$. Combining these gives the total vaccine effectiveness against transmission within households:

$$VT = 1 - (1 - 0.67) \times (1 - 0.11) = 0.71.$$

This means that vaccination reduces an individual's potential for transmitting mumps within the household by 71%. According to this formula, the effectiveness against transmission would be the same if the values of VE and VI were switched, that is, if $VE = 0.11$ and $VI = 0.67$.

The vaccine effectiveness against transmission VT is an individual effect in vaccinees. However, reducing the transmission potential of some individuals by vaccination affects the transmission of infection throughout the entire population, including unvaccinated individuals, who thereby benefit indirectly from the vaccination programme (see Chapters 4 and 5). In the last part of this section, we explore the connection between vaccine effectiveness against transmission, VT, and the impact of the vaccination programme on transmission in the population as a whole. Again, the discussion is primarily conceptual.

The impact of a vaccination programme on transmission of infection in the population may be defined as the relative reduction in the reproduction number of the infection in that population resulting from the vaccination programme. Thus, let R_0 denote the basic reproduction number, and R the effective reproduction number in the presence of a long-standing vaccination programme. (The basic and effective reproductions were introduced in Chapter 4.) The vaccination programme impact on transmission, denoted PT, is therefore:

$$PT = \frac{R_0 - R}{R_0} = 1 - \frac{R}{R_0}.$$

This impact depends on the vaccination coverage within the population, and on the individual vaccine effectiveness against transmission, VT. Under suitable assumptions, for example, that vaccination is randomly administered at birth (Farrington, 2003), the impact measure PT can also be expressed very simply in terms of the vaccine's effectiveness against transmission VT and the vaccine coverage P:

$$PT = P \times VT.$$

Reorganising these last two equations, the critical vaccination coverage P_c required so that $R=1$ (thus achieving the elimination of the infection) is

$$P_c = \frac{1}{VT} \times \left(1 - \frac{1}{R_0}\right).$$

These calculations are based on assumptions that may not be satisfied in practice. Nevertheless, expressions such as these can be used as rules of thumb to investigate the likely consequences of specific vaccination programmes. An illustration is provided in Box 12.17.

Box 12.17 Is elimination of mumps achievable?

Suppose that the mumps vaccine, in a given population, has protective effectiveness $VE = 0.8$ against infection and that its effectiveness against infectiousness is $VI = 0.10$. Thus, the vaccine effectiveness against transmission is

$$VT = 1 - (1-0.8) \times (1-0.1) = 0.82;$$

the contribution of the vaccine effectiveness against infectiousness in this case is small. If the maximum achievable vaccine coverage is $P = 0.95$, then the vaccine programme effectiveness is at most

$$PT = 0.95 \times 0.82 = 0.779.$$

In these circumstances, elimination can only be achieved if the basic reproduction number is less than

$$R_0 = \frac{1}{1-PT} = \frac{1}{1-0.779} = 4.5.$$

This value of R_0 for mumps is on the low side, so it is perhaps unlikely that elimination can be achieved in this population with this vaccine and this vaccine coverage.

In Box 12.17, the expression linking P_c, VT and R_0 was manipulated to obtain R_0 in terms of PT, because R_0 is seldom known with any degree of confidence. Simple calculations such as this are necessarily approximate, but can nevertheless provide useful benchmarks. More realistic calculations generally require mathematical modelling.

Summary

- Vaccine effectiveness (VE) measures individual protection against infection resulting from vaccination in field conditions. It contrasts with vaccine efficacy, established under experimental conditions in randomised clinical trials.

- $VE = 1 - RR$, where RR is the relative risk of infection in vaccinated compared to unvaccinated individuals.
- Vaccine effectiveness may also be assessed for clinical disease or for severe clinical disease. A vaccine may alter the clinical course of disease. This may be measured by effectiveness against disease progression, VP.
- Vaccine effectiveness against a clinical syndrome is usually lower than the effectiveness against a specific infection causing the syndrome, since the syndrome of interest will also include disease not caused by the targeted infection.
- Vaccines may also reduce the infectiousness of infected individuals. This may be quantified using VI, the vaccine effectiveness against infectiousness.
- The measures VE against infection and VI may be combined into a measure of the effectiveness of the vaccine against transmission, VT. VT and the vaccine coverage are related to the impact of the vaccination programme on the reproduction number of the infection.

References

Andrew, M. K., Shinde, V., Ye, L., Hatchette, T., Haguinet, F., Dos Santos, G., ... McNeil, S. (2017). The importance of frailty in the assessment of influenza vaccine effectiveness against influenza-related hospitalisation in elderly people. *Journal of Infectious Diseases, 216*, 405–414.

Armah, G. E., Sow, S. O., Breiman, R. F., Dallas, M. J., Tapia, M. D., Feikin, D. R., ... Neuzil, K. M. (2010). Efficacy of pentavalent rotavirus vaccine against severe rotavirus gastroenteritis in infants in developing countries in sub-Saharan Africa: A randomised, double-blind, placebo-controlled trial. *Lancet, 376*, 606–614.

Barbour, M. L., Mayon-White, R. T., Coles, C., Crook, D. W., & Moxon, E. R. (1995). The impact of conjugate vaccine on carriage of *Haemophilus influenzae* type b. *Journal of Infectious Diseases, 171*, 93–98.

Carter, R. J., Idriss, A., Widdowson, M. -A., Samai, M., Schrag, S. J., Legardy-Williams, J. K., ... Callis, A. (2018). Implementing a multisite clinical trial in the midst of an Ebola outbreak: Lessons learned from the Sierra Leone trial to introduce a vaccine against Ebola. *Journal of Infectious Diseases, 217*(Suppl. 1), S16–S23.

Cortese, M. M., Immergluck, L. C., Held, M., Jain, S., Chan, T., Grizas, A. P., ... Vásquez, M. (2013). Effectiveness of monovalent and pentavalent rotavirus vaccine. *Pediatrics, 132*(1), e25–e33.

Craig, L., Elliman, D., Heathcock, R., Turbill, D., Walsh, B., & Crowcroft, N. (2011). Pragmatic management of programmatic vaccination errors: Lessons learned from incidents in London. *Vaccine, 29*, 65–69.

Fanoy, E. B., Cremer, J., Ferreira, J. A., Dittrich, S., van Lier, A., Hahné, S. J., ... van Binnendijk, R. S. (2011). Transmission of mumps virus from mumps-vaccinated individuals to close contacts. *Vaccine, 29*, 9551–9556.

Farrington, C. P. (2003). On vaccine efficacy and reproduction numbers. *Mathematical Biosciences, 185*, 89–109.

Feikin, D. R., Scott, A. G., & Gessner, B. D. (2014). Use of vaccines as probes to define disease burden. *Lancet, 383*, 1762–1770.

Greenwood, M., & Yule, G. U. (1915). The statistics of anti-typhoid and anti-cholera inoculations, and the interpretation of such statistics in general. *Proceedings of the Royal Society of Medicine (Section of Epidemiology and State Medicine), 8*, 113–194.

Hall, A. J., Inskip, H. M., Loik, F., Day, N. E., O'Conor, G., Bosch, X., ... Parkin, M. (1987). The Gambia hepatitis intervention study. *Cancer Research*, *47*, 5782–5787.

Halloran, M. E., Longini, I. M., & Struchiner, C. J. (1999). Design and interpretation of vaccine field studies. *Epidemiologic Reviews*, *21*(1), 73–88.

Halloran, M. E., Longini, I. M., & Struchiner, C. J. (2010). *Design and analysis of vaccine studies*. New York: Springer.

Henao-Restrepo, A. M., Camacho, A., Longini, I. M., Watson, C. H., Edmunds, W. J., Egger, M., ... Dean, N. E. (2017). Efficacy and effectiveness of an rVSV-vectored vaccine in preventing Ebola virus disease: Final results from the Guinea ring vaccination, open-label, cluster-randomised trial (Ebola Ça Suffit!). *Lancet*, *389*, 505–518.

Im, J., Islam, T., Ahmmed, F., Kim, D. R., Chon, Y., Zaman, K., ... Clemens, J. D. (2019). Use of cholera vaccine as a vaccine probe to determine the burden of culture-negative cholera. *PLoS Neglected Tropical Diseases*, *13*(3), e0007179.

Jackson, L. A., Neuzil, K. M., Yu, O., Benson, P., Barlow, W. E., Adams, A. L., ... Thompson, W. W. (2003). Effectiveness of pneumococcal polysaccharide vaccine in older adults. *New England Journal of Medicine*, *348*, 1747–1755.

McVernon, J., Howard, A. J., Slack, M. P., & Ramsay, M. E. (2004). Long-term impact of vaccination on *Haemophilus influenzae* type b (Hib) carriage in the United Kingdom. *Epidemiology and Infection*, *132*, 765–767.

Ohmit, S. E., Petrie, J. G., Malosh, R. E., Cowling, B. J., Thompson, M. G., Shay, D. K., & Monto, A. S. (2013). Influenza vaccine effectiveness in the community and the household. *Clinical Infectious Diseases*, *56*(10), 1363–1369.

Patel, M., Pedreira, C., De Oliveira, L. H., Tate, J., Leshem, E., Mercado, J., ... Parashar, U. (2016). Effectiveness of pentavalent rotavirus vaccine against a diverse range of circulating strains in Nicaragua. *Clinical Infectious Diseases*, *62*(Suppl. 2), S127–S132.

Pletz, M. W., Maus, U., Krug, N., Welte, T., & Lode, H. (2008). Pneumococcal vaccines: Mechanism of action, impact on epidemiology and adaption of the species. *International Journal of Antimicrobial Agents*, *32*, 199–206.

Préziosi, M. -P., & Halloran, M. H. (2003). Effects of pertussis vaccination on disease: Vaccine efficacy in reducing clinical severity. *Clinical Infectious Diseases*, *37*, 772–779.

Qureshi, H., Gessner, B. D., Leboulleux, D., Hasan, H., Alam, S. E., & Moulton, L. H. (2000). The incidence of vaccine-preventable influenza-like illness and medication among Pakistani pilgrims to the Haj in Saudi Arabia. *Vaccine*, *18*, 2956–2962.

Snijders, B. E., van Lier, A., van de Kassteele, J., Fanoy, E. B., Ruijs, W. L., Hulsof, F., ... Hahné, S. J. (2012). Mumps vaccine effectiveness in primary schools and households, the Netherlands, 2008. *Vaccine*, *30*, 2999–3002.

Tate, J. E., Ngabo, F., Donnen, P., Gatera, M., Uwimana, J., Rugambwa, C., ... Parashar, U. D. (2016). Effectiveness of pentavalent rotavirus vaccine under conditions of routine use in Rwanda. *Clinical Infectious Diseases*, *62*(Suppl. 2), S208–S212.

Thors, V., Morales-Aza, B., Pidwill, G., Vipond, I., Muir, P., & Finn, A. (2016). Population density profiles of nasopharyngeal carriage of 5 bacterial species in pre-school children measured using quantitative PCR offer potential insights into the dynamics of transmission. *Human Vaccines and Immunotherapeutics*, *12*(2).

Treanor, J. J., Talbot, H. K., Ohmit, S. E., Coleman, L. A., Thompson, M. G., Cheng, P. -Y., ... Shay, D. K. (2012). Effectiveness of seasonal influenza vaccines in the United States during a season with circulation of all three vaccine strains. *Clinical Infectious Diseases*, *55*(7), 951–959.

Vesikari, T., Matson, D. O., Dennehy, P., van Damme, P., Santosham, M., Rodriguez, Z., ... Heaton, P. M. (2006). Safety and efficacy of a pentavalent human–bovine (WC3) reassortant rotavirus vaccine. *New England Journal of Medicine*, *354*, 23–33.

Viviani, S., Carrieri, P., Bah, E., Hall, A. J., Kirk, G. D., Mendy, M., ... Hainaut, P. (2008). 20 years into the Gambia hepatitis intervention trial: Assessment of initial hypotheses and prospects for evaluation of protective effectiveness against cancer. *Cancer Epidemiology, Biomarkers and Prevention, 17*(11), 3216–3223.

Zaman, K., Anh, D. D., Victor, J. C., Shin, S., Yunus, M., Dallas, M. J., ... Ciarlet, M. (2010). Efficacy of pentavalent rotavirus vaccine against severe rotavirus gastroenteritis in infants in developing countries in Asia: A randomised, double-blind, placebo-controlled trial. *Lancet, 376*, 615–623.

Chapter 13

Estimating vaccine effectiveness
General methodological principles

This is the first of four chapters about epidemiological study designs that are commonly used for estimating vaccine effectiveness. We focus in these four chapters entirely on methods for estimating field effectiveness for vaccines routinely used in vaccination programmes. General references for the material in the present and next two chapters include Orenstein et al. (1985), Orenstein, Bernier, and Hinman (1988) and Halloran, Longini, and Struchiner (2010).

Assessing efficacy of vaccines used in routine programmes by means of randomised trials with an unvaccinated control group is usually considered to be unethical, since the control group is deprived of a vaccine they would normally be offered. (Non-inferiority trials, in which a new, potentially better vaccine is compared to the existing vaccine, may be acceptable.) Thus, vaccine effectiveness is assessed using observational studies. These share the strengths, but also the shortcomings, of epidemiological studies in other application areas. One such strength is that the vaccine is evaluated in the population for which it is intended, using routine vaccine delivery methods, rather than the more artificial setting of a trial. Also, observational studies can be larger, or of longer duration, than may be possible under experimental conditions and can examine a broader range of outcomes.

Field studies should aspire to retain as much as possible of the rigour that characterises randomised controlled studies. Ideally, they should be based on a study plan or protocol that has been set out in advance. This plan should state the primary and secondary study questions, specify the inclusion and exclusion criteria for the study, define case and exposure definitions and laboratory procedures and describe data collection and analysis methods. Steps should be taken where possible to avoid selection and information biases by using rigorous, validated procedures for case ascertainment and assessment of vaccination histories. Case ascertainment should be independent of vaccination history, and adjustments should be made as required to minimise the impact of potential confounders. Evidence of vaccination status should be documented where possible. Procedures for handling incomplete data should be specified. Nevertheless, however

DOI: 10.4324/9781315166414-14
This Chapter has been made available under a CC-BY-NC-ND license.

carefully planned and executed they are, there is no getting round the fact that field studies of vaccine effectiveness evidently, and fundamentally, differ from randomised studies in one crucial respect: the absence of randomisation, which is the most effective tool to avoid bias.

In this chapter we discuss general methodological issues relevant to field studies of vaccine effectiveness. These include: the choice of case definitions in Section 13.1; biases due to misclassification of disease and vaccination status, and inclusion of prior cases, in Section 13.2; confounding bias including indication bias and healthy vaccine bias in Section 13.3; bias-indicator studies in Section 13.4; and the choice of epidemiologic measures (risks or rates) to calculate vaccine effectiveness and their impact on vaccine effectiveness in Section 13.5. We end with some brief remarks about modelling frameworks in Section 13.6. All of these issues are relevant to the specific designs of vaccination effectiveness studies that are discussed in Chapter 14 to 16.

13.1 Influence of case definitions on vaccine effectiveness estimates

An important early step in any analytical epidemiological study, including vaccination effectiveness studies, is to agree on the criteria that define a case, which may include laboratory as well as clinical components. When assessing protection against disease, the clinical criterion in the case definition is usually chosen towards the more severe end of the clinical spectrum. For example, the effectiveness of influenza vaccines is often evaluated for purely clinical end points or syndromes such as influenza-like illness (ILI) or death. Depending on the aim of the study, the clinical criterion may be combined with laboratory evidence of infection by the pathogen targeted by vaccination. When the aim is to assess vaccine effectiveness against infection, relatively mild clinical symptoms are used to identify potential cases, from whom biological samples are then collected and sent for laboratory confirmation.

When the case definition includes laboratory confirmation, it is important to realise that vaccination may affect the performance of the laboratory method used to confirm cases. Furthermore, if the vaccine modifies the clinical course of disease, different clinical case definitions may produce different vaccine effectiveness estimates, a possibility that should be taken into account when comparing studies that have used different case definitions. The example in Box 13.1 is drawn from the reanalysis of a randomised clinical trial, and shows that, even in such controlled conditions, case definitions can have a large influence on results.

Box 13.1 Pertussis vaccine effectiveness: the influence of case definitions

In 1986–1987, a placebo-controlled randomised trial of acellular pertussis vaccines was undertaken in Sweden. We describe the results for one vaccine containing only pertussis toxin. These were disappointing: the vaccine efficacy was only 54% against culture-confirmed pertussis. However, a reanalysis of the data showed

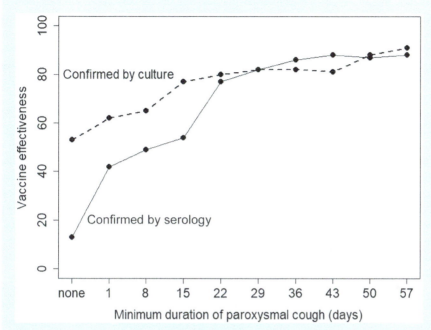

Figure 13.1 **Vaccine effectiveness of acellular pertussis vaccine by confirmation method and duration of paroxysmal cough.**
Source: Adapted from Storsaeter et al. (1990).

that the effectiveness of the vaccine depended very much on the case definition (Storsaeter et al., 1990). Figure 13.1 shows the results of one reanalysis.

If pertussis infection was confirmed by serology, the vaccine effectiveness (VE) increased from 13%, 95% confidence interval (CI) (−28%, 41%) when all cases were included, irrespective of symptoms, to 88%, 95% CI (67%, 95%) for cases with paroxysmal coughs of 57 days or more. If confirmation was done by culture, the effectiveness increased from 53%, 95% CI (24%, 71%) for all cases, irrespective of symptoms, to 87%, 95% CI (66%, 95%) for cases with paroxysmal cough of 57 days or more.

Thus Figure 13.1 shows that, while the vaccine may not offer much protection against infection, it does offer substantial protection ($VE > 80\%$) against typical whooping cough with more than 28 days' paroxysmal cough.

The effectiveness gradient apparent in Figure 13.1 suggests that the vaccine modifies disease: cases in vaccinated individuals tend to be less severe than cases in unvaccinated individuals. Furthermore, the vaccine effectiveness against mild disease depends on the method used for confirming infection. The difference between culture and serological confirmation may be due to lower sensitivity of culture in less severe vaccinated cases, or lack of specificity of the serological criterion in less severe cases (sensitivity and specificity are discussed further in Section 13.2). The authors considered the second possibility to be less likely.

The fact that the vaccine effectiveness may depend on the case definition (irrespective of issues of misclassification, which are discussed in Section 13.2) makes it all the more important that the primary purpose of the study, and the primary case definition to be used to meet that purpose, are agreed in advance. On the other hand, it is often informative to undertake supplementary analyses with different case definitions. As illustrated in Box 13.1, vaccine effectiveness may be better represented by a vaccine effectiveness profile than by a single numerical value.

13.2 Biases due to misclassification and prior infections

Vaccine effectiveness studies involve classifying individuals according to their vaccination status, and according to their disease (or infection) status. Misclassification errors occur when either categorisation is incorrect, and may introduce bias. If the misclassification errors occur at random, they will bias the vaccine effectiveness towards zero. However, if the errors are not random, vaccine effectiveness estimates may be biased up or down. These biases, and their likely impact on vaccine effectiveness in different study designs, are described in De Smedt et al. (2018), who also provide a web-based simulation tool to study them.

To minimise misclassification, evidence of vaccination should be documented where possible, whether from immunisation registers, clinic data or family-held vaccination cards, since information based on recall is likely to be inaccurate. Careful thought should be given as to whether absence of evidence of vaccination constitutes evidence of no vaccination; this is likely to depend on the specific circumstances of each study. An example of the impact on vaccine effectiveness and the source of vaccination data is given in Box 13.2.

Box 13.2 Measles vaccine effectiveness under routine conditions in Tanzania

A study was undertaken to assess the protective effectiveness of measles vaccination in Dar Es Salaam, Tanzania, in 1986–1988. The study was a matched case-control study (see Chapter 15) in children aged 9 months to 8 years. Some 172 cases were obtained from hospital admissions; four age- and sex-matched neighbourhood controls were obtained for each case (Killewo, Makwaya, Munubhi, & Mpembeni, 1991).

Vaccination status of cases and controls was ascertained using two methods: by mother's recall and by vaccination cards; in each case children with missing information were excluded from the analysis. The vaccine effectiveness calculated using recalled vaccination history was VE = 51% with 95% CI (30%, 65%). On the other hand, when the calculation of vaccine effectiveness was based on vaccination cards, VE = 78% with 95% CI (57%, 89%).

The authors surmise that mothers of some measles cases without vaccination cards may have been unwilling to say their children had not been vaccinated, which would bias VE downwards. Random recall error would also result in underestimation of VE.

In the study described in Box 13.2, vaccine effectiveness was calculated using two methods for ascertaining vaccination histories, which allows some assessment to be made of the reliability of the results and the magnitude of possible biases.

For multi-dose vaccines, the vaccinated group might include only those individuals having received a full vaccination course according to the recommended schedule; depending on the aim of the study, it might alternatively include all individuals having received one or more doses of vaccine. Whatever definition is used for the vaccinated group, individuals who have received the vaccine but who do not meet this definition should be excluded. Such exclusions also apply to control groups obtained from coverage surveys or vaccine uptake statistics (as used in the case-cohort and screening methods to be described in Chapter 15).

For some vaccines, vaccinated individuals take some time to mount an immune response, and in this case the follow-up time should begin at this point: the period between vaccination and the time the individual is deemed to be fully protected should not be included in the analysis. Likewise, cases arising in this time interval should be excluded.

Cases should be ascertained independently of vaccination (with vaccination status concealed if possible), using objective criteria. All cases should be ascertained with the same methods, applied with the same intensity irrespective of vaccination status. An example of the bias that may ensue when this is not the case is given in Box 13.3.

Box 13.3 Pertussis vaccine effectiveness and notifications in Wales

A study was undertaken to estimate the effectiveness of pertussis vaccine during an outbreak in the St David's area of Wales in 1987 (Palmer, 1991). The cases arising in children aged 1–6 years in the outbreak area were identified using a parental questionnaire. Cases were children formally notified to the local authority as having pertussis, or children with a cough lasting 2 weeks or more, accompanied by vomiting, whooping or choking. The clinical symptoms of the notified and non-notified cases were similar.

Vaccine effectiveness based on notified cases alone was 88%, with 95% CI (68%, 95%). Based on notified and non-notified cases, VE dropped to 75%, with 95% CI (56%, 89%). The author ascribed the difference to the propensity of local physicians not to formally notify cases whom they knew had been vaccinated. Thus, vaccine effectiveness estimates based on notifications data are likely to be biased upwards owing to differential misclassification of disease status.

As described in Section 13.1, cases are identified using clinical symptoms that define a threshold of clinical severity, and may be confirmed using laboratory methods to identify the causative pathogen. This often leads to a hierarchy of cases according to the degree of diagnostic certainty: for example, cases may be definite, probable or possible. Usually, only definite, or definite and probable, cases are included in vaccine effectiveness calculations.

The degree of misclassification of disease status is often expressed in terms of the sensitivity, specificity and positive predictive value of the case definition in a given population; these quantities were defined in Chapter 8. If the sensitivity or specificity of the case definition differs according to whether individuals are vaccinated or unvaccinated, the ensuing misclassification is said to be differential. Otherwise, it is called non-differential misclassification.

Provided that the case definition is 100% specific, suboptimal sensitivity does not bias vaccine effectiveness unless the sensitivity is related to vaccination, and thus results in differential misclassification. For example, if the vaccine reduces severity of disease, vaccinated cases may be less likely to be detected, leading to overestimation of vaccine effectiveness.

In contrast, low specificity will generally bias vaccine effectiveness towards zero, even with non-differential misclassification. This is because the vaccine affords no protection against cases of disease not attributable to the infection. The bias arises even with 100% sensitivity. If the case definition is less than 100% specific, suboptimal sensitivity further increases the magnitude of the bias.

In vaccine effectiveness studies, the positive predictive value (PPV) is often more readily obtained than the specificity and sensitivity. The PPV may be estimated by laboratory testing of a random subsample of cases meeting the case definition, to estimate the proportion of true cases. The PPV for vaccinated cases depends on vaccine effectiveness (it is zero in vaccinated cases if $VE = 100\%$) and, as a result, the PPV is usually lower in vaccinated compared to unvaccinated cases even for non-differential sensitivity and specificity. The PPV in unvaccinated cases is most useful: a high value is essential to avoid serious bias. These effects are illustrated in Box 13.4.

Box 13.4 Sensitivity, specificity, PPV and bias in vaccine effectiveness

Suppose that there are 1,000 vaccinated and 1,000 unvaccinated children, that the risk of infection is 10% over the study period and that vaccine effectiveness is 80%. So, there are 100 true cases in unvaccinated and 20 true cases in vaccinated children (all such numbers in this example are values expected on average).

Suppose first that the case definition is 100% specific but only 50% sensitive, as might arise when using laboratory confirmation. Of the true cases, 50 are classified as unvaccinated cases and 10 as vaccinated cases; the rest are classified as not meeting the case definition (which might include 'possible' cases). The estimated vaccine effectiveness is

$$VE = 1 - \frac{10/1,000}{50/1,000} = 80\%.$$

Thus, there is no bias, because misclassification due to insensitivity of the case definition was non-differential and the specificity was 100%. Note also that the full denominators were used: possible cases, if any had been so defined, were not excluded.

Now suppose that the case definition is 95% specific and 100% sensitive, as might be the case for a clinical case definition. Then, the 100 true unvaccinated cases and the 20 true vaccinated cases are all classified as cases. But 5% of non-cases in each group are also classified as cases: these include 45 (5% of 900) in the unvaccinated group and 49 (5% of 980) in the vaccinated group. So, the total numbers of cases, according to the case definition, are 145 in the unvaccinated group and 69 in the vaccinated group. The vaccine effectiveness, based on these cases, is

$$VE = 1 - \frac{69/1,000}{145/1,000} = 52\%$$

and so, the vaccine effectiveness is severely biased towards zero, even though the specificity did not depend on vaccination status. This is because the vaccine cannot be expected to protect against clinical symptoms that are not caused by the infection.

In this latter scenario (with 100% sensitivity and 95% specificity) the positive predictive values (denoted PPV) in unvaccinated and vaccinated cases are, respectively,

$$PPV_{unvac} = \frac{100}{145} = 69\%, \quad PPV_{vac} = \frac{20}{69} = 29\%.$$

The PPV is lower for vaccinated cases than for unvaccinated cases, as expected since $VE > 0$. In this example, a PPV of 69% in unvaccinated cases is insufficient to avoid bias in VE.

If the case definition is both 50% sensitive and 95% specific, then there are $50 + 45 = 95$ unvaccinated cases and $10 + 49 = 59$ vaccinated cases. This gives:

$$VE = 38\%, \quad PPV_{unvac} = 53\%, \quad PPV_{vac} = 17\%.$$

Note that low sensitivity compounds the effect of incomplete specificity, resulting in increased bias in VE. The low PPV in unvaccinated cases signals the presence of serious bias.

Case definitions with or without laboratory confirmation of the pathogen involved will generally lead to similar vaccine effectiveness estimates when the incidence is high and the clinical syndrome is both sensitive and highly specific, such as during outbreaks, or in some highly endemic situations, yielding a high PPV in unvaccinated cases. Otherwise, the vaccine effectiveness obtained without laboratory confirmation of cases may be appreciably biased towards zero.

From a public health perspective, it may be relevant to assess effectiveness explicitly relating to a clinically defined syndrome, since it quantifies the contribution a vaccine can make to improving health of a local population. However, vaccine effectiveness estimates against a clinical syndrome obtained in a certain population may not be extrapolated to other populations where the attribution of the syndrome to different pathogens may vary. The choice of case definition is discussed in Box 13.5 in relation to the study of measles in Tanzania discussed in Box 13.2.

> **Box 13.5 Case definition and ascertainment for the Tanzanian measles vaccine study**
>
> The study described in Box 13.2 used cases admitted to hospital with a clinical measles diagnosis based on fever, morbilliform rash, cough, coryza and conjunctivitis. Only cases with all four of these signs or symptoms were included in the study. No serological test was used to confirm the diagnosis, owing to limited availability and cost.
>
> Although the case definition used was entirely based on clinical criteria, the authors comment that non-measles conditions mimicking such strict criteria are rare. Thus, the clinical case definition is highly specific. In addition, measles was endemic in Tanzania. Thus, a sizeable bias due to misclassification of disease status is unlikely in this study.
>
> As noted by the study authors, cases ascertainment from admissions to hospital has the potential to introduce a selection bias, if vaccinated children are more likely to present to hospital than unvaccinated children (perhaps in relation to their socio-economic background). This would tend to bias the vaccine effectiveness downwards.

Whether individuals with prior infections should be excluded is a difficult question, the answer to which depends at least partly on how the vaccine works. In any case, it is often problematic to identify all prior infections, owing to the presence of subclinical or mild infections (as with polio and mumps, for example) and inadequate recall. Including or excluding prior infections does not generally make much difference provided that the risk of infection and cumulative incidence are low. However, when the risk or cumulative incidence is high, as may be the case when the study includes older children, an appreciable bias may arise. This issue will be discussed further in Chapter 16.

Additional analyses, undertaken to quantify the impact of different definitions or different procedures from those used in the primary analysis, are called sensitivity analyses. If a wide range of VE values are obtained under different plausible assumptions, it is difficult to reach firm conclusions. However, sensitivity analyses may also show that the results are robust to variations in definitions and procedures (i.e., the vaccine effectiveness does not vary much according to what choices are made). Such an example is described in Box 13.6.

Box 13.6 Measles vaccine effectiveness in Pakistan

In 1990, a measles outbreak was reported in an area of Pakistan where vaccine coverage was thought to be high. An investigation to assess vaccine effectiveness was undertaken among children aged 9 months to 13 years living in one village within this area (Murray & Rasmussen, 2000).

Vaccination status was determined using vaccination cards; children without cards were classified as unvaccinated provided their parents were sure the children never had been vaccinated. Measles histories were determined from interviews with the parents, and classified as measles during the outbreak, measles before the outbreak and no measles. Four different estimates of vaccine effectiveness were calculated:

(a) risks calculated irrespective of prior measles history;
(b) excluding all children with measles prior to the outbreak;
(c) excluding only children with measles prior to the outbreak in a known outbreak year;
(d) excluding children without a vaccination card.

In addition, the analyses were repeated using only household contacts of primary cases, to control for exposure, thus making eight analyses in total. All analyses were adjusted for age group and religious group.

The adjusted estimates of vaccine effectiveness for these eight analyses ranged from 81%, 95% CI (69%, 89%), to 89%, 95% CI (76%, 91%), providing robust evidence that the vaccine was effective. The measles outbreak was not caused, as had been feared, by a breakdown in the cold chain. The authors found that vaccine coverage was very low among members of a local minority religious group, and that the outbreak began within this community before spreading to the rest of the village.

13.3 Confounding bias

Confounding bias arises in epidemiological studies when the relationship between an exposure and a disease outcome is altered by a third variable (called a confounder), which is associated with both the exposure and the disease. Confounding may introduce a spurious association when there is none, alter the strength or direction of the association or conceal a true association.

In observational studies of vaccine effectiveness, vaccines have not been administered at random within the population. This may result in confounding bias if a variable associated with vaccination is also associated with exposure to a pathogen, or with the probability of infection given exposure or with a clinical outcome of interest. The bias may be in either direction. The numerical example in Box 13.7 was constructed so as to illustrate this important phenomenon.

Box 13.7 Confounding bias in vaccine effectiveness studies

Suppose that 101 of 1,100 vaccinated persons get the infection, compared to 180 of 1,100 unvaccinated persons. The vaccine effectiveness is apparently

$$VE = 1 - \frac{101/1,100}{180/1,100} = 0.4388,$$

or about 44%. But now suppose that the data come from two subgroups, A and B. The subgroups might be different locations, or different age groups, or different socio-economic categories, or some other defined subsets. In subgroup A, there are 1,000 vaccinated persons, 100 of whom get infected, and 100 unvaccinated persons of whom 90 get infected.

So, the vaccine effectiveness in subgroup A is:

$$VE_A = 1 - \frac{100/1,000}{90/100} = 0.8888,$$

or about 89%. In subgroup B, there is just one case among the 100 vaccinated persons and 90 cases among the 1000 unvaccinated persons. So, the vaccine effectiveness in subgroup B is:

$$VE_B = 1 - \frac{1/100}{90/1,000} = 0.8888,$$

or about 89% as in subgroup A. Thus, in both subgroups the vaccine effectiveness is 89%. The value 44% obtained when combining subgroups A and B is biased: the grouping variable confounds the association. This is because vaccination coverage and incidence are both high in subgroup A, and both low in subgroup B, so the group variable is associated both with vaccination and with incidence of infection: it is a confounder.

The correct approach is to adjust for the confounder, which means taking a suitably weighted average of the results stratified by the levels of the confounding variable. In this case, $VE = 89\%$ in each subgroup, so the vaccine effectiveness adjusted for the grouping variable, being a weighted average, is also $VE = 89\%$.

Variables that are strongly associated with both the likelihood of receiving a vaccine and with disease incidence are possible confounders. The standard techniques for handling confounders, provided information is available on them, is to stratify by the confounding variable (as in Box 13.7), or to adjust for them in a multiple regression model. Control of confounding may also be improved by matching, followed by an analysis that adjusts for the matching variables. Other techniques include propensity scores – in which the propensity of each individual to be vaccinated is allowed for in the statistical model.

These statistical techniques are standard tools in epidemiology, but the details lie beyond the scope of this book.

The example in Box 13.7 was constructed to demonstrate how confounding arises. The example in Box 13.8 illustrates just how substantial the impact of such confounders can be in practice.

Box 13.8 Effectiveness of rotavirus vaccination in the United Kingdom

Rotavirus vaccination was introduced in the routine childhood immunisation programme in the United Kingdom in 2013. The oral monovalent vaccine is administered in two doses at 2 and 3 months of age; high vaccination coverage was rapidly achieved.

A 2-year study was undertaken to assess the effectiveness of the vaccine, using the test-negative case-control design (this will be described in Chapter 15). The vaccine effectiveness reported here was calculated for two doses of vaccine, against confirmed wild-type rotavirus infection, using data obtained from an enhanced national surveillance programme, with vaccination information obtained from GPs (Walker et al., 2019). The aggregated raw data are in Table 13.1.

Based on these aggregated data, the vaccine effectiveness is $VE = 45\%$ with 95% CI (28%, 58%); how VE is obtained from these data will be explained in Chapter 15. However, after adjusting for age in months, and for the month and year of onset of symptoms, the adjusted vaccine effectiveness was $VE = 77\%$ with 95% CI (66%, 85%).

Thus, VE would have been seriously underestimated if the confounding effects of age and time had not been adjusted in the analysis.

Table 13.1 **Effectiveness of two doses of rotavirus vaccine against confirmed wild-type infection**

Vaccine doses received	Confirmed cases	Controls
2	277	653
0	133	173

The type of adjustment for measured confounders undertaken in Box 13.8 is standard: age and time are obvious potential confounders, since vaccination and disease are both age- and time-dependent, and they are easily measured. However, some confounders are more difficult to measure, or even to define in a relevant manner. This is especially the case for variables relating to propensity to vaccinate, for example socio-economic status and underlying state of health.

If persons more likely to be infected (or to become ill once infected) are also those more likely to be vaccinated, then VE will be biased downwards. This bias is called bias by indication. On the other hand, if persons less likely to be infected (or to become ill) are those more likely to be vaccinated, then VE will be biased upwards. This bias is sometimes called a healthy vaccinee bias.

Biases due to confounding by indication or healthy vaccinee bias can be difficult to handle. This is illustrated in Box 13.9.

Box 13.9 Does vaccination against seasonal influenza reduce all-cause mortality?

Many studies, undertaken in different countries, have reported that seasonal influenza vaccination is associated with a reduction in all-cause mortality during the influenza season, the vaccine effectiveness against mortality in the elderly being of the order of 50%. However, a systematic review, including 12 studies reporting on all-cause mortality, suggested that both confounding by indication and a healthy vaccinee effect may be present, to varying degree, in many such studies (Remschmidt, Wichmann, & Harder, 2015).

Evidence for confounding by indication comes from the fact that adjustment for measured confounders, including comorbidities, led to an increase in vaccine effectiveness for all-cause mortality in 11 of the 12 studies. The increase was 12% on average.

Evidence for a healthy vaccinee bias comes from the observation that influenza vaccination appears to be associated with a large reduction in mortality even when no influenza virus would be expected to be circulating. This was observed for all 12 studies. For 8, the vaccine effectiveness was statistically significantly greater than zero outside the influenza season.

Confounding both by indication and by healthy vaccinee bias was found to affect studies of other non-specific outcomes, namely all-cause hospitalisation, and ILI. The authors warn against the use of non-specific outcomes in studies of influenza vaccine effectiveness in the elderly.

In observational studies, it is seldom possible to be sure that all confounders have been taken into account. In the next section an alternative approach is described.

13.4 Bias-indicator studies

In some circumstances, an additional analysis may be planned with a specially chosen negative control, in order to verify the validity of the main effectiveness study (Lipsitch, Tchetgen Tchetgen, & Cohen, 2010). Using events outside the influenza season as negative controls in studying the effectiveness of influenza vaccination, as described in Box 13.9, was such an example. This type of study has been described as a bias-indicator study.

The approach is a fruitful one, in that it can provide some evidence of the validity or otherwise of the study design and analysis, including the procedures used for ascertaining vaccination status and disease outcomes. An example is given in Box 13.10.

> ### Box 13.10 Effectiveness and bias-indicator study of oral cholera vaccination in rural Haiti
>
> A reactive cholera vaccination campaign was undertaken in Haiti in 2012, in response to a major cholera epidemic of *Vibrio cholera* O1 that began in 2010. The vaccine used was an oral vaccine administered in two doses. A field evaluation of the effectiveness of the vaccine was subsequently undertaken (Ivers et al., 2015).
>
> Participants were residents of the study areas who were eligible for vaccination during the campaign (over 12 months of age and not pregnant). Two case-control analyses were undertaken, using contrasting end points and verified vaccination status. The first was a vaccine effectiveness evaluation using the end point of acute watery diarrhoea testing culture positive for *Vibrio cholerae* O1. The vaccine effectiveness was 58% with 95% CI (13% to 80%).
>
> The second analysis was a bias-indicator study, using the end point of acute watery diarrhoea testing negative for cholera by culture and by another, rapid, detection method. The vaccine effectiveness was –21%, with 95% CI ranging from –238% to 57%, thus not statistically significant.
>
> This provides some evidence that the first analysis was not biased. If the vaccine had been shown to be effective against this supplementary end point, this would have cast doubt on the validity of the main findings. The results suggest that the vaccine effectiveness estimate of 58% is not obviously biased by artefacts related to the study design.

The example in Box 13.10 was a case-control study, but the same principle may be applied to any study design. The key is to choose a vaccine-event pair for which there should be no association, and for which the same ascertainment procedures and adjustments apply as in the main study. Bias-indicator studies, provided they have sufficient power, can provide some evidence of the validity or otherwise of the main study design. However, while the presence of bias can be identified in this way, the precise source of the bias cannot.

13.5 Vaccine effectiveness based on risks and rates

In Section 13.1, we expressed the vaccine effectiveness in terms of the relative risk (RR) of infection associated with vaccination:

$$VE = 1 - \frac{R_v}{R_u} = 1 - RR,$$

where R_v and R_u denoted the risk of infection in vaccinated and unvaccinated individuals, respectively. However, to keep matters simple at that stage, we did not make it clear over what period these risks are calculated, nor whether only people who are at risk of infection at the start of observation are included. These decisions can influence the estimate of VE that is obtained. It is therefore important to make such decisions explicit and to understand their implications.

We will take the expression 'being at risk of infection' to mean that a person can potentially become infected because of not having acquired immunity from prior infection. In this sense, a vaccinated person is at risk of infection, if they do not benefit from such natural immunity: vaccine-induced immunity does not feature in this definition. Similarly, 'time at risk of infection', or 'time at risk' for short, is time prior to developing immunity through infection. These definitions are particularly relevant when applied to infections that confer lasting immunity.

As it turns out, a range of different but related epidemiological measures can be used to measure the chance of infection, all of which may be used to calculate VE. We will begin by defining these various measures more precisely. Then, we will outline how the choice of measure can influence the estimate of VE that is obtained.

The risk of infection π_T over a defined period between times 0 and T is the probability of infection in this period in individuals at risk of infection. In a sample, it is estimated thus:

$$\pi_T = \frac{Number\ of\ persons\ infected\ between\ 0\ and\ T}{Number\ of\ persons\ at\ risk\ at\ time\ 0}. \quad (13.1)$$

Being a probability, π_T is a number between 0 and 1, and is dimensionless.

The rate of infection (or incidence of infection) between 0 and T, on the other hand, is the expected number of infections per unit time at risk. In a sample it is estimated thus:

$$\lambda_T = \frac{Number\ of\ infections\ between\ 0\ and\ T}{Total\ person\ time\ at\ risk\ between\ 0\ and\ T}. \quad (13.2)$$

The rate λ_T cannot be negative, but can exceed 1, and is expressed as a number per unit of time. Confusingly, the risk of infection is sometimes referred to as the attack rate, when in fact the terms 'risk' and 'rate' refer to different quantities. In practice, the distinction only really matters when the chance of infection is high, so that both risk and rate are high.

The rate λ_T is more precisely an average rate (or average incidence) over the time interval 0 to T. In contrast, the instantaneous incidence rate $\lambda(t)$ at time t is the probability of infection of an individual at risk of infection during a small interval of time after t, divided by the duration of this small time interval. It is also called the hazard, or incidence density, or force of infection.

When we sum this instantaneous incidence rate $\lambda(t)$ over the period from 0 to T, we obtain the cumulative incidence Λ_T (also called cumulative incidence rate) over the period from 0 to T:

$$\Lambda_T = \int_0^T \lambda(t)dt.$$

The integral sign just indicates summation over vanishingly short intervals dt. Like the risk, Λ_T is a dimensionless quantity, but like the rate, it can take non-negative values and, in particular, it can exceed 1. When the instantaneous incidence rate $\lambda(t)$ is constant over the period 0 to T, it equals the average incidence rate λ_T, and then there is a simple relationship between the instantaneous, average and cumulative incidence rates:

$$\lambda(t) = \lambda_T = \frac{\Lambda_T}{T}. \tag{13.3}$$

Finally, there is a very important relationship between risk and cumulative incidence, as follows:

$$\pi_T = 1 - e^{-\Lambda_T}, \text{ or } \Lambda_T = -\log(1 - \pi_T), \tag{13.4}$$

where log is the natural logarithm (in base e), sometimes also written ln. The relationship described in expressions (Equation 13.4) applies to infections that confer long-lasting immunity. When the infection does not confer lasting immunity, so that individuals can become reinfected, the relationship applies to first infections. Box 13.11 illustrates these different quantities.

Box 13.11 Risks and rates

Suppose there are 100 vaccinated and 100 unvaccinated children in a school, all previously uninfected. During an outbreak lasting 8 weeks, 40 of the vaccinated and 80 of the unvaccinated children become infected; once infected, children are no longer at risk of this infection.

Consider the vaccinated group. At least four different epidemiologic measures can be calculated in this example. The *risk* of infection in vaccinated children is

$$\pi_T = 40/100 = 0.40 \text{ (from Equation 13.1)}.$$

The *cumulative incidence* in vaccinated children over the 8 weeks of the outbreak is

$$\Lambda_T = -\log(1 - 0.40) = 0.5108 \text{ (from Equation 13.4)}.$$

If the *instantaneous incidence rate* $\lambda(t)$ is constant over the duration of the outbreak, the *average incidence rate* in vaccinated children is:

$$\lambda_T = \frac{\Lambda_T}{T} = \frac{0.5108}{8} = 0.064 \text{ per week (from Equation 13.3)}.$$

Table 13.2 Numbers infected per week in vaccinated and unvaccinated groups

Week	1	2	3	4	5	6	7	8	Not infected
Vaccinated	15	12	6	3	2	1	0	1	60
Unvaccinated	26	24	11	8	5	3	2	1	20

If the incidence rate $\lambda(t)$ is not constant, then Equation 13.2 is used to calculate the average infection rate. To do this we need to calculate the total person-time at risk. Suppose that the numbers infected in each week of the outbreak are as in Table 13.2.

Consider the vaccinated group. The 60 not infected each contribute 8 full weeks of person-time. The 15 infected in week 1 each contribute 0.5 week, assuming they are infected mid-week on average, and similarly for the other weeks. Thus, the total person-time at risk in vaccinees is:

$$15 \times 0.5 + 12 \times 1.5 + 6 \times 2.5 + 3 \times 3.5 + 2 \times 4.5 + 1 \times 5.5 + 0 \times 6.5 + 1 \times 7.5 + 60 \times 8$$
$$= 553 \text{ person-weeks}.$$

Hence the *average incidence rate* in vaccinated children is

$$\lambda_T = \frac{40}{553} = 0.072 \text{ per week (from Equation 13.2)}.$$

The corresponding values for the unvaccinated group are: risk of infection 0.8; cumulative incidence 1.6094 (calculated using Equation 13.4); total person-weeks at risk 324; average incidence rate 0.247 (calculated using Equation 13.2).

In the example described in Box 13.11, the most natural measure is perhaps the risk of infection, because all individuals are observed over the same relatively brief period. The rate of infection is particularly useful when follow-up times vary between individuals.

The protective vaccine effectiveness (given by the expression $VE = 1 - RR$) may be risk-based, if the relative risk RR is a ratio of risks, or rate-based, if it is a ratio of rates (whether the rate is instantaneous, average or cumulative). Generally, different choices give different results. But if the chance of infection is low over the study period, so that both the risk and the cumulative incidence are small, the difference between the different measures is small. This is illustrated in Box 13.12.

Box 13.12 Risk-based and rate-based vaccine effectiveness

We continue the example from Box 13.11. Over the 8 weeks of the outbreak, the risks in vaccinated and unvaccinated children are:

$$\pi_V = \frac{40}{100} = 0.40, \quad \pi_U = \frac{80}{100} = 0.80,$$

and so the risk-based effectiveness is

$$VE = 1 - \frac{0.40}{0.80} = 0.50,$$

or 50%.

The cumulative incidences are (using natural logs):

$$\Lambda_V = -\log(1 - 0.4) = 0.51083, \quad \Lambda_U = -\log(1 - 0.8) = 1.6094,$$

and so the rate-based vaccine effectiveness (based on cumulative incidences) is

$$VE = 1 - \frac{0.51083}{1.6094} = 0.68,$$

or 68%.

The average incidence rates are:

$$\lambda_V = 0.072, \quad \lambda_U = 0.247,$$

and so the rate-based vaccine effectiveness (based on average incidence rates) is

$$VE = 1 - \frac{0.072}{0.247} = 0.71,$$

or 71%.

The two rate-based effectiveness measures give similar results, but both are appreciably higher than the risk-based effectiveness. The difference arises because the chance of infection in this example is relatively high.

If the risk in this school outbreak was much lower, with only 12 cases of whom 4 were vaccinated and 8 unvaccinated, then $\pi_V = 0.04$, $\pi_U = 0.08$, $\Lambda_V = 0.040822$ and $\Lambda_U = 0.083382$. In this case, the risk-based measure is $VE = 50\%$, whereas the cumulative rate-based measure is $VE = 51\%$. The difference between them is now of no practical importance.

The calculations in Box 13.12 show that risk-based and rate-based measures of vaccine effectiveness can produce different results from the same data when the chance of infection over the study period, and hence the risk and cumulative incidence, are high. Therefore, when comparing vaccine effectiveness across different studies, the measure used to quantify the chance of infection should be taken into account. However, as also illustrated in Box 13.12, risk-based and rate-based measures of VE are similar when the risk (or cumulative incidence) of infection is low. This is the case in most studies involving a short period of follow-up after vaccination and in those where infections are uncommon.

However, when the chance of infection (or of past infection) in the study population is high, the question whether to use risks or rates in vaccine estimation is more important. If follow-up differs between individuals, rate-based measures are likely to be the simplest option. If all individuals have the same follow-up, either type of measure may be used. If comparisons are to be made with other studies, it makes sense to use similar measures where possible, in order to compare like with like.

Further considerations are involved when assessing vaccine effectiveness some years after vaccination, since the risk and cumulative incidence of infection may have accumulated to relatively high levels over the intervening period. This situation arises commonly when assessing vaccine effectiveness in older age groups. In this situation, rate-based and risk-based VE measures may vary over time in different ways, irrespective of any waning effect of the vaccine, which further complicates the analysis. These issues are deferred until Chapter 16.

13.6 Some remarks on modelling frameworks

In the next chapters, we shall review the methods commonly used for estimating vaccine effectiveness. The statistical techniques described there are inherited from those used in non-infectious disease epidemiology, and so make a key assumption, namely that the disease states of different individuals are independent. In the case of infectious diseases, this is clearly not the case. Thus, all the estimation methods to be described should be regarded as approximate. However, in most cases they are perfectly adequate.

Taking full account of the dependencies between individuals, and hence of the process variability as well as the sampling variability, requires modelling the whole infection process. This is generally a demanding enterprise involving stochastic modelling, often requiring rather more data than are commonly available, and some simplifying assumptions. These methods lie well beyond the scope of this book.

Summary

- Vaccine effectiveness estimates may vary according to the case definition used, in particular whether it targets disease or infection, and whether laboratory confirmation is sought.
- Misclassification of vaccination or disease status is likely to bias vaccination effectiveness estimates. Vaccination status should be documented where possible, and cases should be ascertained independently of vaccination status.
- Confounding may arise in the estimation of vaccine effectiveness when a variable

associated with vaccination is also associated with exposure to infection. Common confounders are time and age. When the confounding variable is measured, it can be adjusted for in the analyses. Unmeasured confounding is more difficult to address.
- Confounding by indication and healthy vaccinee effects may also bias vaccination effectiveness estimates and should be adjusted statistically or taken into account in the design of the study.
- Bias indicator studies may provide insights into the robustness of field assessments of vaccine effectiveness.
- Vaccine effectiveness may be based on risks or on rates (instantaneous, average or cumulative). Risk-based and rate-based vaccine effectiveness measures may differ when infections are common.

References

De Smedt, T., Merrall, E., Macina, D., Perez-Vilar, S., Andrews, N., & Bollaerts, K. (2018). Bias due to differential and non-differential disease and exposure misclassification in studies of vaccine effectiveness. *PLoS ONE, 13*(6), e0199180.

Halloran, M. E., Longini, I. M., & Struchiner, C. J. (2010). *Design and analysis of vaccine studies.* New York: Springer.

Ivers, L. C., Hilaire, I. J., Teng, J. E., Almazor, C. P., Jerome, J. G., Ternier, R., ... Franke, M. E. (2015). Effectiveness of reactive oral cholera vaccination in rural Haiti: A case-control study and bias-indicator analysis. *Lancet Global Health, 3*(3), e162–e168.

Killewo, J., Makwaya, C., Munubhi, E., & Mpembeni, R. (1991). The protective effect of measles vaccine under routine vaccination conditions in Dar Es Salaam, Tanzania: A case-control study. *International Journal of Epidemiology, 20*(2), 508–514.

Lipsitch, M., Tchetgen Tchetgen, E., & Cohen, T. (2010). Negative controls: A tool for detecting confounding and bias in observational studies. *Epidemiology, 21*(3), 383–388.

Murray, M., & Rasmussen, Z. (2000). Measles outbreak in a northern Pakistani village: Epidemiology and vaccine effectiveness. *American Journal of Epidemiology, 151*, 811–819.

Orenstein, W. A., Bernier, R. H., Dondero, T. J., Hinman, A. R., Marks, J. S., Bart, K. J., & Sirotkin, B. (1985). Field evaluation of vaccine efficacy. *Bulletin of the World Health Organization, 63*(6), 1055–1068.

Orenstein, W. A., Bernier, R. H., & Hinman, A. R. (1988). Assessing vaccine efficacy in the field: Further observations. *Epidemiologic Reviews, 10*, 212–241.

Palmer, S. R. (1991). Vaccine efficacy and control measures in pertussis. *Archives of Disease in Childhood, 66*, 854–857.

Remschmidt, C., Wichmann, O., & Harder, T. (2015). Frequency and impact of confounding by indication and healthy vaccine bias in observational studies assessing influenza vaccine effectiveness: A systematic review. *BMC Infectious Diseases, 15*, 429.

Storsaeter, J., Hallander, H., Farrington, C. P., Olin, P., Möllby, R., & Miller, E. (1990). Secondary analyses of the efficacy of two acellular pertussis vaccines evaluated in a Swedish phase III trial. *Vaccine, 8*, 457–461.

Walker, J. L., Andrews, N. J., Atchison, C. J., Collins, S., Allen, D. J., Ramsay, M. E., ... Thomas, S. L. (2019). Effectiveness of oral vaccination in England against rotavirus-confirmed and all-cause acute gastroenteritis. *Vaccine, X*(1), 100005.

Chapter 14

Estimating vaccine effectiveness
Cohort and household contact studies

Cohort studies to assess vaccine effectiveness involve following a defined group of individuals (the cohort) over a predetermined time interval, and recording their vaccination and disease histories. Cohort studies may be undertaken in many different settings: during outbreaks, within population-based surveillance systems or within pre-existing databases. Some cohort studies are done in real time; others are undertaken retrospectively, after the study time has elapsed.

In Section 14.1, we consider cohort studies with parallel vaccinated and unvaccinated groups, in which all individuals are followed for the same period of time. Then in Section 14.2 we consider cohort studies in which follow-up times may vary between individuals. In Section 14.3 we discuss cohort studies undertaken within households; such studies are also called household contact studies. A summary table is provided at the end of the chapter, listing the various designs and some of their key properties.

Throughout, we give formulas and worked examples for vaccine effectiveness and its 95% confidence interval (CI) only in the simplest instances. Very often, more complicated (but standard) statistical methods are required, usually involving some form of regression technique. These methods are described in general terms, with some inevitably technical references to the models, but without extensive explanations or any details of their implementation, which require statistical knowledge that lies beyond the scope of this book.

14.1 Cohort studies with parallel groups and identical follow-up

We consider a cohort design involving two or more groups of individuals defined by their vaccination status (e.g., vaccinated and unvaccinated) that are followed over a defined time interval from 0 (the start of the study) to some predetermined time T. We discuss vaccine effectiveness based on risks and rates separately; these measures were discussed in Chapter 13, Section 13.5.

DOI: 10.4324/9781315166414-15
This Chapter has been made available under a CC-BY-NC-ND license.

14.1.1 Risk-based vaccine effectiveness

Suppose that there are two groups, comprising n_v vaccinated and n_u unvaccinated individuals. Suppose also that, by time T, r_v vaccinated cases have occurred within the vaccinated group, and r_u unvaccinated cases have occurred within the unvaccinated group. The estimated risks, or attack rates, in the two groups are then:

$$R_v = \frac{r_v}{n_v}, \quad R_u = \frac{r_u}{n_u}.$$

The estimated relative risk is

$$RR = \frac{r_v / n_v}{r_u / n_u}$$

and the estimated (risk-based) vaccine effectiveness is

$$VE = 1 - RR = 1 - \frac{r_v / n_v}{r_u / n_u}.$$

Approximate 95% confidence limits for VE are given by

$$VE^- = 1 - RR^+, \quad VE^- = 1 - RR^-,$$

with

$$RR^- = RR \times \exp(-1.96 \times \sigma), \quad RR^+ = RR \times \exp(+1.96 \times \sigma)$$

where σ is the standard error of the log relative risk,

$$\sigma = \sqrt{\frac{1}{r_v} - \frac{1}{n_v} + \frac{1}{r_u} - \frac{1}{n_u}}.$$

Cohort studies with parallel groups often arise in the context of outbreaks. Box 14.1 describes one example.

Box 14.1 Effectiveness of post-exposure measles vaccination in Catalonia

A retrospective cohort study was undertaken to assess the effectiveness of measles vaccination after exposure to measles during a school outbreak of measles in Catalonia (Barrabeig et al., 2011). It is recommended that a susceptible person (unvaccinated and not having had measles) exposed to measles is vaccinated within 72 hours of exposure. The study cohort included 75 susceptible contacts of 10 unvaccinated primary cases; a contact is a child who had shared the same classroom as the primary case for at least 1 day during the infectious period of the case (4 days before rash onset to 4 days after).

Of the 75 susceptible contacts, 54 were vaccinated post-exposure and 21 were not vaccinated. There were 13 secondary cases among unvaccinated contacts (attack rate 13/21 or 62%) and 12 among vaccinated contacts, including 1 case among the 17 (1/17 or 5.9%) who were vaccinated within 72 hours of exposure and 11 among the 37 (11/37 or 30%) vaccinated later.

The estimated relative risk of measles for vaccination within 72 hours of exposure versus no post-exposure vaccination is

$$RR = \frac{1/17}{13/21} = 0.095023.$$

Note that full accuracy (here, to five significant figures) should be kept in intermediate calculations, any rounding taking place at the end. Thus, the vaccine effectiveness is

$$VE = 1 - 0.095023 = 0.90498,$$

or 90% as a percentage, after rounding.

To obtain an approximate 95% CI, first obtain

$$\sigma = \sqrt{\frac{1}{1} - \frac{1}{17} + \frac{1}{13} - \frac{1}{21}} = 0.98513.$$

Hence, the 95% confidence limits for the relative risk are

$$RR^- = 0.095023 \times \exp(-1.96 \times 0.98513) = 0.013781,$$

$$RR^+ = 0.095023 \times \exp(+1.96 \times 0.98513) = 0.65522,$$

and so the 95% confidence limits for VE are

$$VE^- = 1 - 0.65522 = 0.34, VE^+ = 1 - 0.013781 = 0.99.$$

Thus, the (risk-based) vaccine effectiveness for prophylactic vaccination within 72 hours of exposure is 90%, with 95% CI (34% to 99%).

Corresponding calculations for vaccination after 72 hours post-exposure yield $RR = 0.48025$, $\sigma = 0.30526$, $RR^- = 0.26401$, $RR^+ = 0.87359$. Thus, the vaccine effectiveness is 52%, with 95% CI (13% to 74%).

In conclusion, this study provides some evidence that measles vaccination within 72 hours of exposure gives good protection; later vaccination may provide only partial protection.

The expressions for the confidence limits used in Box 14.1 are approximations. However, they cannot be used when there are 0 cases in either group. Nevertheless, confidence intervals can still be obtained, and should be quoted. But more advanced statistical methods for obtaining confidence limits are required in such situations. One such example is described in Box 14.2.

Box 14.2 Rubella vaccine effectiveness in Guangzhou, China

An outbreak of rubella occurred in 2014 in a school in Guangzhou city, China. An outbreak investigation was undertaken to assess which factors might have contributed to the outbreak, and to estimate the effectiveness of the rubella vaccines in use (Chang et al., 2015).

In one vaccine effectiveness calculation, school students who had been vaccinated less than 12 years prior to the outbreak were compared to those never vaccinated. There were 0 cases among the 15 vaccinated children and 65 cases among the 171 unvaccinated children. Thus, the relative risk is

$$RR = \frac{0/15}{65/171} = 0$$

and hence the vaccine effectiveness is $VE = 100\%$. However, the method described above for calculating the 95% CI cannot be used, because 0 cases were observed in the vaccinated group. The upper 95% confidence limit for VE must be 100%, because it cannot be any higher; and the lower limit is less than 100% – but how much less? Using the profile likelihood method (McCullagh & Nelder, 1989), an approximate value for the lower 95% confidence limit may be calculated to be 68%. Thus, the 95% CI for VE is 68% to 100%.

While the calculations for the example described in Box 14.1 are straightforward, there is often a need to adjust for possible confounders in the analysis (see Chapter 13). This requires more elaborate statistical methods known as generalised linear models (Davison, 2003; McCullagh & Nelder, 1989).

For studies involving parallel groups with identical follow-up, the risk-based estimate of VE and its confidence interval, adjusted for potential confounders, may be obtained using a suitable statistical model. This is typically a generalised linear model with binomial error and log link function. The response variable is the number of cases, the binomial index is the cohort size, both cross-classified by vaccination status and other covariates. The log link is required because we seek to estimate relative risks. Thus, the parameters of the model are log relative risks $\beta = \log(RR)$, vaccine effectiveness being obtained as $VE = 1 - \exp(\beta)$. An example is described in Box 14.3.

Box 14.3 Effectiveness of adolescent booster acellular pertussis vaccination in Maine

This retrospective cohort study was undertaken in 2011 in two schools in Maine, USA, in which large outbreaks of pertussis were reported (Terranella et al., 2016). Students included in the study were aged 11–19 years, had full immunisation histories available and had completed their primary pertussis vaccination course in childhood.

Students were classified as vaccinated if they had received tetanus, diphtheria and acellular pertussis (Tdap) booster vaccine at age 11 years at least 2 weeks before the start of the outbreak, and as unvaccinated if not. Overall, 314 students across the two schools were included in the study. Table 14.1 shows the full data for the two schools.

For school A,

$$VE = 1 - \frac{5/77}{9/41} = 0.70,$$

whereas for school B,

$$VE = 1 - \frac{3/82}{12/114} = 0.65.$$

The vaccine effectiveness is similar for the two schools, so it makes sense to average them in some way. However, if we were just to combine the two tables into one, we would obtain

$$VE = 1 - \frac{(5+3)/(77+82)}{(9+12)/(41+114)} = 0.63$$

which is less than the estimate for either school. This anomaly is due to confounding, by school, of the association between vaccination and pertussis: there are many more unvaccinated students in school B, but the pertussis attack rate is

Table 14.1 **Numbers of vaccinated and unvaccinated students and cases**

	School A		School B	
	Cases	Students	Cases	Students
Vaccinated	5	77	3	82
Unvaccinated	9	41	12	114

higher in school A, and these imbalances make the vaccine appear slightly worse than it really is when the data are aggregated across schools.

To adjust for confounding, a binomial model with logarithmic link is used, which includes the school and vaccination variables. This model produces a suitably weighted average of the results from the two schools and thus gives an estimate of the combined vaccine effectiveness, which removes the confounding effect:

$$VE = 0.68, 95\%\,CI(0.30, 0.86).$$

The overall vaccine effectiveness is 68%, with 95% CI (30%, 86%). The authors comment that booster vaccination in adolescents was moderately effective in preventing pertussis.

The binomial model in Box 14.3 adjusts for the school effect, thus removing confounding due to that variable. This statistical modelling approach is very flexible, very widely used and is recommended. Several potential confounders may be handled together, and effect modification can be investigated using appropriate interaction terms in the model. Some more details of this modelling approach are deferred to Box 14.6.

Where possible, the binomial assumption should be verified by checking for overdispersion, that is, greater variability in the numbers of cases than expected under the binomial model, perhaps due to unmeasured heterogeneity. In this case a quasi-binomial model can be used instead. However, these and other statistical modelling issues lie beyond the scope of this book.

A further application of the risk-based estimation methods described in this section is to the estimation of the vaccine effectiveness against disease progression; this was defined in Chapter 12, Section 12.3. An example is shown in Box 14.4.

Box 14.4 Mumps vaccine effectiveness against orchitis in the Netherlands

In 2011 the Centre for Infectious Disease Control for the Netherlands advised that university students who were unvaccinated or had received only one dose of vaccine in the past should be vaccinated against mumps. To support this policy, a study to evaluate the effectiveness of mumps vaccination against progression to orchitis (VP) was undertaken, based on data from mumps notifications in 2009–2011 (Hahné, Whelan, van Binnendijk, Boot, & de Melker, 2012).

In this study, the mumps cases deemed severe are those with orchitis. We describe the results obtained for two doses of mumps, measles and rubella (MMR) vaccine (compared to 0 doses). Of the 338 male vaccinated mumps cases in the study, 31 had orchitis; of the 86 male unvaccinated cases, 20 had orchitis. Thus,

$$VP = 1 - \frac{31/338}{20/86} = 0.60562,$$

or 61%. This means that vaccination reduces the risk of mumps progressing to orchitis by 61%. The 95% CI for VP is obtained using

$$\sigma = \sqrt{\frac{1}{31} - \frac{1}{338} + \frac{1}{20} - \frac{1}{86}} = 0.26014,$$

and is (34%, 76%).

The published analysis used a different measure of relative risk, the odds ratio (to be discussed in Chapter 15) and adjusted for age. The adjusted VP was 74%, with 95% confidence limits (49%, 87%). These results show that two doses of MMR vaccine in men reduces the risk of mumps progressing to orchitis.

14.1.2 Vaccine effectiveness based on the cumulative incidence

We now consider the rate-based measure of vaccine effectiveness using cumulative incidences; see Chapter 13 for details. Such an estimate may be preferred over the risk-based measure if, for example, a direct comparison is to be made with rate-based estimates obtained in other studies.

The setting is as before: there are two groups, comprising n_v vaccinated and n_u unvaccinated individuals. By some time T, r_v vaccinated cases have occurred within the vaccinated group, and r_u unvaccinated cases have occurred within the unvaccinated group. The estimated cumulative incidences are $\Lambda_v = -\log(1 - r_v / n_v)$ in the vaccinated group and $\Lambda_u = -\log(1 - r_u / n_u)$ in the unvaccinated group.

The estimated cumulative incidence ratio is

$$CIR = \frac{\Lambda_v}{\Lambda_u} = \frac{-\log(1 - r_v / n_v)}{-\log(1 - r_u / n_u)}$$

and the estimated (rate-based) vaccine effectiveness is

$$VE = 1 - CIR = 1 - \frac{\Lambda_v}{\Lambda_u} = 1 - \frac{-\log(1 - r_v / n_v)}{-\log(1 - r_u / n_u)}.$$

Approximate 95% confidence limits for VE are given by

$$VE^- = 1 - CIR^+, \ VE^+ = 1 - CIR^-,$$

with

$$CIR^- = CIR \times \exp(-1.96 \times \sigma), \ CIR^+ = CIR \times \exp(+1.96 \times \sigma)$$

COHORT AND HOUSEHOLD CONTACT STUDIES 271

where σ is the standard error of the log CIR,

$$\sigma = \sqrt{\frac{r_v/\Lambda_v^2}{n_v(n_v - r_v)} + \frac{r_u/\Lambda_u^2}{n_u(n_u - r_u)}}.$$

The calculations are illustrated in Box 14.5, using the data previously described in Box 14.1.

Box 14.5 Rate-based measles vaccine effectiveness in Catalonia outbreak

We use the data on prophylactic measles vaccination within 72 hours previously described in Box 14.1. The cumulative incidences are:

$$\Lambda_v = -\log\left(1 - \frac{1}{17}\right) = 0.060625, \quad \Lambda_u = -\log\left(1 - \frac{13}{21}\right) = 0.96508$$

and so the cumulative incidence ratio is $CIR = \dfrac{0.060625}{0.96508} = 0.062819$ and the rate-based vaccine effectiveness is

$$VE = 1 - CIR = 1 - 0.062819 = 0.93718$$

or 94%, slightly higher than the 90% risk-based vaccine effectiveness.

To obtain an approximate 95% CI, first obtain

$$\sigma = \sqrt{\frac{1/0.060625^2}{17(17-1)} + \frac{13/0.96508^2}{21(21-13)}} = 1.0408$$

Hence, the 95% confidence limits for the cumulative incidence ratio are

$$CIR^- = 0.062819 \times \exp(-1.96 \times 1.0408) = 0.0081685,$$

$$CIR^+ = 0.062819 \times \exp(+1.96 \times 1.0408) = 0.48310,$$

and so the 95% confidence limits for VE are

$$VE^- = 1 - 0.48310 = 0.52, \quad VE^+ = 1 - 0.0081685 = 0.99.$$

Thus, the rate-based vaccine effectiveness for prophylactic vaccination within 72 hours of exposure is 94%, with 95% CI (52% to 99%).

272 VACCINE EFFECTIVENESS

Estimates and 95% confidence intervals can also readily be obtained by statistical modelling, with the added advantage that confounders may be adjusted. In this case, the model is a generalised linear model with binomial error and complementary log–log link. The responses are the numbers of cases, the binomial indices are the group sizes, both cross-classified by vaccination status and other covariates. The complementary log–log link function CLL applied to a proportion p is defined as follows:

$$CLL(p) = \log(-\log(1-p)).$$

The parameters β represents contrasts on the CLL scale, so that $VE = 1 - \exp(\beta)$ just as for the binomial model with log link.

In Box 14.6, we contrast the rate-based and risk-based vaccine effectiveness estimates obtained with the pertussis example in Box 14.3.

Box 14.6 Rate-based and risk-based vaccine effectiveness estimates for pertussis vaccine

We return to the data described in Box 14.3 on pertussis vaccination in two schools. To obtain the rate-based estimate of pertussis vaccine effectiveness for schools A and B combined, we fit a binomial model with complementary log–log link, and include the variables for school and vaccine (coded 0 for unvaccinated, 1 for vaccinated). The vaccine effect parameter (which is the log CIR) is $\beta = -1.2176$, with standard error $\sigma = 0.4261$. Thus, the rate-based vaccine effectiveness is

$$VE = 1 - \exp(\beta) = 0.70.$$

The 95% confidence limits are

$$VE^- = 1 - \exp(\beta + 1.96 \times \sigma) = 1 - \exp(-1.2176 + 1.96 \times 0.4261) = 0.32$$

$$VE^+ = 1 - \exp(\beta - 1.96 \times \sigma) = 1 - \exp(-1.2176 - 1.96 \times 0.4261) = 0.87$$

Thus, the rate-based vaccine effectiveness is 70%, with 95% CI (32%, 87%).

The risk-based vaccine effectiveness described in Box 14.3 was obtained in a similar manner, but using a binomial model with log link. The vaccine parameter in this case was the log relative risk $\beta = -1.1538$, with standard error $\sigma = 0.4046$. Thus, the risk-based vaccine effectiveness was

$$VE = 1 - \exp(\beta) = 0.68,$$

or 68%, and the 95% CI, obtained as above, was (30%, 86%).

For the example described in Box 14.6 there is little difference between the risk-based and rate-based vaccine effectiveness estimates, essentially because the attack rates are relatively low. Only when attack rates are higher are relevant differences likely to arise.

14.2 Cohort studies with arbitrary follow-up times

For many cohort studies, particularly population-based studies, different individuals may be followed for different periods of time, and so there is not a unique time period of follow-up to calculate risks and risk-based vaccine effectiveness. Study time prior to vaccination may also be available. In such circumstances, vaccine effectiveness based on rates may be estimated. We distinguish two situations, which require different methods: grouped data, and individual data.

14.2.1 Cohort studies with grouped person-time

In this setting, person-time at risk in the study is grouped into discrete categories. For example, suppose there are just two groups, vaccinated and unvaccinated. A vaccinated individual followed up for 1 year after vaccination would contribute 1 year of person-time to the vaccinated group; an unvaccinated person followed up for 6 months would contribute 0.5 years to the unvaccinated group. This allocation of person-time is done for all individuals in the cohort, who can contribute person-time to both the unvaccinated and vaccinated groups if they are vaccinated during follow-up. The total person-time in each group is obtained by adding up the individual contributions. In such a two-group setting, there are r_v cases and t_v person-time units in the vaccinated group, and r_u cases and t_u person-time units in the unvaccinated group. The average incidence rates in each group are then

$$R_v = \frac{r_v}{t_v}, \quad R_u = \frac{r_u}{t_u}.$$

These rates are averaged over the person-time available. The estimated incidence rate ratio is

$$IRR = \frac{r_v / t_v}{r_u / t_u}$$

and the (rate-based) vaccine effectiveness is

$$VE = 1 - IRR = 1 - \frac{r_v / t_v}{r_u / t_u}.$$

Approximate 95% confidence limits for VE are given by

$$VE^- = 1 - IRR^+, \quad VE^- = 1 - IRR^-,$$

with

$$IRR^- = IRR \times \exp(-1.96 \times \sigma), \; IRR^+ = IRR \times \exp(+1.96 \times \sigma)$$

where σ is the standard error of the log incidence rate ratio,

$$\sigma = \sqrt{\frac{1}{r_v} + \frac{1}{r_u}}.$$

These expressions for the confidence limits cannot be used when there are 0 cases in either group; more advanced statistical methods for obtaining confidence limits are required in such situations; these include the profile likelihood method applied in Box 14.2.

A key aspect of studies involving person-time is how time at risk is defined. For non-recurrent events (or first-incident events), time at risk typically ends at the earliest of time of event, end of record or death, end of study or some other prespecified occurrence. The method is illustrated in Box 14.7.

Box 14.7 Effectiveness of group B meningococcal vaccine in New Zealand

In 2004, vaccination against group B meningococcal disease was introduced in New Zealand. This study was undertaken to estimate the effectiveness of the vaccine in children aged 6 months to 5 years (Galloway, Stehr-Green, McNicholas, & O'Hallahan, 2009). Cases were children notified with meningococcal disease, confirmed as group B. Vaccination status was determined using a vaccination register: a child was deemed to be vaccinated if they had received three correctly spaced doses of vaccine, unvaccinated if they had received no doses. Person-time for each child started 12 weeks after eligibility for a third dose for children aged 6 months to 5 years. It ended at the earliest of 24 months after start of follow-up, time of event, receipt of a fourth dose of vaccine and age 5 years.

In the vaccinated group there were 12 cases and 101,936,906 days of person-time. In the unvaccinated group there were 9 cases and 15,286,382 days of person-time. Thus, the incidence rate ratio is:

$$IRR = \frac{12/101936906}{9/15286382} = 0.19995$$

and the vaccine effectiveness is

$$VE = 1 - 0.19995 = 0.80.$$

To obtain 95% confidence limits, first obtain

$$\sigma = \sqrt{\frac{1}{12} + \frac{1}{9}} = 0.44096.$$

Then the 95% confidence limits of the incidence rate ratio are

$$IRR^- = 0.19995 \times \exp(-1.96 \times 0.44096) = 0.084250,$$

$$IRR^+ = 0.19995 \times \exp(+1.96 \times 0.44096) = 0.47454.$$

Hence the 95% confidence limits for vaccine effectiveness are

$$VE^- = 1 - 0.47454 = 0.53 \,,\, VE^+ = 1 - 0.084250 = 0.92.$$

Thus, the vaccine effectiveness is 80%, with 95% CI (53%, 92%).

Sometimes, more complex analyses than that described in Box 14.7 are required, notably to control for potential confounders and study effect modification. Poisson modelling provides a flexible framework for studying vaccine effectiveness using grouped cohort data, provided that the confounding variables are categorical, so that the cases and person-time can be grouped into discrete categories, including vaccination status. This gives rise to a generalised linear model with Poisson error and logarithmic link. The responses are the counts, cross-classified by vaccination status and other covariates. The logarithms of the person-time within each group are specified as offsets. The parameters of the model are then log incidence rate ratios.

An example of this modelling approach, and how it may be used to identify an effect modifier, is described in Box 14.8.

Box 14.8 Effectiveness of herpes zoster vaccination in elderly people in the United Kingdom

Vaccination against herpes zoster was introduced in the United Kingdom in 2013 for people over the age of 70 years. A study was undertaken in the Clinical Practice Research Datalink (CPRD) database to evaluate the effectiveness of the vaccine (Walker et al., 2018).

For individuals included in the study, follow-up started at the latest of the date zoster vaccination was introduced, and the end of any previous zoster episode. End of follow-up was the earliest of end of the CPRD record, end of the study or date of the first-incident zoster episode. Thus, although herpes zoster is potentially recurrent, the present analysis only included first cases within the follow-up period.

Table 14.2 Cases and person-time by vaccination status and prior history of zoster

	With prior history		No prior history	
	Cases	Person-years	Cases	Person-years
Vaccinated	70	14,784	365	123,185
Unvaccinated	861	88,358	7,145	821,116

The analysis was by Poisson regression, and adjusted for many potential confounders. In this example we focus on comparing vaccine effectiveness in persons without a prior history of zoster, and persons with a prior history. The data are in Table 14.2.

A Poisson model with log link was defined with counts as responses and log person-times as offsets, including factors for vaccine (reference category: unvaccinated) and prior history. The interaction between vaccination and prior history was statistically significant: the chi-squared test statistic was 6.43 on 1 degree of freedom, $p = 0.011$. This indicates that vaccine effectiveness differs according to prior history: prior history is an effect modifier. Suitably parameterised, the interaction model yielded parameters for the two effect measures (which are log incidence rate ratios) simultaneously, β_0 (no prior history) and β_1 (with prior history), and their standard errors σ_0 and σ_1:

$$\beta_0 = -1.07729, \quad \sigma_0 = 0.05366; \quad \beta_1 = -0.72175, \quad \sigma_1 = 0.12429.$$

Thus, in persons with no prior history of zoster,

$$VE = 1 - \exp(-1.07729) = 0.66,$$

with 95% confidence limits

$$VE^- = 1 - \exp(-1.07729 + 1.96 \times 0.05366) = 0.62,$$

$$VE^+ = 1 - \exp(-1.07729 - 1.96 \times 0.05366) = 0.69.$$

So the vaccine effectiveness in this group was 66%, with 95% CI (62%, 69%). Similar calculations for persons with a prior history of zoster yield

$$VE = 1 - \exp(-0.72175) = 0.51,$$

or 51%, with 95% CI (38%, 62%).

The published analysis also adjusted for age and calendar time, and obtained marginally lower vaccine effectiveness in each group (64% and 47%) than those presented here. The authors surmise that the difference in VE between the two groups may be due to differences in the immune systems of persons with and without a prior history of zoster.

When there are sufficient cases, the validity of the Poisson assumption may be examined by checking for overdispersion, that is, variability in excess of that expected under the Poisson model. If this is present, a quasi-Poisson approach with adjusted standard errors can be used.

14.2.2 Cohort studies with individual exposure and event histories

In some situations, it is not possible or not desirable to group the data into a relatively small number of distinct categories, for example in order to avoid discretising continuous covariates such as age. The data then comprise the records of individual exposure and event histories, from the time an individual enters the study to the time they leave it or experience the event of interest.

For such data, the many techniques of survival analysis can be applied, the most common being the Cox proportional hazards model. This provides an estimate of the hazard ratio

$$HR = \frac{\lambda_v(t)}{\lambda_u(t)}$$

where $\lambda_v(t)$ and $\lambda_u(t)$ are the incidence rates in vaccinated and unvaccinated persons (see Chapter 13, Section 13.5). An assumption of this model is that the hazard ratio is time-invariant; time-varying hazard ratios will be considered in Chapter 16. The (rate-based) vaccine effectiveness is then

$$VE = 1 - \frac{\lambda_v(t)}{\lambda_u(t)}.$$

The Cox proportional hazards model involves comparing the exposure history of each case with the exposure histories of those in the risk set associated with that case; the risk set comprises all cohort members who are at risk just before the event time of the case. One advantage of the Cox proportional hazards model is that time-varying exposures (such as additional vaccinations) can be taken into account in a very flexible manner. An application is described in Box 14.9.

Box 14.9 Effectiveness of vaccination in pregnancy to prevent infant pertussis

It has been recommended that pregnant women are vaccinated with the tetanus toxoid, reduced diphtheria toxoid, acellular pertussis (Tdap) vaccine, in order to protect their infant in the first months of life, before they receive their primary three-dose diphtheria, tetanus, acellular pertussis (DTaP) vaccine course. This study was undertaken to investigate simultaneously the effectiveness of Tdap vaccination in pregnancy, and the effectiveness of the primary DTaP course in infants (Baxter, Bartlett, Fireman, Lewis, & Klein, 2017).

The study was conducted within a large health maintenance organisation in the United States, and included infants born between 2010 and 2015, who were followed from birth to age 1 year. In addition to Tdap vaccination of the mother during pregnancy, Tdap vaccination of the mother before and after pregnancy were also considered as exposures. Vaccination of infants with successive doses of the DTaP vaccine were specified as time-varying exposures, with an 8-day delay to allow time for the immune response to develop. A Cox proportional hazards model, stratified on year and month of birth, was applied with these exposures, adjusting for several other variables including sex and ethnicity.

The study included 148,981 newborns; there were 103 pertussis cases (confirmed by polymerase chain reaction (PCR)) by age 12 months (17 by age 2 months). The vaccine effectiveness of Tdap during pregnancy was 91%, 95% CI (19%, 99%) for the first 2 months of life of the infant, and 69% (44%, 83%) for the full 12-month follow-up. The effectiveness of maternal Tdap vaccination for infants prior to their DTaP vaccination was 88% (41%, 98%); after three DTaP doses it was 66% (4%, 88%). Maternal Tdap vaccination prior to pregnancy was also found to be effective; post-pregnancy vaccination was not. The effectiveness of three doses of DTaP vaccine in infants was 87% (69%, 94%).

The study confirms the effectiveness of maternal Tdap vaccination in pregnancy for protecting infants during the first months of life. Indeed, it shows that it provides additional protection over and above that resulting from primary DTaP vaccination of the child.

As illustrated in Box 14.9, the Cox proportional hazards model enables very complex exposure patterns, with different vaccines and possible interactions between them, or different vaccination schedules, to be investigated in a flexible manner.

14.3 Household contact studies

The types of cohort studies discussed so far all involve following individuals over time and documenting if and when they become infected and thus become cases. However, no information may be available on who infected these cases. In contrast, household contact studies are cohort studies undertaken within a collection of households that have experienced at least one case. When the first individual within a given household is infected (the primary case), the risk of infection to other members of the household from this first case during their infectious period may be estimated: this risk is called the secondary attack rate (even though it is actually a risk, not a rate) and denoted SAR:

SAR = probability of infection, given exposure in the household.

Accurate data on the timing of symptoms, and some information on the latent and infectious periods of the infection studied, are required to define primary and secondary cases, as well as co-primary cases (these are cases infected soon after the primary case, but not by the primary case). The advantage of a household study design is that we know that contacts of the primary case have been exposed, and most likely in a similar manner, which reduces the potential for confounding. Another advantage is that household study designs may allow the estimation not only of the protective effectiveness of the vaccine, VE, but also its effectiveness against infectiousness, VI. We consider both in turn.

14.3.1 Protective effectiveness in household studies

In a household study, the (risk-based) vaccine effectiveness may be obtained as

$$VE = 1 - \frac{SAR_v}{SAR_u},$$

where SAR_v is the secondary attack rate in vaccinated household members and SAR_u is the secondary attack rate in unvaccinated household members.

Only secondary cases should be counted in the secondary attack rates; primary and co-primary cases should be excluded from numerators and denominators. The secondary attack rates are estimated by aggregating the data over different households. Suppose there are n_v vaccinated exposed household members of whom r_v become secondary cases during the infectious period of the primary cases, and n_u unvaccinated exposed household members of whom r_u become cases, then

$$SAR_v = \frac{r_v}{n_v}, \quad SAR_u = \frac{r_u}{n_u}$$

and

$$VE = 1 - \frac{r_v/n_v}{r_u/n_u}.$$

This is of the same form as the risk-based vaccine effectiveness for a cohort study with identical follow-up times, and so the same formulas for confidence intervals may be used (see Box 14.1 for an illustration). An example of such a study is in Box 14.10.

Box 14.10 Household study of measles vaccine effectiveness in Bavaria

This study was undertaken during a large measles outbreak that occurred in 2001–2002 in Coburg, Bavaria (Arenz, Schmitt, Tischer, & von Kries, 2005). Primary cases were the first household members with measles, according to a clinical case definition including rash and fever. Co-primary cases were defined as measles cases with fever within 4 days after the onset of rash in the primary case. Secondary cases were measles cases that developed a fever within 5–25 days after the onset of rash in the primary case. Household contacts were defined as persons less than 19 years of age who had come into contact with the primary case during their infectious period. Only contacts who became secondary cases or who did not have a history of measles were included.

There were 38 primary cases and no co-primaries. A total of 43 contacts were included in the study, including 17 who had received at least one dose of measles vaccine and 26 who had not received any measles vaccine. There was 1 case among the vaccinated contacts and 19 cases among the unvaccinated contacts.

Thus, the secondary attack rates and relative risk are:

$$SAR_v = \frac{1}{17}, \quad SAR_u = \frac{19}{26}, \quad RR = \frac{1/17}{19/26} = 0.080495,$$

giving a vaccine effectiveness for one or more doses of vaccine $VE = 1 - RR = 0.92$, or 92%. In view of the small numbers, the authors used an exact statistical method to calculate the 95% CI (48%, 98%). Alternatively, the approximate method described in Box 14.1 gives

$$\sigma = \sqrt{\frac{1}{1} - \frac{1}{17} + \frac{1}{19} - \frac{1}{26}} = 0.97742,$$

and so

$$VE^- = 1 - 0.080495 \times \exp(+1.96 \times 0.97742) = 0.45,$$

$$VE^+ = 1 - 0.080495 \times \exp(-1.96 \times 0.97742) = 0.99,$$

yielding the approximate 95% CI (45%, 99%).

As illustrated in Box 14.10, household studies require explicit definitions of primary, co-primary and secondary cases, taking into account prior knowledge about the infectious period and latent period of the infection. The analysis described in Box 14.10 could be stratified by covariates using the log-linear binomial model described in Section 14.1.1. In particular, it could be stratified according to the vaccination status of the primary case, an issue we shall return to in Section 14.3.3.

Note finally that exposures within the household are likely to be more intense than within the community. For that reason, the estimates of vaccine effectiveness obtained from households may differ from those obtained in other circumstances, if VE depends on exposure dose.

14.3.2 Vaccine effectiveness against infectiousness

The effectiveness of vaccination against infectiousness may be estimated by comparing the secondary attack rates for household contacts exposed to vaccinated and unvaccinated primary cases. Thus, let SAR_{vp} denote the secondary attack rate for household contacts exposed to a vaccinated primary case, and SAR_{up} the secondary attack rate for household contacts exposed to an unvaccinated primary case. Then the vaccine effectiveness against infectiousness is:

$$VI = 1 - \frac{SAR_{vp}}{SAR_{up}}.$$

Only households without co-primary cases should be included in the calculation of these secondary attack rates. Suppose there are r_{vp} secondary cases among the n_{vp} contacts of a vaccinated primary case, and r_{up} cases among the n_{up} contacts of an unvaccinated primary case. Then we estimate

$$SAR_{vp} = \frac{r_{vp}}{n_{vp}}, \quad SAR_{up} = \frac{r_{up}}{n_{up}}$$

and

$$VI = 1 - \frac{r_{vp}/n_{vp}}{r_{up}/n_{up}}.$$

Again, this is of the same form as the risk-based vaccine effectiveness for a cohort study with identical follow-up times, and so the same formulas for confidence intervals may be used, as described in Box 14.1. An example is in Box 14.11.

Box 14.11 Effectiveness against infectiousness of pertussis vaccine in Senegal

This study also featured in Chapter 12. It was undertaken in Niakhar, Senegal, during 1993, an epidemic year for whooping cough. Cases of pertussis were identified using a clinical case definition, and confirmed by culture or serology.

Primary cases were identified within compounds. Co-primary cases were those with onset of cough less than 7 days after that of the primary case. Contacts were children aged under 15 years old living in the same compound other than primary or co-primary cases, without a history of pertussis. Secondary cases were contacts with pertussis whose cough started 7 to 28 days after that of the primary case.

This example is based on primary cases in 109 compounds with no co-primaries. There were 444 contacts of wholly unvaccinated primary cases, of whom 93 became cases; and 194 contacts of fully vaccinated (three doses of pertussis vaccine) primary cases, of whom 6 became cases. Thus,

$$SAR_{vp} = \frac{6}{194}, \quad SAR_{up} = \frac{93}{444}, \quad RR = \frac{6/194}{93/444} = 0.1477,$$

so that the effectiveness of three doses of pertussis vaccine against infectiousness is

$$VI = 1 - RR = 0.8523,$$

or 85%. An approximate 95% CI may be obtained as in Box 14.1, and is (67%, 93%). This value for VI suggests that a full three-dose course of pertussis vaccination substantially reduces infectiousness (Préziosi & Halloran, 2003).

If required, a stratified analysis could be undertaken using the log-linear binomial model described in Section 14.1.1. In particular, it is advisable to stratify according to the vaccination status of the secondary cases. This is the topic of the next section.

14.3.3 Joint estimation of vaccine effectiveness estimates from household studies

The analysis described in Section 14.3.1 was not stratified by vaccination status of the primary cases; that of Section 14.3.2 was not stratified by vaccination status of the contacts. In general, it is advisable to stratify by both types of vaccination status, since the vaccination status of the primary and secondary cases may be related. Furthermore, a fully stratified analysis allows both the protective effectiveness and the effectiveness against infectiousness of the vaccine to be estimated jointly. In addition, how the two effectiveness estimates interact may also be studied. When VE measures protection against infection, VE and VI may be combined to derive the effectiveness of the vaccine against transmission. Such analyses should be undertaken in households with no co-primary cases.

The most convenient way to undertake such an analysis is with a binomial statistical model. This is a generalised linear model with log link function. The number of cases in each category is the response, and the number of contacts is the binomial index. In a first analysis, two factors are included in the model, representing the vaccination status of the primary case, and the vaccination status of the contacts, both coded with the unvaccinated groups as reference. Box 14.12 illustrates the impact of this type of adjustment.

Box 14.12 Joint estimation of mumps vaccine effectiveness measures in the Netherlands

This example, previously described in Chapter 12, relates to a household contact study undertaken during a large mumps outbreak in the Netherlands in 2007 (Snijders et al., 2012). In a first analysis, the vaccine effectiveness measures were estimated without adjustment, using the methods described in Sections 14.3.1 and 14.3.2. The results were $VE = 69\%$ and $VI = 62\%$.

In a further analysis, the vaccine effectiveness measures were estimated jointly, adjusting vaccination status of the primary case and vaccination status of the contact. Age of the contact was also adjusted. The results were $VE = 67\%$ and $VI = 11\%$.

The big change in VI, from 66% to 11%, suggests that the adjustment was necessary to control for confounding. Such confounding would arise if vaccinated contacts tended to cluster within households where the primary case was vaccinated.

The analysis involved in jointly estimating the protective vaccine effectiveness and the vaccine effectiveness against infectiousness, as well as the total effectiveness against transmission that combines both of these measures as described in Chapter 12, Section 12.5, is described in Box 14.13.

Box 14.13 Joint estimation of pertussis vaccine effectiveness measures in Senegal

The data for this example, from Niakhar in Senegal, were described in Box 14.11. The data, stratified by the vaccination status of both primary cases and contacts, are in Table 14.3. These data were obtained from Halloran, Préziosi, and Chu (2003).

The first two columns of Table 14.3 define the factors describing the vaccination status of the primary case and of the contacts respectively, with No coded as 0 and Yes as 1, so that the reference categories correspond to the unvaccinated groups. A binomial model is then fitted with log link, and the two factors as covariates.

The model parameters for the two vaccine effect measures (subscripted p for protective effectiveness and i for effectiveness against infectiousness) and their standard errors are as follows:

$\beta_p = -0.4641, \quad \sigma_p = 0.1812,$

$\beta_i = -1.8637, \quad \sigma_i = 0.4123.$

Table 14.3 Numbers of pertussis cases and contacts by vaccination status

Primary case vaccinated	Contacts vaccinated	Number of cases	Number of contacts
No	No	52	198
No	Yes	41	246
Yes	No	3	67
Yes	Yes	3	127

These values yield $VE = 1 - \exp(\beta_p) = 0.37$ or 37% with 95% CI (10%, 56%) for the protective effectiveness, and $VI = 1 - \exp(\beta_i) = 0.84$ or 84% with 95% CI (65%, 93%) for the effectiveness against infectiousness. This latter value does not differ much from the unstratified value obtained in Box 14.11, indicating that confounding is not an issue here. In what follows, we will assume that VE represents protection against pertussis infection, in conditions of household exposure.

To calculate the effectiveness against transmission VT, we must first check that the effectiveness measures for protection and infectiousness are independent, that is, that there is no interaction between them. This is achieved by including an interaction term in the model and testing its statistical significance. It turns out not to be statistically significant: the chi-squared test statistic is 0.05 on 1 degree of freedom, $p = 0.82$. The total effectiveness against transmission and its standard error, subscripted by t, are:

$$\beta_t = \beta_p + \beta_i = -2.3279, \quad \sigma_t = 0.4407.$$

The standard error may be obtained from the covariance matrix of the estimated parameters, or directly by reparametrising the model.

Thus, the vaccine effectiveness against transmission is $VT = 1 - \exp(\beta_t) = 0.90$ or 90%, with 95% CI (77%, 96%). The vaccine thus reduces transmission of infection by 90%.

In the pertussis example in Box 14.13, the vaccine effectiveness against infectiousness was found to be larger than its protective effectiveness; both contribute to reducing transmission.

Establishing whether there is an interaction between a vaccine's protective effectiveness and its effectiveness against infectiousness is important: when there is such an interaction, it is much less straightforward to estimate any of these quantities. Box 14.14 describes an example where this is an issue.

Box 14.14 Varicella vaccination in California: the effects of interaction

This study was based on data collected between 1997 and 2001 in Antelope Valley, California (Seward, Zhang, Maupin, Mascola, & Jumaan, 2004). Children aged 1 to 14 years were included. A primary case is the first within the household, by date of rash. Co-primary cases are those with rash onset up to 9 days after that of the primary case, and secondary cases are those with rash onset 10 to 21 days after that of the primary case.

The stratified data are in Table 14.4. These data include prior cases of varicella; similar results are obtained if prior cases are excluded. Households with co-primary cases were not excluded; the authors state that excluding them did not greatly affect the secondary attack rates.

An analysis taking into account both the vaccination status of primary and secondary cases is undertaken by fitting a binomial model with log link. The model includes the two factors for vaccination of the primary case and of the contacts, respectively. However, this model indicates that there is a statistically significant interaction between these two factors: the chi-squared test statistic is 14.3 on one degree of freedom, $p < 0.001$.

The presence of an interaction is clear from Table 14.4. On the one hand, the secondary attack rate in unvaccinated contacts of vaccinated primary cases is 25%, which is lower than the 49.9% attack rate in unvaccinated contacts of unvaccinated primary cases. This suggests vaccinees are less infectious. However, the secondary attack rate in vaccinated contacts of vaccinated primary cases is 22.3%, which is higher than the 13.5% attack rate in vaccinated contacts of unvaccinated primary cases. This suggests vaccinees are more infectious. Hence, the effectiveness of the vaccine against infectiousness differs depending on the vaccination status of the contacts.

This interaction induces heterogeneity in the vaccine effectiveness estimates. From the attack rates in Table 14.4, we obtain $VE = 73\%$ in households where the primary case is unvaccinated, but $VE = 11\%$ in households where the

Table 14.4 **Numbers of varicella cases, contacts and secondary attack rate by vaccination status**

Primary case vaccinated	Contacts vaccinated	Number of cases	Number of contacts	Secondary attack rate (%)
No	No	1,170	2,345	49.9
No	Yes	25	185	13.5
Yes	No	27	108	25.0
Yes	Yes	21	94	22.3

primary case is vaccinated. Similarly, VI depends on the vaccination status of the contacts: $VI = 50\%$ for unvaccinated contacts, but $VI = -65\%$ for vaccinated contacts.

In view of this interaction it is not meaningful to calculate summary values of VE, VI or VT. Instead, further work is required to uncover the underlying reasons for the heterogeneity. It may be due, for example, to misclassification of cases (a clinical case definition was used) or vaccination status (in some instances this was based on parental recall), or to confounding associated with individual characteristics (such as age) or with household characteristics (such as intensity of contacts).

The example described in Box 14.14 serves as a reminder that summary measures of vaccine effectiveness are only useful when there is no underlying heterogeneity due to interaction.

Summary

- Cohort methods for evaluating VE include a variety of different designs and a range of different analysis methods, yielding both risk-based and rate-based estimates of VE.
- Generalised linear modelling, using binomial or Poisson models, provides a flexible framework for obtaining vaccine effectiveness estimates and adjusting them for potential confounders.
- Household studies may enable the estimation of the vaccine effectiveness against infectiousness VI as well as the protective effectiveness VE. When VE measures protection against infection, VE and VI may be combined to obtain an estimate of vaccine effectiveness against transmission, VT.
- In household studies, interaction between vaccination of primary cases and of contacts may preclude the calculation of summary effectiveness measures.
- The cohort study designs described in the present chapter are summarised in Table 14.5.

Table 14.5 **Summary table**

Design	What can be estimated	Essential data for all members of the cohort	Typical uses
Parallel groups with identical follow-up	VE based on risks or rates VP	• Case status • Vaccination status	Outbreak investigations in schools
Arbitrary follow-up, with grouped person-time	VE based on rates VP	• Case status • Vaccination status • Person-time of observation for vaccinated and unvaccinated individuals	Community studies Database studies
Arbitrary follow-up, with individual histories	VE based on rates VP	• Case status • Vaccination status • Person-time of observation per individual • Event time (for survival analyses)	Community studies Database studies
Household contact studies	VE based on risks VI and VT VP	• Household identifier • Case status • Vaccination status • Date of onset	Outbreak investigations Community studies

References

Arenz, S., Schmitt, H. -J., Tischer, A., & von Kries, R. (2005). Effectiveness of measles vaccination after household exposure during a measles outbreak. *Pediatric Infectious Disease Journal*, *24*(8), 697–699.

Barrabeig, I., Rovira, A., Rius, C., Muñoz, P., Soldevila, N., Batalla, J., & Domínuez, À. (2011). Effectiveness of measles vaccination for control of exposed children. *Pediatric Infectious Disease Journal*, *30*(1), 78–80.

Baxter, R., Bartlett, J., Fireman, B., Lewis, E., & Klein, N. P. (2017). Effectiveness of vaccination during pregnancy to prevent infant pertussis. *Pediatrics*, *139*(5), e20164091.

Chang, C., Mo, X., Hu, P., Liang, W., Ma, H., An, Z., ... Zheng, H. (2015). Effectiveness of rubella vaccine in a rubella outbreak in Guangzhou city, China, 2014. *Vaccine*, *33*, 3223–3227.

Davison, A. C. (2003). *Statistical models*. Cambridge, UK: Cambridge University Press.

Galloway, Y., Stehr-Green, P., McNicholas, A., & O'Hallahan, J. (2009). Use of an observational cohort study to estimate the effectiveness of the New Zealand group B meningococcal vaccine in children aged under 5 years. *International Journal of Epidemiology*, *38*, 413–418.

Hahné, S., Whelan, J., van Binnendijk, R., Boot, H., & de Melker, H. (2012). Mumps vaccine effectiveness against orchitis. *Emerging Infectious Diseases*, *18*(1), 191–192.

Halloran, M. E., Préziosi, M. -P., & Chu, H. (2003). Estimating vaccine efficacy from secondary attack rates. *Journal of the American Statistical Association, 98*(461), 38–46.

McCullagh, P., & Nelder, J. A. (1989). *Generalized linear models* (2nd ed.). London: Chapman & Hall.

Préziosi, M. -P., & Halloran, M. H. (2003). Effects of pertussis vaccination on transmission: Vaccine efficacy for infectiousness. *Vaccine, 21,* 1853–1861.

Seward, J. F., Zhang, J. X., Maupin, T. J., Mascola, L., & Jumaan, A. O. (2004). Contagiousness of varicella in vaccinated cases: A household contact study. *Journal of the American Medical Association, 292*(6), 704–708.

Snijders, B. E., van Lier, A., van de Kassteele, J., Fanoy, E. B., Ruijs, W. L., Hulsof, F., ... Hahné, S. J. (2012). Mumps vaccine effectiveness in primary schools and households, the Netherlands, 2008. *Vaccine, 30,* 2999–3002.

Terranella, A., Rea, V., Griffith, M., Manning, S., Sears, S., Farmer, A., ... Patel, M. (2016). Vaccine effectiveness of tetanus toxoid, reduced diphtheria toxoid, and acellulatr pertussis vaccine during a pertussis outbreak in Maine. *Vaccine, 34,* 2496–2500.

Walker, J. L., Andrews, N. J., Amirthalingam, G., Forbes, H., Langan, S. M., & Thomas, S. L. (2018). Effectiveness of herpes zoster vaccination in an older United Kingdom population. *Vaccine, 36,* 2371–2377.

Chapter 15

Estimating vaccine effectiveness
Case-control and screening studies

A disadvantage of cohort studies, particularly those involving uncommon infections, is that they can require large samples. In the present chapter, we focus on case-control studies, and their many variants. These generally require more modest sample sizes and are in many settings more practicable than cohort studies, especially when no suitable population databases are available.

We begin in Section 15.1 with traditional case-control studies, in which the controls are chosen among non-cases. Then in Section 15.2 we consider variants of the case-control method in which controls can also be or become cases. In Section 15.3 we discuss two special case-control methods: the test-negative and indirect cohort methods. In Section 15.4 we describe the screening method, in which controls are replaced by vaccine coverage data, which makes the method particularly easy to apply provided reliable coverage data are available. A summary table is provided at the end of the chapter, listing the various case-control designs and some of their key properties.

All case-control studies involve an odds ratio. Like probabilities, odds are measures of chance. If an event occurs with probability p, then the odds of the event is the ratio $p/(1-p)$. For example, the odds of vaccination is the probability of being vaccinated, divided by the probability of not being vaccinated. Whereas in cohort studies the focus is the relative risk or relative rate, in case-control studies it is the odds ratio OR, which is the ratio of the odds of vaccination in cases to the odds of vaccination in controls:

$$OR = \frac{\text{odds of vaccination in cases}}{\text{odds of vaccination in controls}}.$$

How this odds ratio OR relates to relative risks or relative rates, and hence to vaccine effectiveness, differs according to how controls are selected; this raises subtle methodological issues, discussed in Rodrigues and Kirkwood (1990). We shall consider the different types of case-control study in turn. A general reference on case-control methods in vaccine evaluation is Rodrigues and Smith (1999).

15.1 Retrospective case-control studies with exclusive control groups

These studies follow the traditional methodology of retrospective case-control studies: exposures are compared in a sample of cases and controls, the latter being chosen among individuals who had not become cases by the end of the study period. Thus, the control group excludes cases. We distinguish two settings: unmatched and matched studies.

15.1.1 Unmatched case-control studies

Unmatched studies are appropriate when the population in which the cases arise is well defined, so that controls may readily be sampled from it. Suppose there are r cases (r_v vaccinated and r_u unvaccinated) and m controls (m_v vaccinated and m_u unvaccinated). The odds ratio is then

$$OR = \frac{r_v / r_u}{m_v / m_u}.$$

Provided the infection is rare, the odds ratio approximates the relative risk: this is sometimes called the rare disease assumption. In these circumstances, the vaccine effectiveness may be estimated as

$$VE = 1 - OR = 1 - \frac{r_v / r_u}{m_v / m_u}.$$

This approximates the risk-based estimate of vaccine effectiveness. If the infection is not rare, this estimate of VE will differ from that obtained with the relative risk (it will produce values more extreme, that is, further away from 0), but it will only equal zero if the risk-based effectiveness is zero. To obtain a 95% confidence interval (CI), first obtain 95% confidence limits for the odds ratio:

$$OR^- = OR \times \exp(-1.96 \times \sigma), \quad OR^+ = OR \times \exp(+1.96 \times \sigma),$$

where σ is the standard error of the log odds ratio:

$$\sigma = \sqrt{\frac{1}{r_v} + \frac{1}{r_u} + \frac{1}{m_v} + \frac{1}{m_u}}.$$

Then the 95% CI for VE is $(1 - OR^+, 1 - OR^-)$.

When potential confounders need to be taken into account, as is very often the case, the analysis proceeds using a binomial generalised linear model with logistic link, also called logistic regression. The responses are the numbers vaccinated, and the binomial denominators are the numbers of cases or controls; the data are cross-classified by case/control status and other covariates. An example is discussed in Box 15.1.

Box 15.1 Influenza vaccine effectiveness in Malaysian pilgrims attending the Hajj

This study was undertaken in five hotels used by Malaysian pilgrims attending the Hajj in Mecca, Saudi Arabia, in 2000 (Mustafa et al., 2003). Cases were recruited from pilgrims presenting at the hotel clinics with influenza-like respiratory illness, defined as sore throat with either raised temperature or cough. Controls were recruited among pilgrims staying in the same hotels, who had not attended any clinic. Vaccination histories were based on vaccination cards (required for entry to Saudi Arabia) where possible.

There were 820 cases and 600 controls; 513 cases and 530 controls were vaccinated, so the odds ratio is

$$OR = \frac{513/(820-513)}{530/(600-530)} = \frac{513/307}{530/70} = 0.22070.$$

The vaccine effectiveness is therefore

$$VE = 1 - 0.22070 = 0.78.$$

To obtain the 95% CI, we first calculate

$$\sigma = \sqrt{\frac{1}{513} + \frac{1}{307} + \frac{1}{530} + \frac{1}{70}} = 0.14622.$$

The 95% confidence limits for VE are then

$$VE^- = 1 - 0.22070 \times \exp(+1.96 \times 0.14622) = 0.70605,$$

$$VE^+ = 1 - 0.22070 \times \exp(-1.96 \times 0.14622) = 0.83429.$$

Thus, the vaccine effectiveness is 78% against influenza-like respiratory illness, with 95% CI (71%, 83%). Adjusting for age, gender and hotel using logistic regression only had a small impact on the results: the adjusted vaccine effectiveness was 77%, 95% CI (69%, 83%). The authors note that this is an unusually high VE, and discuss possible biases, including possibly lower propensity to attend hotel clinics among vaccinated cases. On the other hand, the vaccine was found not to be effective against upper respiratory tract illness that did not meet the case definition: adjusted VE = 20%, 95% CI (–24%, 49%).

In the example described in Box 15.1, the total population from which cases and controls were selected was about 10,000 (2,000 per hotel), so the attack rate was less than 10%: this is sufficiently low to avoid serious bias from using odds ratios to estimate relative risks in this setting.

15.1.2 Matched case-control studies

Matching is typically used to avoid imbalances between cases and controls with respect to potential confounders, so that they may be controlled more effectively in the analysis. Matching may also be used for convenience in selecting controls. In a matched study, one or more controls are selected for each case, which have the same attributes as the case for selected matching variables such as age or date of birth (often within predetermined categories), sex, location or other characteristics. It is important that the matching variables should be taken into account in the analysis, as the matching process may otherwise introduce bias.

Two methods of analysis may be used for matched case-control studies. A logistic regression model, explicitly controlling for the matching variables, may be applied as described in Section 15.1.1. This method of analysis is appropriate especially when the matching is done on broad categories. However, a different method of analysis, called conditional logistic regression, is required if the matching results in many sparse strata, as is usually the case for closely individually matched studies. (A standard logistic regression explicitly adjusting for matching can produce biased results in such circumstances.) In a conditional logistic regression, the matching is taken account of implicitly, the estimation being undertaken within matched sets. When there is just one control per case there are simple formulas for the matched odds ratio and its confidence interval, which we now describe.

Suppose there are n matched case-control pairs, and that among these pairs there are n_{10} in which the case is vaccinated and the matched control is unvaccinated, and n_{01} in which the case is unvaccinated and the matched control is vaccinated. These are called discordant pairs. It then turns out that the odds ratio in the matched analysis takes the following simple form:

$$OR = \frac{n_{10}}{n_{01}},$$

so that the vaccine effectiveness is

$$VE = 1 - \frac{n_{10}}{n_{01}}.$$

To obtain a 95% CI for VE, first obtain the 95% confidence limits for OR:

$$OR^- = OR \times \exp(-1.96 \times \sigma), \quad OR^+ = OR \times \exp(+1.96 \times \sigma),$$

where σ is the standard error of the log odds ratio for matched pairs:

$$\sigma = \sqrt{\frac{1}{n_{10}} + \frac{1}{n_{01}}}.$$

The 95% CI for VE is then $(1 - OR^+, 1 - OR^-)$. These calculations are illustrated in Box 15.2.

Box 15.2 Pneumococcal vaccine effectiveness in high-risk patients

This retrospective case-control study was motivated by controversy over the effectiveness of pneumococcal vaccination in high-risk patients in the United States (Shapiro & Clemens, 1984). Cases and controls were hospitalised patients with at least one indication for pneumococcal vaccination prior to admission. Some 90 cases with confirmed systemic pneumococcal infection were individually matched to controls who had never presented with a pneumococcal infection. Matching was on age, date of hospitalisation and severity and duration of the indication for the vaccine prior to hospitalisation. Vaccination status was determined by written records.

Among the 90 matched case-control pairs, 5 included a vaccinated case and unvaccinated control, and 15 included an unvaccinated case and a vaccinated control. Thus, $n_{10} = 5$ and $n_{01} = 15$ and

$$OR = \frac{5}{15} = 0.33333,$$

and so the vaccine effectiveness is $VE = 0.67$, or 67%. To obtain a 95% CI for VE, we first calculate

$$\sigma = \sqrt{\frac{1}{5} + \frac{1}{15}} = 0.51640.$$

Then the 95% confidence limits for VE are

$$VE^{-} = 1 - 0.33333 \times \exp(+1.96 \times 0.51640) = 0.083,$$

$$VE^{+} = 1 - 0.33333 \times \exp(-1.96 \times 0.51640) = 0.88.$$

Hence the vaccine effectiveness against systemic pneumococcal infection is 67%, with 95% CI (8.3%, 88%); the authors applied a continuity correction, giving a slightly narrower CI. Further analyses of these data to control for potential confounding variables (such as gender, ethnic group, presence of additional indications for vaccination) did not substantially alter the results.

In the example described in Box 15.2, the overall incidence of infection was low, and so the odds ratio closely approximates the relative risk. This study therefore provides an estimate of risk-based vaccine effectiveness.

Several controls can be matched to each case in order to increase the power of the study; beyond four controls per case there is little further gain in power. Matching can also help to specify a systematic way of identifying suitable controls, when the population from which the cases are sampled cannot readily be described precisely or enumerated in advance. Each case becomes the focus of a control selection strategy that can be described precisely and applied systematically. For this reason, matched case-control studies are particularly useful in settings where there are no convenient databases from which to sample controls. Box 15.3 provides two contrasting examples of control selection strategies.

Box 15.3 Control selection for vaccine studies in outbreaks in Vietnam and Tanzania

These two matched case-control studies were undertaken to assess the effectiveness of cholera vaccination and measles vaccination, respectively, during outbreaks. One study used hospital controls, the other neighbourhood controls.

- *Hospital controls*: during a cholera outbreak in Hanoi, Vietnam, cases aged over 10 years resident in the areas of interest were identified from admission records of selected hospitals, using a clinical case definition. For each case, admission records of patients admitted for non-diarrhoeal conditions, matched with the case on age (in broad age groups), date of admission (within 5 days of the case), gender and district of residence were identified, and the first one listed was selected as a control. The persons selecting cases and controls were unaware of their vaccination status (Anh et al., 2011).
- *Neighbourhood controls*: after an outbreak of measles in Dar Es Salaam in 2006–2007, cases aged up to 18 years were identified from case reports, registers and discussions with local leaders. Controls were selected using a carefully planned procedure, incorporating random elements. The authors describe the method as follows:

Controls were selected from households in the vicinity of cases using a random walk from case households, based on a generated list of random starting directions (right or left) and random numbers (5–25) of households to be passed. Once a household was chosen, one control was randomly selected from a list of all household members aged 0–18 years with no history of measles in 2006.

(Goodson et al., 2010, p. 5981)

Control selection strategies vary greatly and are tailored to each study. In general, whatever the type of case-control study that is being undertaken, the aim is, as far as possible, to select controls that are representative of the population from which the cases arose. As for case-control studies in other areas of epidemiology, it is important to avoid overmatching cases and controls on variables that may be related to the exposure (which in the present context is vaccination).

15.2 Case-control studies with non-exclusive control groups

In Section 15.1 we considered case-control methods in which the control groups exclude cases. These studies may be analysed by logistic regression or conditional logistic regression (if matched), and yield an estimate of risk-based vaccine effectiveness, provided that the incidence of disease is sufficiently low that the relative risk is approximated by the odds ratio: this is the rare disease assumption.

In the present section we consider two other types of case-control study, in which controls can potentially include cases or future cases. For these designs, the rare disease assumption is not necessary: the odds ratio is identical to the relative risk or the relative rate, which may therefore be estimated directly.

15.2.1 Concurrent and nested case-control studies

In a concurrent case-control study, matched controls for each case are chosen among individuals who are still at risk of becoming cases at the time of onset of the case. The design may be thought of as nested within a time-to-event cohort study, with controls randomly selected from the risk set of each case. Indeed, when a cohort has been defined explicitly, the design is known as a nested case-control study. A control may thus, at some later time during the study, also become a case. Several analysis methods exist, the most commonly used being conditional logistic regression (see Section 5.1.2). In this situation the odds ratio is identical to the hazard ratio, and so the estimate of vaccine effectiveness is a rate-based one. Further discussion of this and other designs, with some references to vaccination, may be found in Rodrigues and Kirkwood (1990). An example is in Box 15.4

Box 15.4 Vaccine effectiveness of a cholera vaccine during a cholera outbreak in Guinea

A cholera outbreak was declared in Guinea in 2012, triggering outbreak response measures supplemented in two prefectures by mass vaccination campaigns with two doses of the Sanchol oral cholera vaccine. A matched case-control study was undertaken to evaluate the short-term effectiveness of the vaccine (about 6 months after the end of the vaccination campaigns) in these two areas (Luquero et al., 2014).

The study included 40 cases with confirmed cholera aged over 1 year and satisfying some residency requirements. For each case, four persons were selected as controls among neighbours of the same age group as the case, who had not sought treatment for diarrhoea by the onset date of the case.

Thus, this study was matched on age and location. Vaccination status of cases and controls was ascertained by face-to-face interviews and vaccination cards. The analysis used conditional logistic regression, adjusted for possible confounders: these included number of people living in the household, whether drinking water was treated and whether a latrine was shared with a person who had cholera. The adjusted vaccine effectiveness for full (two-dose) vaccination was 87%, 95% CI (57%, 96%). The authors concluded that timely vaccination campaigns can help in controlling cholera outbreaks.

The example in Box 15.4 is a concurrent case-control study because matched controls were selected among non-cases at the time of onset of the case. As a result, the odds ratio equals the hazard ratio. However, because cholera was not common in this population during the study period, the distinction between risk-based and rate-based measures of effectiveness is not important.

15.2.2 Case-cohort studies

In a case-cohort study, the controls are chosen from within the population at risk at the start of the study, so as to be representative of that population (such as a random sample). Thus, controls can become cases at any time. In effect, the controls are used to estimate the proportion vaccinated in the underlying population from which the cases emerge. Indeed, this type of study has also been called a case-coverage study, involving a sample of cases and a vaccination coverage survey.

In a case-cohort study, a range of different analysis methods can be used. If data on the time to event of the cases are available, then a case-cohort version of the Cox proportional hazards model may be applied; this yields hazard ratios, and hence rate-based vaccine effectiveness measures. This approach, with a focus on vaccine effectiveness, is discussed in Moulton, Wolff, Brenneman, and Santosham (1995). If time to event data are not available, odds ratios may be calculated: in the present context they are identical to relative risks and hence yield risk-based effectiveness measures, without the need for the rare disease assumption; the details of the models lie beyond the scope of this book. An example of a case-cohort study is described in Box 15.5.

Box 15.5 Effectiveness of cholera vaccination during an outbreak in South Sudan

A targeted vaccination campaign with a single dose of oral cholera vaccine was deployed in 2015 during a cholera outbreak in Juba, South Sudan. The campaign was targeted towards high-risk areas, owing to limited vaccine supplies. The short-term effectiveness of vaccination was evaluated in a case-cohort study, which was not limited to the targeted areas (Azman et al., 2016).

Cases included persons aged 1 year and older at the start of the vaccination campaign who sought medical care for diarrhoea, who met clinical and residence criteria and in whom cholera was confirmed. The population cohort was selected using multistage random spatial sampling. The city was partitioned into density-weighted grid cells using aerial imagery. Then grid cells, households within cells and one individual within each household were selected at random. Vaccination histories were obtained from cases and cohort members using a standardised questionnaire and vaccination cards where available. The analysis was undertaken using a case-cohort proportional hazards model to estimate the hazard ratio, starting from the end of the vaccination campaign.

There were 34 confirmed cases of cholera, of whom 2 were vaccinated. The coverage cohort included 898 individuals (373 vaccinated). The unadjusted (rate-based) vaccine effectiveness was 80%, 95% CI (62% to 100%). After adjusting for potential confounders (including age, sex, household size, water treatment), $VE = 87\%$, 95% CI (70%, 100%). The authors commented that single-dose vaccination provides short-term (2-month) protection against cholera in an outbreak setting.

15.3 Test-negative and indirect designs

In this section we discuss two case-control designs in which controls are selected from individuals who share similar clinical symptoms with the case, but who are not infected with the organism targeted by vaccination. These are the test-negative design, most commonly used to evaluate influenza vaccine effectiveness, and the indirect method (also called the Broome method) for evaluating the effectiveness of vaccines against multi-strain infections.

15.3.1 The test-negative design

This method was proposed in order to provide an efficient method for evaluating influenza vaccine effectiveness within a sentinel surveillance system (Skowronski et al., 2007). Patients presenting with influenza-like illness (ILI) are categorised as cases if they test positive for influenza virus, and as controls if they test negative for influenza. The vaccine effectiveness is then

$$VE = 1 - \frac{\text{odds of vaccination in test-positive cases}}{\text{odds of vaccination in test-negative cases}}.$$

Thus, VE aims to estimate the relative reduction in the odds of vaccination in infected versus non-infected persons with disease-like symptoms. The case-control analysis is as described in Section 15.1, adjusting for possible confounders and including matching as required. The method yields an odds ratio that is equal to the relative risk, provided that the probability that a test-negative case is vaccinated is the same as the vaccine coverage in the population. Thus, the method yields a risk-based vaccine effectiveness measure.

An advantage of the method is that the same procedures are used to ascertain cases and controls. A further benefit, it has been argued, is that the method can help to avoid confounding in situations where vaccination is associated with health-seeking behaviour

(Lipsitch, Jha, & Simonsen 2016), though the method can still be prone to this and other types of bias (Ainslie, Shi, Haber, & Orenstein, 2017). Variables associated with vaccination coverage, such as calendar time and location, may be confounders and if so should be adjusted. A further issue is the accuracy of the test; it has been shown that imperfect test sensitivity and specificity, within realistic ranges, have only a modest impact on the results, high specificity being more important than high sensitivity (Jackson & Rothman, 2015). Box 15.6 describes an application of the method, including a comparison with a traditional case-control study.

Box 15.6 Effectiveness of inactivated quadrivalent influenza vaccine in Japan

This study was conducted in one hospital in a district of Tokyo during the 2005–2006 influenza season (Kimiya et al., 2018). The target population included children aged 6 months to 15 years admitted with a fever (a temperature $\geq 38°C$), who received an influenza rapid detection test.

There were 112 confirmed influenza A cases, of whom 33 had received at least one dose of influenza vaccine, 70 influenza B cases (32 vaccinated) and 149 with neither influenza A nor B (85 vaccinated) who served as controls. For influenza A, the odds ratio is

$$OR = \frac{33/(112-33)}{85/(149-85)} = \frac{33/79}{85/64} = 0.31452$$

and so the vaccine effectiveness is

$$VE = 1 - 0.31452 = 0.68548.$$

Thus $VE = 69\%$, with 95% CI (47%, 81%), calculated as set out in Box 15.1. For influenza B,

$$VE = \frac{32/(70-32)}{85/(149-85)} = 1 - \frac{32/38}{85/64} = 0.36594,$$

so $VE = 37\%$ with 95% CI (−12%, 64%). Adjustment for covariates including age and comorbidities did not substantially affect the results.

A traditional case-control study was also conducted, with cases and controls recruited among persons admitted as outpatients to the same hospital. The vaccine effectiveness was lower in this second study (44% for influenza A, 24% for influenza B). The authors discuss possible sources of bias, including differential healthcare-seeking behaviour according to vaccination status in the traditional case-control study.

The test-negative design was developed specifically for estimating influenza vaccine effectiveness, but it has wider application. For example, Khagayi et al. (2020) use the method with rotavirus vaccination in Kenya, and show that while the vaccine gives good protection in well-nourished children, no protection could be demonstrated in malnourished children.

15.3.2 The indirect (Broome) method

The indirect method, also called the Broome method after its originator (Broome, Facklam, & Fraser, 1980), was developed to estimate the effectiveness of pneumococcal vaccines. The method is similar in spirit to the test-negative case-control design, and may be used to estimate the effectiveness of vaccines containing only some of the serotypes of the pathogen of interest. The cases are selected among patients with disease caused by strains included in the vaccine (the vaccine-type patients). Controls are selected among patients with the same disease, but caused by strains not included in the vaccine (non-vaccine-type patients). The vaccine effectiveness is thus

$$VE = 1 - \frac{\text{odds of vaccination in vaccine-type patients}}{\text{odds of vaccination in non-vaccine-type patients}}.$$

As with the test-negative design, the data may be analysed using standard methods for case-control studies, including logistic regression. Box 15.7 provides an illustration.

Box 15.7 Effectiveness of a 13-valent pneumococcal conjugate vaccine in Germany

This is a study of the effectiveness of the 13-valent pneumococcal conjugate vaccine in Germany, using data obtained from a national surveillance programme for invasive pneumococcal disease (IPD) for children under the age of 16 years (Weinberger, van der Linden, Imöhl, & von Kries, 2016).

All IPD patients in the study were positive for pneumococci. After removing patients with incomplete vaccination or serotyping information, there were 117 IPD patients in whom only non-vaccine strains were identified: these were the controls. Of these, 99 received at least one dose of PCV13 vaccine, and 18 were unvaccinated. There were 47 IPD patients in whom a serotype included in the vaccine was isolated: these were the cases. Of these, 18 were vaccinated and 29 unvaccinated. The unadjusted Broome odds ratio was thus

$$OR = \frac{18/29}{99/18} = 0.11285.$$

Thus, the vaccine effectiveness was 89%, with 95% CI (76%, 95%), calculated as set out in Box 15.1. Adjusting for covariates using logistic regression did not alter these estimates.

> The authors also estimated vaccine effectiveness against the serotypes included in the 7-valent vaccine ($VE = 91\%$ for at least one vaccine dose), against the additional serotypes included in the 13-valent vaccine ($VE = 88\%$), and for different vaccination schedules.

As illustrated in Box 15.7, the method enables vaccine effectiveness to be evaluated for specific strains, or groups of strains.

The method assumes that the vaccine provides no protection against serotypes not included in the vaccine (also called cross-protection, see Chapter 2). A further potential difficulty with the indirect method is that vaccination may increase the probability of carriage of non-vaccine serotypes, compared to unvaccinated individuals. This would result in overestimation of VE. If VE is the true vaccine effectiveness, VE_B is the Broome vaccine effectiveness, VE_C is the vaccine effectiveness against carriage (all three being expressed as numbers less than 1), and p is the proportion of carriage that is of vaccine type in the unvaccinated, then under the assumption of complete strain replacement in carriage,

$$VE = 1 - (1 - VE_B) \times \left(1 + VE_C \times \frac{p}{1-p}\right).$$

This expression is derived from Andrews et al. (2011), and may be used for undertaking sensitivity analyses. A practical application is described in Box 15.8.

Box 15.8 Effectiveness of the 7-valent pneumococcal vaccine in England and Wales

This study was undertaken using a database of cases of invasive pneumococcal disease with confirmed *Streptococcus pneumoniae* infection (Andrews et al., 2011). There were 919 patients with non-vaccine types, of whom 825 received at least one dose of vaccine, and 153 patients with vaccine types, of whom 74 were vaccinated. The unadjusted Broome vaccine effectiveness was thus

$$VE_B = 1 - \frac{74/79}{825/94} = 0.89327.$$

So $VE = 89\%$; the 95% CI was (84%, 93%). Adjustment by logistic regression for age, sex, period and cohort reduced this to 79%, 95% CI (67%, 87%).

To investigate sensitivity to vaccine-induced changes in carriage, the authors suggest values for VE_C in the range 0.3 to 0.5, and $p = 0.4$ based on external data. Thus with $VE_C = 0.4$, a Broome effectiveness of $VE_B = 0.79$ would correspond to a true effectiveness of

$$VE = 1-(1-0.79)\times\left(1+0.4\times\frac{0.4}{1-0.4}\right) = 0.734.$$

Thus, if there were complete serotype replacement, the true vaccine effectiveness might be about 6% lower than that measured by the Broome method.

15.4 The screening method

The screening method involves comparing the proportion of cases that are vaccinated to the vaccine coverage in the underlying population from which the cases arose. The method may be applied when accurate vaccine coverage data are available, and only requires a sample of cases. For this reason, the method is easy to use as part of a routine surveillance system, and is commonly employed in studies of vaccine effectiveness for infections controlled by routine vaccination programmes. Further details of the method may be found in (Farrington, 1993).

Suppose that a sample of cases is available, of whom r_v are vaccinated and r_u are unvaccinated. Suppose furthermore that the vaccine coverage in the cohort from which the cases are drawn is π; individuals with incomplete or unknown vaccination status are excluded. The screening odds ratio is then

$$OR_S = \frac{r_v/r_u}{\pi/(1-\pi)},$$

and the screening vaccine effectiveness is

$$VE = 1-OR_S = 1-\frac{r_v/r_u}{\pi/(1-\pi)}.$$

Note that only r_v and r_u are estimated, using all or a random sample of cases: the vaccine coverage π is known. All quantities should relate to the exposure of interest. For example if, in a multi-dose vaccination schedule, only full vaccination is being evaluated, then r_v is the number of fully vaccinated cases, r_u is the number of wholly unvaccinated cases and π is the proportion of the population fully vaccinated among those fully vaccinated or wholly unvaccinated (i.e., excluding individuals who are only partially vaccinated). The 95% confidence limits for the screening odds ratio are

$$OR_S^- = OR_S \times \exp(-1.96\times\sigma),\quad OR_S^+ = OR_S \times \exp(+1.96\times\sigma)$$

where σ is the standard error of the log odds of vaccination in cases,

$$\sigma = \sqrt{\frac{1}{r_v}+\frac{1}{r_u}},$$

from which the 95% CI for the vaccine effectiveness is obtained:

$$VE^- = 1 - OR_S^+, \quad VE^+ = 1 - OR_S^-.$$

Conceptually, the method shares some similarities with a case-cohort method, in which the cohort data are replaced by a census of the entire population. The screening odds ratio is equal to the relative risk (no rare disease assumption needed), and so the screening vaccine effectiveness is a risk-based measure.

The screening method may be used in two ways: as a screening tool and as a more elaborate estimation method, adjusting for confounders by means of a statistical model. We consider the two approaches in turn.

15.4.1 Screening studies

These are the applications initially envisaged for the screening method, from which it derives its name. In a screening study, the vaccine effectiveness is estimated rapidly (and often approximately) in order to determine whether there is a problem with the vaccine that may require further action, for example within an outbreak investigation. Box 15.9 describes such an application.

Box 15.9 Measles vaccine effectiveness in South Africa

Additional measures to control measles in South Africa were introduced from 1996. After a period in which measles was well controlled, a large outbreak occurred in 2003–2005. An investigation, including a screening estimation of vaccine effectiveness, was carried out in two districts in Gauteng and Eastern Cape (McMorrow et al., 2009). Vaccine effectiveness was estimated in children aged 12–59 months. Based on provincial measles first-dose vaccination coverage, the vaccine coverage was taken as 80% in both districts. As similar effectiveness was found in the two districts, the analysis presented here is based on the combined data.

There were 49 confirmed measles cases, of whom 16 were vaccinated. The screening odds ratio is

$$OR_S = \frac{16/33}{0.80/(1-0.80)} = 0.12121.$$

The estimated vaccine effectiveness is therefore

$$VE = 1 - 0.12121 = 0.87879,$$

or 88%. To obtain a 95% CI, first obtain

$$\sigma = \sqrt{\frac{1}{16} + \frac{1}{33}} = 0.30464.$$

The 95% confidence limits for the screening odds ratio are then

$$OR_S^- = 0.12121 \times \exp(-1.96 \times 0.30464) = 0.066715,$$

$$OR_S^+ = 0.12121 \times \exp(+1.96 \times 0.30464) = 0.22022.$$

Hence the 95% confidence limits for the vaccine effectiveness are

$$VE^- = 1 - 0.22022 = 0.78, \quad VE^+ = 1 - 0.066715 = 0.93.$$

Thus, the screening vaccine effectiveness for one dose of measles vaccine is 88%, 95% confidence limits (78%, 93%). This does not suggest that the outbreak was caused by primary or secondary vaccine failure. Further investigations were undertaken in HIV positive and HIV negative cases, and to evaluate the sensitivity of the results to the vaccine coverage value of 80%.

The screening method also provides a convenient monitoring tool for real-time vaccine effectiveness surveillance based on case notifications and vaccine coverage data. Such an application, to influenza vaccine effectiveness, is described in Box 15.10.

Box 15.10 Surveillance of influenza vaccine effectiveness in France

This application relates to a real-time system for monitoring the effectiveness of the seasonal influenza vaccine in France (Vilcu et al., 2018). In the 2015–2016 influenza season, cases of ILI were ascertained through the nationwide *Sentinelles* network of sentinel general practitioners. Vaccine coverage data were obtained from the CNAMTS, a national health insurance database.

Vaccine effectiveness monitoring began at the start of the influenza epidemic and stopped 2 weeks after it ended. We shall restrict attention to individuals aged 65 years or older.

Figure 15.1 shows the weekly trace of the VE estimate, estimated from cumulative cases using the screening method. This shows that the vaccine effectiveness estimate stabilised at around 40% by week 6 of 2016, the confidence intervals narrowing thereafter as cases accrue.

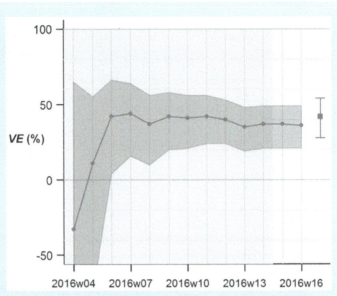

Figure 15.1 **Weekly VE estimate for ILI in persons aged 65 years or older.**
Note: The shaded areas represent the epidemic period (light shade) and the 95% confidence intervals (dark shade).
Source: Reproduced with permission from Vilcu et al. (2018).

By the end of the influenza season, 337 ILI cases had been ascertained in persons aged 65 years or older, of whom 126 had been vaccinated. The vaccine coverage in this age group was 50.8%. The effectiveness of the vaccine over the whole period, obtained with the screening method, was 42%, with 95% CI (28%, 54%). This overall estimate, and its 95% CI, is shown to the right in Figure 15.1. Further analyses were undertaken in other age groups, with confirmed cases and for specific influenza types.

In the application described in Box 15.10, data from different age groups were also analysed together to obtain a single combined *VE* estimate. How this is done, and more generally how potential confounders are allowed for with this method, is described in the next section.

15.4.2 Control of potential confounders with the screening method

Adjustment for covariates with the screening method is possible provided that the data, including the coverage data, are stratified by these covariates. In this way, some degree of confounder control is possible. For example, vaccine coverage data are often available by age, birth cohort and location, and so associations with these variables can readily be controlled.

To apply the screening method to data of this type, the statistical modelling approach described by Farrington (1993) should be used. This is a binomial generalised linear model with logistic link; the number of vaccinated cases in each stratum is the response, and the binomial index is the number of cases. In addition, the log-odds of the vaccination coverage is declared as an offset. Thus, if in stratum i the vaccine coverage is π_i, then $\log\{\pi_i/(1-\pi_i)\}$ is the offset for that stratum. Nested models may be fitted and interactions tested in the usual way. The overall adjusted vaccine effectiveness is obtained by fitting a model with no covariates.

In such analyses, care is required to ensure that the coverage figures relate to the cases in each category. An application is described in Box 15.11.

Box 15.11 Effectiveness of Hib vaccine in England and Wales

The *Haemophilus influenzae* type b (Hib) conjugate vaccine was introduced in the United Kingdom in 1992, and initially resulted in a large drop in the incidence of invasive Hib disease. Subsequently, the incidence began rising again, and a vaccine effectiveness study using the screening method was undertaken to explore the reasons for this increase (Ramsay, McVernon, Andrews, Heath, & Slack, 2003).

In the study period, and in birth cohorts eligible for routine (three doses at 2, 3, 4 months of age) or catch-up (one dose after 12 months of age) Hib vaccination, there were 443 reported cases of Hib with known vaccination status. Of these, 363 were fully vaccinated, 19 were partially vaccinated and 61 were unvaccinated. Only the 363 + 61 = 424 fully vaccinated or unvaccinated cases were used in the calculations. Information on vaccine coverage was obtained from routine statistics on the proportions of children receiving complete courses of vaccination for each birth cohort and age group. These values were adjusted to exclude the proportion partially vaccinated, estimated in a separate survey.

The screening method was applied using logistic regression to the data on cases and coverage, cross-classified by birth cohort and time since vaccination. The overall vaccine effectiveness was 57%, 95% CI (43%, 67%), but was found to be lower in children vaccinated under 6 months of age, and in older children for whom 2 years had elapsed since vaccination.

The key requirement of a screening analysis, exemplified by the Hib vaccine study described in Box 15.11, is to make sure that the vaccine coverage relates to the population from which the cases arise.

When vaccine coverage varies over time, age or birth cohort, the analysis should be stratified so that the cases and coverage in each stratum reflect such variation. When there are few cases, these may need to be individually paired with the corresponding vaccine coverages, as was done by Parikh et al. (2016) in their analysis of the effectiveness of meningitis B vaccination in England.

Summary

- A range of case-control methods are available to estimate vaccine effectiveness VE. These include standard unmatched and matched designs, as well as concurrent or nested case-control studies and case-cohort studies.
- The test-negative and indirect cohort (Broome) methods may be used in certain circumstances to mitigate certain types of bias.
- The screening method may be used to provide a rapid assessment of vaccine effectiveness, or more detailed analyses when reliable coverage data are available.
- All methods may be adjusted for potential confounders, provided data on these are available.

The study designs described in the present chapter differ primarily in terms of the different strategies used for selecting controls. These designs are summarised in Table 15.1.

Table 15.1 Summary table

Design	Controls	VE calculated from odds ratio	Essential data for cases and controls	Typical uses
Traditional case control	Non-cases over the study period, unmatched or matched	Approximates VE calculated from relative risk when events are rare	• Vaccination status	Outbreak investigations, community studies
Concurrent or nested	Non-cases at time of each case	Equals VE calculated from relative rate	• Vaccination status • Date of onset	Time-to-event studies
Case cohort	Population sample	Equals VE calculated from relative risk or relative rate	• Vaccination status	Population sample available
Test negative	Symptomatic individuals testing negative	Equals VE calculated from relative risk	• Vaccination status	Influenza, rotavirus, cholera vaccines
Broome	Non vaccine serotypes	As above	• Vaccination status	Pneumococcal vaccines
Screening	Entire population (vaccine coverage)	As above	• Cases: vaccination status • Population: vaccine coverage	Rapid evaluations or more detailed studies with good coverage data

References

Ainslie, K. E. C., Shi, M., Haber, M., & Orenstein, W. A. (2017). On the bias of estimates of influenza vaccine effectiveness from test-negative studies. *Vaccine, 35*, 7297–7301.

Andrews, N., Waight, P. A., Borrow, R., Ladhani, S., George, R. C., Slack, M. P. E., & Miller, E. (2011). Using the indirect cohort design to estimate the effectiveness of the seven valent pneumococcal conjugate vaccine in England and Wales. *PLoS One, 6*(12), e28435.

Anh, D. D., Lopez, A. L., Thiem, V. D., Grahek, S. L., Duong, T. N., Park, J. K., ... Clemens, J. D. (2011). Use of oral cholera vaccines in an outbreak in Vietnam: A case control study. *PLoS Neglected Tropical Diseases, 5*(1), e1006.

Azman, A. S., Parker, L. A., Rumunu, J., Tadesse, F., Grandesso, F., Deng, L. L., ... Luquero, J. (2016). Effectiveness of one dose of oral cholera vaccine in response to an outbreak: A case-cohort study. *Lancet Global Health, 4*, e856–e863.

Broome, C. V., Facklam, R. R., & Fraser, D. W. (1980). Pneumococcal disease after pneumococcal vaccination: An alternative method to estimate the efficacy of pneumococcal vaccine. *New England Journal of Medicine, 303*, 549–552.

Farrington, C. P. (1993). Estimation of vaccine effectiveness using the screening method. *International Journal of Epidemiology, 22*(4), 742–746.

Goodson, J. L., Perry, R. T., Mach, O., Manyanga, D., Luman, E. T., Kitambi, M., ... Cairns, L. (2010). Measles outbreak in Tanzania, 2006–2007. *Vaccine, 28*, 5979–5985.

Jackson, M. L., & Rothman, K. J. (2015). Effects of imperfect test sensitivity and specificity on observational studies of influenza vaccine effectiveness. *Vaccine, 33*, 1313–1316.

Khagayi, S., Omore, R., Otieno, G. P., Ogwel, B., Ochieng, J. B., Juma, J., ... Verani, J. R. (2020). Effectiveness of monovalent rotavirus vaccine against hospitalization with acute rotavirus gastroenteritis in Kenyan children. *Clinical Infectious Diseases, 70*(11), 2298–2305.

Kimiya, T., Shinjoh, M., Anzo, M., Takahashi, H., Sekiguchi, S., Sugaya, N., & Takahashi, T. (2018). Effectiveness of inactivated quadrivalent influenza vaccine in the 2015/2016 season as assessed in both a test-negative case-control study design and a traditional case-control study design. *European Journal of Pediatrics, 177*, 1009–1017.

Lipsitch, M., Jha, A., & Simonsen, L. (2016). Observational studies and the difficult quest for causality: Lessons from vaccine effectiveness and impact studies. *International Journal of Epidemiology, 45*(6), 2060–2074.

Luquero, F. J., Group, L. Ciglenecki, I., Sakoba, K., Traore, B., Heile, M., ... Grais, R. F. (2014). Use of Vibrio cholerae vaccine in an outbreak in Guinea. *New England Journal of Medicine, 370*(22), 2111–2120.

McMorrow, M. L., Gebremedhin, G., van den Heever, J., Kezaala, R., Harris, B. N., Nandy, R., ... Cairns, K. L. (2009). Measles outbreak in South Africa, 2003–2005. *South African Medical Journal, 99*(5), 314–319.

Moulton, L. H., Wolff, M. C., Brenneman, G., & Santosham, M. (1995). Case-cohort analysis of case-coverage studies of vaccine effectiveness. *American Journal of Epidemiology, 142*(9), 1000–1006.

Mustafa, A. N., Gessner, B. D., Ismail, R., Yusoff, A. F., Abdullah, N., Ishak, I., ... Merican, M. I. (2003). A case-control study of influenza vaccine effectiveness among Malaysian pilgrims attending the Haj in Saudi Arabia. *International Journal of Infectious Diseases, 7*, 210–214.

Parikh, S. R., Andrews, N. J., Beebeejaun, K., Campbell, H., Ribeiro, S., Ward, C., ... Ladhani, S. N. (2016). Effectiveness and impact of a reduced infant schedule of 4CMenB vaccine against group B meningococcal disease in England: A national observational cohort study. *Lancet, 388*, 2775–2782.

Ramsay, M. E., McVernon, J., Andrews, N. J., Heath, P. T., & Slack, M. P. (2003). Estimating *Haemophilus influenzae* type b vaccine effectiveness in England and Wales by use of the screening method. *Journal of Infectious Diseases, 188*, 481–485.

Rodrigues, L. C., & Kirkwood, B. R. (1990). Case-control designs in the study of common diseases: Updates on the demise of the rare disease assumption and the choice of sampling scheme for controls. *International Journal of Epidemiology, 19*(1), 205–213.

Rodrigues, L. C., & Smith, P. G. (1999). Use of the case-control approach in vaccine evaluation: Efficacy and adverse effects. *Epidemiologic Reviews, 21*(1), 56–72.

Shapiro, E. D., & Clemens, J. D. (1984). A controlled evaluation of the protective efficacy of pneumococcal vaccine for patients at high risk of serious pneumococcal infections. *Annals of Internal Medicine, 101*, 325–330.

Skowronski, D. M., Masaro, C., Kwindt, T. L., Mak, A., Petric, M., Li, Y., … De Serres, G. (2007). Estimating vaccine effectiveness against laboratory-confirmed influenza using a sentinel physician network: Results from the 2006–2006 season of dual A and B vaccine mismatch in Canada. *Vaccine, 25*, 2842–2851.

Vilcu, A. -M., Souty, C., Enouf, V., Capai, L., Turbelin, C., Masse, S., … Falchi, A. (2018). Estimation of seasonal influenza vaccine effectiveness using data collected in primary care in France: Comparison of the test-negative design and the screening method. *Clinical Microbiology and Infection, 24*(4), 431.e5–431.e12.

Weinberger, R., van der Linden, M., Imöhl, M., & von Kries, R. (2016). Vaccine effectiveness of PCV13 in a 3+1 vaccination schedule. *Vaccine, 34*, 2062–2065.

Chapter 16

Waning vaccine effectiveness and modes of vaccine action

In this chapter we turn to the issue of waning of vaccine effectiveness over time since vaccination. We dedicate a separate chapter to waning effectiveness since it commonly arises, is of public health importance and because assessing it is associated with specific methodological challenges.

In this chapter, we shall refer to age-specific vaccine effectiveness as the effectiveness of the vaccine when evaluated at a specified age, often some years after the vaccine was administered. This notion of age-specific vaccine effectiveness is particularly relevant for vaccines given in childhood according to a fixed schedule and is closely related to the issue of waning effectiveness over time since vaccination. It differs from the notion of vaccination-age-specific vaccine effectiveness (also often called age-specific effectiveness), which relates to the effectiveness of the vaccine when administered at a specified age.

We begin in Section 16.1 with situations in which the incidence of infection is low. In such situations, estimating age-specific vaccine effectiveness, and effects of time since vaccination to assess the presence of waning of vaccine-induced protection, is straightforward.

When the incidence of infection over the study period is not low, assessing the presence and extent of waning immunity is more complicated. In Section 16.2 we show why, if the incidence of infection is higher, problems of interpretation may arise: vaccine effectiveness may appear to vary according to the time interval over which it is measured, suggesting that age-specific effectiveness may also change, even when the vaccine (or the response of vaccinees to it) does not vary in any biological sense. In order to draw correct inferences about vaccine effectiveness over time in this setting, it is necessary to take into account the mode of action of the vaccine. This is discussed in greater detail in Section 16.3. In Section 16.4 we briefly touch upon how the mode of action of the vaccine might be determined. In Section 16.5 we discuss the estimation of age-specific vaccine effectiveness and in particular whether prior infections should be included or excluded. Finally, in Section 16.6 we discuss how to evaluate waning effectiveness when the incidence of infection is high and present some practical examples.

16.1 Assessing waning vaccine effectiveness when the incidence of infection is low

Assessing whether vaccine effectiveness wanes over time since vaccination (and hence at older ages, if vaccination is administered in childhood) requires vaccine effectiveness VE to be estimated some time (possibly a long time) after the vaccine was administered. In this section, we assume infections acquired in the intervening period can be ignored, because their incidence is low, or because they are not an issue for other reasons (e.g., if infection confers no lasting immunity).

In this situation, any of the methods described in Chapters 14 and 15 may be applied to evaluate the protective effectiveness of the vaccine in some older age group, or at some specified time since vaccination. The vaccine effectiveness at time t since vaccination, is defined as:

$$VE(t) = 1 - RR(t),$$

where $RR(t)$ is the relative risk or relative rate of infection or infection-related disease in a short time interval starting at time t after vaccination. Alternatively, for vaccines administered close to birth, t may represent age, in which case $VE(t)$ is the age-specific vaccine effectiveness at age t, estimated in a short time interval after age t. To be specific, suppose that n_u and n_v are the numbers of cases in unvaccinated and vaccinated individuals, respectively, occurring between t and $t+d$, for some small value d. For example, we might choose $d = 1$ year. The vaccine effectiveness at t is then

$$VE(t) = 1 - \frac{n_v / D_v}{n_u / D_u},$$

where D_u, D_v are person (for risk-based effectiveness) or person-time (for rate-based effectiveness) denominators. Generally, how to adjust these denominators to take account of prior cases, that is, cases that have arisen before age t, requires special attention. But when infections are uncommon the issue is not critical. Box 16.1 demonstrates this with a practical example.

> ### Box 16.1 Calculating age-specific vaccine effectiveness
>
> Suppose that we wish to estimate vaccine effectiveness against an immunising infection at age 10, in a population of 20,000 10-year-olds of whom 50% were vaccinated close to birth. We shall assume the infection incidence rate is 0.02 per

year in unvaccinated children and 0.004 per year in vaccinated children; the true vaccine effectiveness is thus 80% and does not vary over time. Based on these infection rates, there would have been (on average) 1,813 cases before age 10 and 162 aged 10 (i.e., in their 11th year) in unvaccinated children; and 392 cases prior to age 10 and 38 aged 10 in vaccinated children (Box 16.2 gives details of these calculations).

The age-specific vaccine effectiveness at age 10 years excluding prior cases (assuming these are known) using the risk-based cohort method is obtained as follows:

$$VE(10) = 1 - \frac{38/(10,000 - 392)}{162/(10,000 - 1813)} = 0.800.$$

To obtain the rate-based estimate while excluding prior cases, we first calculate the person-time at risk during the 11th year of age. Assuming that the cases in 10-year-olds arose halfway through their 11th year on average, the person-times at risk (in person-years) are (see Chapter 13):

$$D_u = (10,000 - 1813 - 162) \times 1 + 162 \times 0.5 = 8,106,$$

$$D_v = (10,000 - 392 - 38) \times 1 + 38 \times 0.5 = 9,589,$$

and so the rate-based cohort estimate of age-specific vaccine effectiveness at age 10 years, excluding prior cases, is:

$$VE(10) = 1 - \frac{38/9,589}{162/8,106} = 0.802.$$

If prior cases are not excluded, perhaps because they were not documented, the calculations are as follows. For the risk-based estimate,

$$VE(10) = 1 - \frac{38/10,000}{162/10,000} = 0.765.$$

Similarly, the screening method, using 50% vaccine coverage in the original birth cohort, yields:

$$VE(10) = 1 - \frac{38/162}{0.50/(1 - 0.50)} = 0.765.$$

The rate-based estimate is obtained without removing prior cases from the person-time denominators, as follows:

$$D_u = (10,000 - 162) \times 1 + 162 \times 0.5 = 9,919,$$

$$D_v = (10,000 - 38) \times 1 + 38 \times 0.5 = 9,981,$$

and so the rate-based age-specific vaccine effectiveness is

$$VE(10) = 1 - \frac{38/9{,}981}{162/9{,}919} = 0.767.$$

All methods result in similar estimates, close to the true value of 80%. This is because the underlying incidence rate (0.02 per year in unvaccinated) is low. In particular, it matters little whether or not prior cases are excluded from person or person-time denominators. Confidence intervals are calculated as described in Chapters 14 and 15, and are also similar for the different methods.

For completeness, we set out in Box 16.2 the calculations of numbers of cases in Box 16.1.

Box 16.2 Details of calculations of cases in Box 16.1

The expected numbers of cases are obtained using Equation 13.4 from Chapter 13. The numbers of cases by age 10 in the unvaccinated and vaccinated groups are, respectively:

$$N_u = 10{,}000 \times \left(1 - e^{-0.02 \times 10}\right) = 1813, \quad N_v = 10{,}000 \times \left(1 - e^{-0.004 \times 10}\right) = 392.$$

The expected numbers of cases arising at age 10 years (in the 11th year) are, respectively:

$$n_u = (10{,}000 - 1813) \times \left(1 - e^{-0.02}\right) = 162, \quad n_v = (10{,}000 - 392) \times \left(1 - e^{-0.004}\right) = 38.$$

As shown in Box 16.1, when the cumulative incidence of infection up to time t is low, prior infections arising before t may be ignored when estimating $VE(t)$. What to do when prior infections are common is deferred until Section 16.4. We illustrate the approach with two examples. The first, in Box 16.3, uses the screening method.

Box 16.3 Waning of mumps vaccine effectiveness in England and Wales

This study included cases reported during the 2004–2005 mumps epidemic in England and Wales (Cohen et al., 2007). This epidemic followed several years of very low mumps incidence. The screening method was used. Only cases aged

Table 16.1 **Mumps vaccine effectiveness (%, with 95% CI) by age group and number of vaccine doses**

Number of doses	Age group (years)				
	2	5–6	7–8	9–10	11–12
One dose	96 (81, 99)	94 (84, 98)	90 (81, 95)	87 (75, 93)	66 (30, 83)
Two doses	NA	99 (97, 100)	96 (93, 98)	92 (88, 95)	87 (74, 93)

2 years or 5–12 years were included, as accurate vaccine coverage data were only available for these cohorts. Vaccine effectiveness by age was estimated separately for one dose of measles, mumps and rubella (MMR) vaccine (administered before age 2 years) and two doses of MMR vaccine (the second dose being given before age 5). The results are in Table 16.1.

These results suggest that mumps vaccine effectiveness soon after vaccination (at age 2 years for a single dose, and at 5–6 years for two doses) is very high. Subsequently it wanes with age for both the one-dose and the two-dose regimes, an impression that is confirmed by formal statistical tests of trend ($p<0.001$ for each dosage). However, the extent of waning is relatively small by age 12 years for the two-dose regime compared to the one-dose regime.

As the incidence of mumps prior to the study was very low, the results in Box 16.3 are not substantially affected by prior infections, which can thus be ignored. The second example, in Box 16.4, uses an adaptation of the case-cohort method described in Chapter 15, Section 15.2.2.

Box 16.4 Duration of BCG protection in England

This is a study of the effectiveness of Bacille Calmette-Guérin (BCG) vaccination against tuberculosis in adulthood. In England, BCG vaccination was administered to children aged 12–13 years from the 1950s until the programme was discontinued in 2005. The vaccination histories of adult cases of tuberculosis were compared to those of a sample of the general population: an application of the case-cohort method (Mangtani et al., 2018). The study was restricted to white people born in the United Kingdom. Vaccination status was determined using a combination of inspection of the BCG scar and self-report. The data were analysed using Cox regression, the hazard ratio being estimated as a smooth function of time since vaccination. The results for one model are presented in Figure 16.1.

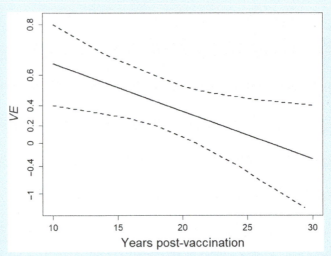

Figure 16.1 BCG vaccine effectiveness (with 95% confidence bands) by time since vaccination.
Source: Adapted from Mangtani et al. (2018).

Figure 16.1 shows that BCG vaccination still offered substantial protection against tuberculosis 10 years after vaccination, but then waned over the following 20 years. The results were robust, as evidenced by the similar results obtained using sensitivity analyses to explore different assumptions about vaccination status, and adjustment for several covariates.

Again, the low incidence of tuberculosis in England means that the analysis is not materially affected by prior cases of tuberculosis, and so the occurrence of these cases has not biased the estimated extent of waning of vaccine effectiveness.

16.2 Risk-based and rate-based vaccine effectiveness revisited

In Chapter 13, Section 13.5 we discussed risk-based and rate-based measures of vaccine effectiveness, and showed that they could produce different estimates of the vaccine effectiveness VE, even when calculated from the same data. Such discrepancies may arise when the incidence of infection over the study period is not low and when infection results in at least partial immunity.

In this section we explore the behaviour of risk-based and rate-based measures of vaccine effectiveness over time. We begin by showing that if one measure of vaccine effectiveness (rate-based or risk-based) is constant whatever the duration of the study, the other may not be. This is important because it has implications for the interpretation of VE estimates over time since vaccination, as to whether these indicate the presence of waning age-specific vaccine effectiveness. It also motivates our discussion of vaccine action models in Section 16.3.

Our focus in this section is not age-specific vaccine effectiveness, but how VE may depend on study duration. Accordingly, we define the vaccine effectiveness in the time interval from 0 to t after vaccination, or in the age group 0 to t, as

$$VE(0,t) = 1 - RR(0,t)$$

where $RR(0,t)$ is the relative risk or relative rate in the post-vaccination time or age interval from 0 to t. Thus here, t denotes the duration of the study. Note that this differs from the vaccine effectiveness at t, $VE(t)$, defined in Section 16.1. We shall assume, for the remainder of this section, that we are studying an infection and a vaccine that induce immunity that does not wane over time, and that vaccine effectiveness is evaluated over the time interval 0 to t.

Suppose first that the rate-based measure of vaccine effectiveness is constant, whatever the duration of the study or the cumulative incidence over the period. This corresponds to a situation in which the vaccine reduces the rate of infection in each vaccinee by the same fixed amount compared to the rate in unvaccinated individuals (this will be explored further in Section 16.3). Then it can be shown that the risk-based VE necessarily declines as the duration of the study increases (or equivalently, as the cumulative incidence over the study period increases). The decline is very substantial when the cumulative incidence is high (a high cumulative incidence can arise over a short time interval when the incidence is high, or over a longer time interval when the incidence is moderate). This effect is illustrated in Box 16.5.

Box 16.5 Risk-based vaccine effectiveness when the rate-based VE is constant

Figure 16.2 shows the rate-based and risk-based vaccine effectiveness $VE(0,t)$ plotted against the cumulative incidence over the study period when the rate-based measure is constant.

Figure 16.2 shows that, when the cumulative incidence is low, as in the left panel of the figure, there is little difference between rate-based and risk-based vaccine effectiveness. However, when the cumulative incidence is high, the two measures diverge rapidly: the rate-based VE is higher than the risk-based VE. The risk-based VE declines as the cumulative incidence (or equivalently, the time since vaccination) increases, falsely suggesting there is considerable waning.

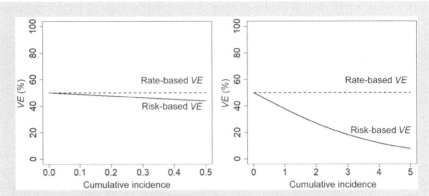

Figure 16.2 Rate-based and risk-based vaccine effectiveness for constant rate-based *VE* equal to 50%. Left: low cumulative incidences; right: high cumulative incidences.

The reason for the discrepancy between risk-based and rate-based VE in Box 16.5 is as follows. We assumed that the rate-based VE was constant over time: thus, the rates in vaccinated and unvaccinated individuals are always in a constant proportion. This implies that, over time, all individuals eventually become infected, whether or not they are vaccinated. So the risks of infection in both groups tend to 1, and the risk-based VE tends to 0, as observed in Box 16.5.

Now suppose that it is the risk-based measure of vaccine effectiveness that is constant, whatever the duration of the study or the cumulative incidence. This corresponds to a situation in which the vaccine protects a fixed proportion of vaccinated individuals completely, so they never get infected, but leaves the remaining vaccinees unprotected (this will be further discussed in Section 16.3). It then turns out that rate-based VE measures increase as the duration of the study increases (or equivalently, as the cumulative incidence over the study period increases). The increase is substantial when the cumulative incidence is high. This effect is illustrated in Box 16.6.

Box 16.6 Rate-based vaccine effectiveness when the risk-based *VE* is constant

Figure 16.3 shows the rate-based and risk-based vaccine effectiveness $VE(0,t)$ plotted against the cumulative incidence over the study period when the risk-based measure is constant.

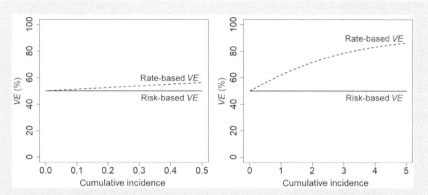

Figure 16.3 **Rate-based and risk-based vaccine effectiveness for constant risk-based VE equal to 50%. Left: low cumulative incidences; right: high cumulative incidences.**

Figure 16.3 shows that, when the cumulative incidence is low, there is little difference between rate-based and risk-based VE. However, when the cumulative incidence is high, the two measures of VE diverge: the rate-based VE is higher than the risk-based VE. The rate-based measure of VE increases as the cumulative incidence (or equivalently, the time since vaccination) increases, falsely suggesting that VE improves over time.

The reason for the pattern observed in Box 16.6 is as follows. Because the risks of infection in vaccinated and unvaccinated individuals are in a constant ratio, not all vaccinees can eventually become infected. For if they did, the risk-based measure would eventually drop to zero, as in Box 16.5. So, some vaccinees can never become infected. As time goes on, these fully protected individuals force the infection rate in uninfected vaccinees to zero, and hence the rate-based VE tends to 100% over time.

The discrepancies highlighted in Boxes 16.5 and 16.6 can invite incorrect inferences about possible changes in the effectiveness of the vaccine over time. For example, if the rate-based VE is constant over time but the risk-based measure is used to estimate VE, the effectiveness of the vaccine will appear to decline when measured over increasing time intervals, according to the accumulating cumulative incidence as shown by Figure 16.2 in Box 16.5. This may suggest that the vaccine effectiveness wanes over time, when in fact it does not. Similarly, as shown in Figure 16.3 in Box 16.6, if the risk-based measure of VE is constant, but a rate-based measure is used to estimate VE, then the effectiveness of the vaccine will appear to increase when measured over increasing time intervals, when in reality it remains unchanged.

The temporal effects displayed in Boxes 16.5 and 16.6 are unrelated to any change in the protection afforded by the vaccine, which, as we assumed, remains constant throughout. Thus, there is no waning of vaccine effectiveness in any biological sense, irrespective of what the graphs show. These results may at first sight appear disconcerting, in that which measure of vaccine effectiveness is used (risk-based or rate-based) should not lead to different conclusions about whether or not the vaccine effectiveness wanes (or increases) over time.

To resolve this conundrum, we need to study more closely the way the vaccine actually works, that is, the vaccine's mode of action. This in turn will determine in what sense vaccine effectiveness can be said to wane over time, and how to estimate it. Vaccine action modes is the topic of the next section.

16.3 Modes of vaccine action

In Section 16.2 we investigated the implications of assuming that the rate-based measure of VE was constant, or, alternatively, that the risk-based measure of VE was constant. It was shown that, in each case, the other measure is not constant. We noted that the constant rate assumption corresponded to the situation in which the infection rate was reduced by the same constant amount in all vaccinees. In contrast, the constant risk assumption corresponded to the situation in which a proportion of vaccinees are completely protected, but the remaining vaccinated individuals are unprotected.

Thus, the two scenarios explored in Section 16.2 relate to different modes of vaccine action in the absence of waning of vaccine-induced protection. The key distinction between the two modes is what happens under repeated exposures: in the first mode, vaccinated individuals eventually become infected following repeated exposure, albeit at a lower rate than if they had not been vaccinated. In the second mode of vaccine action, some vaccinated individuals never become infected, however many exposures they encounter, whereas the rest are wholly unprotected. These notions are made more precise in what follows; each mode of action is represented by a particular model of how vaccine-induced protection operates.

The assumption that the rate-based measure of vaccine effectiveness is constant over time corresponds to a model of vaccine action known as the partial protection model (sometimes also called the leaky model). In this model of vaccine action, vaccination does not confer complete immunity to any vaccinee, but reduces the infection rate of all vaccinees by some constant factor θ. Thus, under repeat exposures, all vaccinees eventually acquire infection. Let Λ_u denote the cumulative incidence of infection in unvaccinated individuals over the period 0 to t. The cumulative incidence in vaccinees is $\Lambda_v = \theta \Lambda_u$ and so the relative rate over the period $(0,t)$ is:

$$RR(0,t) = \frac{\Lambda_v}{\Lambda_u} = \theta.$$

This is also called the proportional hazards model; the relative rate does not depend on t. The rate-based vaccine effectiveness is then constant: $VE(0,t) = 1 - \theta$. This is the model implied in Box 16.5. As there is no change over time, the age-specific vaccine effectiveness is also constant with $VE(t) = 1 - \theta$.

In contrast, the assumption that the risk-based measure of vaccine effectiveness is constant over time, corresponds to a model of vaccine action called the all-or-nothing model. In this model, vaccination confers no protection to a proportion θ of vaccinees, and complete protection to the remaining proportion $1 - \theta$ of vaccinees. Thus, under repeat exposures, a proportion of vaccinees never acquire infection. Let π_u denote the risk of infection in unvaccinated individuals over some specified period 0 to t. For a randomly chosen vaccinated individual, the risk of infection is thus π_u with probability θ and 0 with probability $1-\theta$, so that the risk of infection π_v in vaccinated individuals over the period is

$$\pi_v = \theta \times \pi_u + (1-\theta) \times 0 = \theta \times \pi_u.$$

The risk of infection in vaccinees is then $\pi_v = \theta \times \pi_u$ and so, over the period from 0 to t,

$$RR(0,t) = \frac{\pi_v}{\pi_u} = \theta.$$

This does not depend on the duration of the period from 0 to t. Thus, the risk-based effectiveness is constant and equal to $VE(0,t) = 1-\theta$. This is the model implied in Box 16.6. As there is no change over time, the age-specific vaccine effectiveness is also constant with $VE(t) = 1-\theta$.

The two modes of vaccine action discussed above represent contrasting opposites. Clearly, it is possible to envisage other, more complex, modes of action. These various possibilities are discussed schematically in Box 16.7.

Box 16.7 Partial protection, all-or-nothing protection and other modes of vaccine action

The partial protection and all-or-nothing modes of vaccine action are represented schematically in Figure 16.4. Black represents complete protection and white complete lack of protection, while grey represents partial protection.

Under the partial protection mode, all vaccinated individuals have the same level of protection, whereas under the all-or-nothing mode, the level of protection is dichotomous (complete protection or none) across individuals. Thus, under the

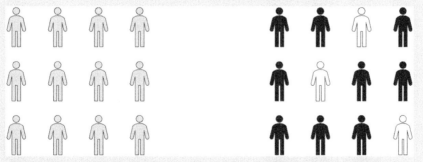

Figure 16.4 Individual protection in vaccinated individuals. Left: partial protection mode. Right: all-or-nothing mode. The greyscale shading represents degree of protection (see text).

partial protection model, protection is homogeneous across individuals, whereas under the all-or-nothing model it is heterogeneous. Using this schematic representation, it is possible to envisage other modes of action by combining black, white and grey (of different shades) in different proportions. Such more complex models of vaccine action will not be considered in this book.

These models of vaccine action, and their implications for rate-based and risk-based measures of VE, were first explored by Smith, Rodrigues, and Fine (1984). How they impact on the estimation of age-specific vaccine effectiveness was highlighted by Farrington (1992). As shown in Section 16.2, the behaviour of the risk-based and rate-based measures over increasing study durations differs for the two models. The key point, however, is that the biological action of the vaccine or the response of vaccinees to it does not change over time in either model. Thus, an appropriate measure of vaccine effectiveness should not wane or increase over time either.

These observations have the following practical consequences for vaccine effectiveness studies. If the effectiveness of a vaccine is to be investigated over a prolonged study interval or age range $(0,t)$, over which the cumulative incidence in unvaccinated individuals is substantial, the measure of vaccine effectiveness used to estimate $VE(0,t)$ may need to take account of the likely vaccine action model. If the vaccine has a partial protection mode of action, a rate-based measure should be used. If the vaccine has an all-or-nothing mode of action, then a risk-based measure should be preferred. Any apparent changes in $VE(0,t)$ with t should be interpreted in the light of these observations. Exceptions include outbreaks with cases spanning a wide age range, in settings where the past incidence of infection was low. Box 16.8 provides an illustration.

Box 16.8 Long-term effectiveness of varicella vaccine

A 14-year prospective cohort study was undertaken in the United States to evaluate the effectiveness of varicella vaccine. The cohort comprised 7,585 vaccinees; incident cases of varicella were actively sought and person-time at risk was calculated every 6 months after vaccination. Retention over the 14 years was 97%; there were 174 varicella cases in the first year after vaccination, and 1,425 over the 14-year period as a whole. Comparable data for unvaccinated children were obtained from two historical, pre-vaccination studies denoted NHIS and Kentucky (Baxter et al., 2013).

The average rates for the first year and for the entire 14-year follow-up, along with the rate-based vaccine effectiveness obtained by the authors, are shown in Table 16.2.

The authors note that (rate-based) vaccine effectiveness appeared to increase over the study duration: the vaccine effectiveness is higher when measured over 0–14 years than when measured over 0–1 year. They comment that such

Table 16.2 **Average incidence rates of varicella (per 1,000 person-years) in vaccinated and unvaccinated children, and rate-based vaccine effectiveness, by study period**

Follow-up	Rate in vaccinees	Rate in unvaccinated		Vaccine effectiveness	
		NHIS	Kentucky	vs NHIS	vs Kentucky
0–1 year	26.6	97	120	73%	78%
0–14 years	15.9	140.1	158.9	89%	90%

Table 16.3 **Risks of varicella in vaccinated and unvaccinated children, and risk-based vaccine effectiveness, by study period**

Follow-up	Risk in vaccinees	Risk in unvaccinated		Vaccine effectiveness	
		NHIS	Kentucky	vs NHIS	vs Kentucky
0–1 year	0.02625	0.09244	0.1131	72%	77%
0–14 years	0.1996	0.8593	0.8919	77%	78%

an increase may appear counter-intuitive. They suggest it may be due to herd immunity, the unvaccinated comparators not being concurrent with the vaccinees.

An alternative explanation is that varicella vaccine has an all-or-nothing mode of action, and that the increase in the rate-based measure is spurious, as described in Box 16.6. To explore this, we calculated risks and risk-based vaccine effectiveness. These are shown in Table 16.3.

From Table 16.3, the risk-based vaccine effectiveness remains constant, unlike the rate-based estimates. Thus, the data are consistent with an all-or-nothing model of vaccine action with constant vaccine effectiveness of about 75%.

The risks in Table 16.3 were calculated using Equation 13.4 linking risks and cumulative incidences given in Chapter 13. For example, the 0–14-year risk in NHIS is $1 - \exp(-140.1 \times 14 / 1,000)$.

For completeness, Box 16.9 provides the mathematical formulas for VE, which were used to draw Figures 16.2 and 16.3.

Box 16.9 Some mathematical formulas

These formulas are provided solely for completeness. For a partial protection vaccine, the rate-based measure is $VE_{rate} = 1 - \theta$. The cumulative incidence is Λ_u in unvaccinated individuals, and $\Lambda_v = \theta \Lambda_u$ in vaccinated individuals. So, using Equation 13.4 from Chapter 13, the risks in unvaccinated and vaccinated individuals are

$$\pi_u = 1 - e^{-\Lambda_u}, \quad \pi_v = 1 - e^{-\theta \Lambda_u},$$

so the risk-based vaccine effectiveness is:

$$VE_{risk} = 1 - \frac{1 - e^{-\theta \Lambda_u}}{1 - e^{-\Lambda_u}}.$$

Figure 16.2 shows VE_{rate} and VE_{risk} plotted against Λ_u for a partial protection vaccine.

For an all-or-nothing vaccine, the risk-based measure is $VE_{risk} = 1 - \theta$. The risk in the vaccinated group is $\pi_v = \theta \pi_u$, the cumulative incidence in vaccinated individuals is

$$\Lambda_v = -\log\left(1 - \theta\left(1 - e^{-\Lambda_u}\right)\right),$$

and hence the rate-based effectiveness, based on cumulative incidences, is:

$$VE_{rate} = 1 - \frac{-\log\left(1 - \theta\left(1 - e^{-\Lambda_u}\right)\right)}{\Lambda_u}.$$

Figure 16.3 shows VE_{risk} and VE_{rate} plotted against Λ_u for an all-or-nothing vaccine.

16.4 Determining the vaccine action model

Clearly, the partial protection and all-or-nothing vaccine models are probably oversimplified. Actual vaccines are unlikely to conform exactly to either model. Nor are these two models the only possible ones: for example, it is perfectly possible to envisage models that combine aspects of both all-or-nothing and partial protection models (Halloran, Haber, & Longini, 1992). In addition, we have assumed that natural infection confers lifelong immunity, which may not be the case in practice.

An all-or-nothing model may apply, approximately at least, if there is a protective antibody threshold above which individuals are protected against infection. In this case, the vaccine effectiveness is the proportion of vaccinated individuals whose antibody levels are above the threshold, and who are therefore protected. Box 16.10 provides an example in which such a threshold might exist.

Box 16.10 Protective antibody threshold for measles

An outbreak of 100 measles cases among students occurred in 1985 at Boston University, shortly after a campaign for blood donations had taken place. This coincidence enabled researchers to obtain measles antibody levels prior to exposure in samples of cases and non-cases (Chen et al., 1990). The tests used included the highly sensitive plaque reduction neutralisation (PRN) test.

Of nine blood donors with PRN titres less than or equal to 120 mIU/ml, eight met the clinical criteria for measles. In contrast, there were no cases of classical measles among the 71 donors with pre-exposure PRN titres greater than 120 mIU/ml.

These data suggest that a PRN titre > 120 mIU/ml is protective against measles, and that a PRN titre ≤ 120 mIU/ml confers virtually no protection. Thus, vaccination may provide all-or-nothing protection, according to whether post-vaccination titres achieve this level.

More recently, however, measles cases have been found to occur in persons with PRN titres above 120 mIU/ml, so the all-or-nothing model is most likely only an approximation to the true mechanism of vaccine action (Hahné et al., 2016). In particular, the threshold, if there is one, may depend on the intensity of exposure.

When there is a protective antibody threshold, waning of vaccine effectiveness may result from the natural decline of antibody levels over time. Individuals are then protected for as long as their antibody levels remain above the threshold level. The proportion of unprotected individuals at time t since vaccination (or at age t) is $\theta(t)$, which may rise as t increases, resulting in a decline of the vaccine effectiveness $VE(t) = 1 - \theta(t)$.

For some vaccines, there may not be a protective antibody threshold, though antibody levels may be correlated with the degree of protection. For some such vaccines, a partial protection model might be relevant. In this case, vaccine effectiveness quantifies the degree of protection shared by all vaccinated individuals. Box 16.10 describes a possible candidate.

Box 16.11 Serological correlate of protection for *Bordetella pertussis*

Acellular vaccines against *Bordetella pertussis* comprise a variety of antigens involved in mounting an immune response to infection by this bacterium. However, there does not appear to be a threshold above which the corresponding antibody levels, alone or in combination, provide complete protection against infection. Nevertheless, a study of clinical whooping cough following exposure

> in the household found evidence of a positive association between the degree of protection and the presence of high antibody levels for pertussis toxin, pertactin and fimbriae (Storsaeter, Hallander, Gustaffson, & Olin, 1998). This serological correlate of protection was subsequently validated by Kohberger, Jemiolo, and Fernando (2008).
>
> This suggests that vaccinated individuals benefit from partial protection, depending on their antibody profile. This is consistent with a version of the partial protection model of vaccine action: vaccination reduces the incidence rate by some random quantity Z for each individual in line with their antibody response, the parameter θ denoting the mean of Z, which depends on the average antibody levels in vaccinees.

For the partial protection model, waning vaccine effectiveness may result from a decline in the level of protection afforded to all vaccinated individuals over time, which is also represented by a vaccine effectiveness at time or age t of the form $VE(t) = 1 - \theta(t)$ where $\theta(t)$ increases over time. But the vaccine action model differs from the all-or-nothing model: $\theta(t)$ is not the proportion of individuals completely protected, because under the partial protection model all vaccinated individuals have a degree of protection, which reduces with time.

More tentatively, it could be suggested that the choice of vaccine action model should be determined by the importance played by cellular immunity in protecting against infection: the greater the role played by cellular immunity, the more appropriate the partial protection model is likely to be. According to this hypothesis, for infections for which a serological correlate for protection has not been established (despite attempts to find one), cellular immunity is probably important in protecting against infection, and the partial immunity model should be preferred. Conversely, for infections for which immunoglobulins are effective in preventing infection (e.g., hepatitis A and B, measles or chickenpox), an all-or-nothing vaccine model is likely to be most appropriate.

Most often, the mode of vaccine action is not known with any degree of certainty. This does not matter provided that the cumulative incidence of infection is low. But it cannot be ignored when the incidence is high, and this may complicate the interpretation of changes in vaccine effectiveness over time. This is discussed in the next section.

16.5 Assessing waning vaccine effectiveness when the incidence of infection is high

We now consider the problem of assessing the effectiveness $VE(t)$ of a vaccine at some time t (in effect, over a short time interval after t) after vaccination, or the age-specific vaccine effectiveness at age t, when the incidence in the intervening period from time 0 to t is high and the infection confers immunity. In particular, we discuss how one might decide whether the vaccine effectiveness wanes over time. In this situation it is necessary to take account of the depletion of susceptibles (i.e., uninfected individuals) up to time t. How to do this depends on the assumed mode of vaccine action.

Recall from Section 16.1 that vaccine effectiveness at time t after vaccination, or at age t, is

$$VE(t) = 1 - \frac{n_v / D_v}{n_u / D_u}.$$

The n_u and n_v are the numbers of cases in unvaccinated and vaccinated individuals, respectively, occurring between t and $t + d$, for some small value d; and D_u, D_v are person (for risk-based effectiveness) or person-time (for rate-based effectiveness) denominators. The key issue is how to take account of prior cases in the denominators.

If the vaccine works by proportionately reducing the infection rate (as is the case with the partial protection model), then individuals infected before time t should be *excluded* from person or person-time denominators when calculating risks or rates in a short time interval after t.

However, if the vaccine works by proportionately reducing the risk of infection (as is the case with the all-or-nothing model), then individuals infected before time t should be *included* in person or person-time denominators (as if they had not been infected) when calculating risks or rates in a short time interval after t.

Note that whether $VE(t)$ is calculated using a risk or rate-based measure (i.e., whether D_u, D_v are person or person-time denominators) does not matter provided that the incidence is low in the short time interval after t in which the age-specific vaccine effectiveness at t is evaluated. What matters is how infections in the possibly long interval prior to t are handled. These procedures are illustrated in Boxes 16.12 and 16.13.

Box 16.12 Estimating VE(t) with high incidence: partial protection mode of vaccine action

We return to the scenario described in Box 16.1, but now assume a much higher incidence. The vaccine has a partial protection mode of action, and there is no waning. Suppose that we wish to estimate the vaccine effectiveness at age 10 years, in a population of 20,000 10-year-olds of whom 50% were vaccinated close to birth. We now assume the infection rate is 0.2 per year in unvaccinated children and 0.04 per year in vaccinated children. This corresponds to a partial protection model with constant rate-based $VE = 80\%$. With these infection rates, there would have been (on average) 8,647 cases before age 10 and 245 aged 10 (i.e., in the 11th year) in unvaccinated children; and 3,297 cases prior to age 10 and 263 aged 10 in vaccinated children (the calculations are similar to those in Box 16.2).

If prior cases are not removed from the denominators, the age-specific vaccine effectiveness at age 10 obtained using the risk-based cohort method would be:

$$VE(10) = 1 - \frac{263/10,000}{245/10,000} = -0.073$$

or −7%. The same result would have been obtained with the screening method applied with 50% vaccine coverage of the birth cohort. Similarly, the rate-based method applied without prior cases being removed from the denominators would yield (the person-time calculations are similar to those described in Box 16.1):

$$VE(10) = 1 - \frac{263/9{,}868.5}{245/9{,}877.5} = -0.074.$$

These estimates are very heavily biased and may suggest, incorrectly, that vaccine effectiveness wanes with increasing age. In fact, the true age-specific effectiveness at age 10 is 80%.

If prior cases are removed, the risk-based cohort method yields:

$$VE(10) = 1 - \frac{263/(10{,}000 - 3{,}297)}{245/(10{,}000 - 8{,}647)} = 0.783,$$

or 78%, which is close to the correct value. Similarly, the rate-based cohort method with person-time corresponding to prior cases removed (as illustrated in Box 16.1) gives

$$VE(10) = 1 - \frac{263/6{,}571.5}{245/1{,}230.5} = 0.799,$$

or 80%. Thus, with prior cases or person-time removed from the denominators, the correct age-specific vaccine effectiveness is obtained.

The example in Box 16.12 shows that, if the partial protection model applies and the incidence is high, it is essential to remove prior cases and person-time from the denominators to calculate age-specific effectiveness. Note that it does not matter much, when calculating age-specific VE, whether risk-based or rate-based measures are used, provided the time interval in which the age-specific VE is evaluated is brief (in Box 16.12, it is 1 year). What does matter, for a partial protection vaccine, is that prior cases should be removed: otherwise, the estimates may be seriously biased. However, as shown in Box 16.13, exactly the reverse is true when the all-or-nothing model applies.

Box 16.13 Estimating $VE(t)$ with high incidence: all-or-nothing mode of vaccine action

We use the same context as in Box 16.12, with an infection rate of 0.2 per year in unvaccinated children, but now with an all-or-nothing vaccine with constant risk based VE of 80%. This means that, of the 10,000 vaccinees, 8,000 are wholly protected (irrespective how often they are exposed) and have an infection rate of 0, while the remaining 2,000 are unprotected and have an infection rate of 0.2 per year. With these infection rates, there would have been (on average) 8,647 cases before age 10 and 245 aged 10 years (i.e., in the 11th year) in unvaccinated children; and 1,729 cases before age 10 and 49 aged 10 in the vaccinated group.

Without removing prior cases from the denominators, the age-specific vaccine effectiveness at age 10 years obtained using the risk-based cohort method is then:

$$VE(10) = 1 - \frac{49/1,000}{245/10,000} = 0.800,$$

or 80%. This is the correct value; the same would have been obtained using the screening method with 50% coverage. On the other hand, if we had removed prior cases from the denominators, we would have obtained:

$$VE(10) = 1 - \frac{49/(10,000-1,729)}{245/(10,000-8,647)} = 0.967,$$

or 97%. This value is severely biased upwards. Similar results are obtained with rate-based measures. Thus, if prior cases are not removed when calculating person-time denominators (the calculation is illustrated in Box 16.1),

$$VE(10) = 1 - \frac{49/9,975.5}{245/9,877.5} = 0.802,$$

or 80%: this is the correct value. However, if we do remove prior cases when calculating person-time denominators, we obtain:

$$VE(10) = 1 - \frac{49/8,246.5}{245/1,230.5} = 0.970,$$

or 97%, which is severely biased. Thus, for an all-or-nothing vaccine, prior cases should not be excluded from person or person-time denominators, but should be treated as if they were still at risk of infection when assessing age-specific vaccine effectiveness.

Note once again, as in Box 16.13, similar results are obtained with risk-based and rate-based measures of $VE(t)$, provided the time interval over which the age-specific effectiveness is assessed is brief. What does matter is that, for an all-or-nothing vaccine, prior cases should not be excluded.

The procedures illustrated in Boxes 16.12 and 16.13 ensure that, if the vaccine effectiveness $VE(t)$ does not wane over time, its estimated effectiveness at time t will be constant over time, that is $VE(t) = VE$. Thus, we circumvent the distorting effects discussed in Section 16.2 and displayed in Boxes 16.5 and 16.6. These distorting effects may suggest that changes in vaccine effectiveness over time are occurring when in fact there are none. If, on the other hand, the effectiveness of the vaccine does wane over time, this should be apparent from the estimated values of $VE(t)$, which will progressively decline as t increases. For completeness, the mathematical rationale for these recommendations is set out in Box 16.14.

Box 16.14 How to handle prior infections: mathematical rationale

Suppose first that the vaccine reduces the infection rate by a constant factor θ, as in the partial protection model. The expected number of cases arising in a short interval $[t, t + dt)$ is $N \exp\{-\theta \Lambda_u(t)\} \theta \lambda_u(t) dt$ in N vaccinated individuals and $N \exp\{-\Lambda_u(t)\} \lambda_u(t) dt$ in N unvaccinated individuals, where $\lambda_u(t)$ and $\Lambda_u(t)$ are the instantaneous and cumulative incidence rates at t, respectively. The person-time at risk in $[t, t + dt)$, excluding prior cases, is $N \exp\{-\theta \Lambda_u(t)\} dt$ in vaccinated and $N \exp\{-\Lambda_u(t)\} dt$ in unvaccinated individuals. The rate ratio in $[t, t + dt)$ with this person-time is thus $RR(t) = \theta$ and so $VE(t) = 1 - \theta$ is constant.

Now suppose that the vaccine reduces the risk (probability) of infection by a constant factor θ, as in the all-or-nothing model. The expected number of cases arising in a short interval $[t, t + dt)$ is $N \theta \{1 - \pi_u(t)\} \lambda_u(t) dt$ in N vaccinated individuals and $N \{1 - \pi_u(t)\} \lambda_u(t) dt$ in N unvaccinated individuals, where $\pi_u(t)$ is the probability that an unvaccinated individual became a case by t. Without excluding prior cases, the denominator in each group is N. The risk ratio in $[t, t + dt)$ with these denominators is thus $RR(t) = \theta$ and so $VE(t) = 1 - \theta$ is constant.

16.6 Evaluating age-specific vaccine effectiveness in practice when infections are common

When prior infections are frequent, the recommended procedure for vaccines operating according to the all-or-nothing protection model is not to remove prior infections. This is usually straightforward; in particular, results obtained using the screening method with vaccine coverage relating to the age groups studied will be valid.

In contrast, the recommended procedure for vaccines operating according to the partial protection model is to remove all individuals with prior infections occurring before time t when estimating $VE(t)$. This can be problematic when ascertainment of infections is incomplete, or a high proportion of infections are subclinical, because all prior infections might not be observed. In this case, sensitivity analyses may be undertaken to assess the robustness of the results to different assumptions about the completeness of reporting of prior infections.

In such sensitivity analyses the following adjusted vaccine effectiveness $VE(t)^*$ may be useful, when the partial protection model is thought to apply, prior infections have not been excluded and the vaccine effectiveness is presumed not to wane over time:

$$VE(t)^* = 1 - [1 - VE(t)] \times S(t)^{1-\theta}. \qquad (16.1)$$

In this expression, $VE(t)$ is the risk-based estimate of vaccine effectiveness at age t, obtained without excluding prior infections, $S(t)$ is the probability than an unvaccinated person remains susceptible at age t, and θ is the amount by which vaccination reduces the incidence of infection in the partial protection model. Then, provided the assumptions are correct, we should observe

$$VE(t)^* = 1 - \theta, \qquad (16.2)$$

that is, $VE(t)^*$ should be constant over time. Equations 16.1 and 16.2 follow from the developments in Box 16.14. They can be used when the partial protection model is thought to apply, but vaccine effectiveness has been calculated using a risk-based measure, as with the screening method or a risk-based cohort method.

The procedure set out above is essentially a hypothesis-testing framework, the null hypothesis being no waning. Estimating the degree to which a vaccine may wane over time (as distinct from investigating whether waning is likely to be present or not) is not straightforward; a model-based approach is described by Kanaan and Farrington (2002).

We end this section with two examples in which the waning of vaccine effectiveness is assessed in conditions where the cumulative incidence cannot be assumed to be low.

The first example relates to rubella vaccine effectiveness in China. The data for this example were previously discussed in Chapter 14. The example is described in Box 16.15.

Box 16.15 Rubella vaccine effectiveness and time since vaccination in Guangzhou, China

These data, previously described in Chapter 14, relate to an outbreak of rubella in a middle school in Guangzhou City, China, in early 2014 (Chang et al., 2015). The schoolchildren were born in 1998–2001 and were thus aged between 12 and 16 years. Vaccine effectiveness (of a single dose of vaccine, usually administered in the second year of life) was estimated using secondary attack rates in classrooms. These were 65/171 for unvaccinated children, 0/15 for children vaccinated less than 12 years previously and 2/70 for children vaccinated 12 or more years previously. There is no compelling reason to assume that incidence of rubella was low prior to the outbreak. Vaccine effectiveness VE was calculated from these risks.

In Chapter 14, the vaccine effectiveness in children vaccinated less than 12 years previously was shown to be 100% with 95% confidence interval (CI) 68% to 100%. For children vaccinated more than 12 years ago, VE = 92% with 95% CI (70% to 98%). The authors concluded that rubella vaccination imparts solid protection for at least 12 years.

Under the all-or-nothing model of vaccine action, which is a reasonable one for rubella vaccine (Plotkin, 2008), the interpretation of the results in Box 16.15 is straightforward because VE was estimated using a risk-based measure and prior cases (i.e., cases occurring before the outbreak) were not excluded. Cases in vaccinees only arose 12 or more years post-vaccination: this suggests that the vaccine offers complete protection for 12 years, and that VE may then drop a little. However, the confidence intervals are wide, so there is no compelling evidence of a decline in vaccine effectiveness beyond 12 years post-vaccination.

However, because VE is so close to 100%, the mode of vaccine action is not important in this instance. Indeed, if $VE(t)=1$ in Equation 16.1 then $VE(t)^* = 1$ as well. So even if the partial protection model were to apply, VE would still be 100% up to 12 years. Thereafter the true VE may be a little higher than the estimated 92% value. So, in this example there is little doubt about the interpretation of the results.

The example given in Box 16.16 relates to whole-cell pertussis vaccine age-specific effectiveness.

Box 16.16 Whole-cell pertussis vaccine age-specific effectiveness in England and Wales

Following a large drop in vaccine coverage in the 1970s, pertussis incidence increased and whooping cough epidemics reappeared in the United Kingdom. This study was undertaken to assess the effectiveness of the whole-cell vaccine, prior to a change in the vaccination schedule. The original schedule involved three doses of diphtheria, tetanus and pertussis (DTP) vaccine with a whole-cell pertussis component, administered at 3, 5 and 8–11 months of age (Ramsay, Farrington, & Miller, 1993). The data are in Kanaan and Farrington (2002).

Vaccine effectiveness for a full three-dose course was estimated using the screening method, for cases aged 1–9 years of age arising outside an epidemic period. The results are displayed in Table 16.4.

The estimated age-specific vaccine effectiveness drops from 95% at age 1 year to 78% at age 9 years. However, the authors urge caution in interpreting this apparent decline as 'a fall in efficacy with age may be observed, even if the protective effect of the vaccine remains constant' (Ramsay et al., 1993, p. 46).

Table 16.4 **Effectiveness of pertussis vaccine by age (years), with 95% CI**

Age (t)	1	2	3	4	5	6	7	8	9
$VE(t)$%	95	92	93	93	90	94	91	85	78
95% CI	92–97	87–95	88–96	88–96	84–93	88–97	78–96	64–94	46–91

The results in Box 16.16 suggest that whole-cell pertussis vaccine effectiveness remains broadly constant at ages 1–4 years (these ages correspond, roughly, to 0 to 4 years after the third dose of whole-cell pertussis vaccine), but then wanes.

If the pertussis vaccine behaves like an all-or-nothing vaccine, then we can definitely conclude that the effectiveness wanes over time: if it did not wane, we would observe a constant effectiveness with this model of vaccine action, since the screening VE values are risk-based and prior infections are not removed from the risk denominators.

However, the partial protection model is perhaps a more reasonable one for pertussis vaccine (see Box 16.11). But the risk-based estimate of vaccine effectiveness in each age group provided by the screening method uses vaccine coverage data for the entire cohort, and thus includes prior cases. When applied to a partial protection type vaccine, risk-based estimates using whole cohort denominators may be biased when, as is the case here, the incidence is relatively high. This bias was illustrated in Box 16.5: if the partial protection model holds and the vaccine effectiveness does not wane, then the rate-based VE is constant but the risk-based VE measure may decline over time. The same applies to age-specific effectiveness $VE(t)$.

To avoid bias, individuals with prior pertussis infections should be removed from the calculation of vaccine coverage values used in the screening method. For example, to evaluate the vaccine effectiveness at age 9 (i.e., during the 10th year of life), the vaccine coverage in susceptible individuals reaching their 9th birthday should be used. But this is not possible: first, because the notification data used in this study are incomplete and, second, because in any case a large number of infections are likely to be mild or inapparent, and thus unlikely to be notified.

The best that can be done is to undertake a sensitivity analysis to assess the likely impact of this possible bias, using the expressions in Equations 16.1 and 16.2. We assume that the vaccine effectiveness is a constant value and investigate what incidences of past infection, if any, are consistent with this assumption. The method is described in Box 16.17.

Box 16.17 Sensitivity analysis for the whole-cell pertussis vaccine data

We shall assume that the vaccine effectiveness under the partial protection model is a constant value 95% (corresponding to that observed at age 1 in Table 16.4). We then adjust the observed vaccine effectiveness $VE(t)$ using Equation 16.1 to obtain

$$VE(t)^* = 1 - \left[1 - VE(t)\right] \times S(t)^{1-\theta}$$

with $1 - \theta = 0.95$ and $S(t) = e^{-0.15t}$, this value corresponding to an annual incidence of 0.15. This adjustment gives the results shown in Figure 16.5.

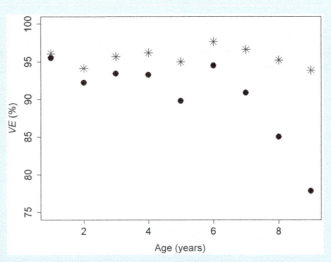

Figure 16.5 Age-specific effectiveness of whole-cell pertussis vaccine. Dots: estimated values. Stars: adjusted for prior infections.

The dots in Figure 16.5 correspond to the $VE(t)$ estimates in Table 16.4. The stars correspond to the adjusted values $VE(t)^*$. With this adjustment, there is no longer any evidence of waning: at age 1 year, $VE^* = 96\%$ and at 9 years, $VE^* = 94\%$, broadly in line with Equation 16.2.

Thus, if the annual incidence rate of pertussis infection is of the order of 0.15, the observed waning is likely to be spurious (assuming a partial protection model of vaccine action). If it is substantially less than 0.15 per year, the observed waning is most likely genuine.

In Box 16.17 we found that, if pertussis vaccine conforms to the partial protection model, then the vaccine effectiveness could indeed be constant, provided that the average annual incidence in unvaccinated children was about 0.15 up to age 9 years. This would imply that, by age 9 years, about 75% of unvaccinated children would have been infected. Further contextual information, for example from surveillance or seroprevalence studies, is then required to assess whether this is a reasonable value.

As shown in this example, the assessment of vaccine effectiveness long after vaccination has taken place, when the incidence of infection in the intervening period is high, may not be straightforward. We have outlined a strategy based on critical appraisal of the data in context, supplemented by sensitivity analyses. The main characteristics of this strategy are set out in Box 16.18.

Box 16.18 Assessing *VE* long after vaccination when prior infections are common

- Begin, if possible, by identifying which model of vaccine action (partial protection or all-or-nothing) is likely to be closest to the true vaccine mechanism. If this is not possible, consider each model in turn; the model determines whether prior infections should be included or excluded.
- If the preferred vaccine action model is all-or-nothing, include individuals who are prior cases in person or person-time denominators, as if they had not been infected. If the preferred vaccine action model is partial protection, consider whether all prior immunising infections (not just clinical cases) can be excluded. If they can, then do so.
- If they cannot all be excluded (e.g., because they cannot all be identified), then include prior cases and undertake a sensitivity analysis with a range of assumptions about the infection rate in unvaccinated individuals and the vaccine effectiveness, here presumed constant. This sensitivity analysis can be undertaken using the adjustment in Equations 16.1 and 16.2.
- Assess the results of these sensitivity analyses in context in the light of what is known about the epidemiology of the infection and the vaccine, and in terms of the internal consistency of the sensitivity analyses.
- Provide a full description of the sensitivity analyses and the assumptions underpinning them.

Summary

- Studies to evaluate the effectiveness of a vaccine long after vaccinations have been administered may need to take account of infections arising in the intervening period.
- When the infection rate is low, prior infections may be ignored, and standard methods may be applied, for example to assess whether vaccine effectiveness wanes over time.
- When the infection rate is high, different measures of *VE* may diverge over time. It then becomes necessary to take into account the mode of action of the vaccine.
- Models for vaccine action include the partial protection model and the all-or-nothing model. The characteristics of these models are summarised in Table 16.5. Often, sensitivity analyses, varying the inclusion of prior cases, are required to explore the likely effectiveness of the vaccine long after vaccination.

Table 16.5 **Summary table**

Vaccine model	Direct effect in vaccinees	Temporal effects (in the absence of waning)	Possible immunological mechanisms
All-or-nothing protection	Complete protection for a proportion of vaccinees and none for the rest	Risk-based VE constant Rate-based VE increases	Serological threshold established
Partial protection	Infection rate reduced proportionally in all vaccinees	Risk-based VE decreases Rate-based VE constant	Cellular immunity predominates

References

Baxter, R., Ray, P., Tran, T. N., Black, S., Shinefield, H. R., Coplan, P. M., … Saddler, P. (2013). Long-term effectiveness of varicella vaccine: A 14-year, prospective cohort study. *Pediatrics*, *131*(5), e1389–e1396.

Chang, C., Mo, X., Hu, P., Liang, W., Ma, H., An, Z., … Zheng, H. (2015). Effectiveness of rubella vaccine in a rubella outbreak in Guangzhou city, China, 2014. *Vaccine*, *33*, 3223–3227.

Chen, R. T., Markowitz, L. E., Albrecht, P., Stewart, J. A., Mofenson, L. M., Preblud, S. R., & Orenstein, W. A. (1990). Measles antibody: Reevaluation of protective titers. *Journal of Infectious Diseases*, *162*(5), 1036–1042.

Cohen, C., White, J. M., Savage, E., Glynn, J. R., Choi, Y., Brown, D., … Ramsay, M. E. (2007). Vaccine effectiveness estimates, 2004–2005 mumps outbreak, England. *Emerging Infectious Diseases*, *13*(1), 12–17.

Farrington, C. P. (1992). The measurement and interpretation of age-specific vaccine efficacy. *International Journal of Epidemiology*, *21*(5), 1014–1020.

Hahné, S. J., Nic Lochlainn, L. M., van Burgel, N. D., Kerkhof, J., Sane, J., Bing Yap, K., & van Binnendijk, R. S. (2016). Measles outbreak among previously immunized healthcare workers, the Netherlands, 2014. *Journal of Infectious Diseases*, *214*, 1980–1986.

Halloran, M. E., Haber, M., & Longini, I. M. (1992). Interpretation and estimation of vaccine efficacy under heterogeneity. *American Journal of Epidemiology*, *136*(3), 328–343.

Kanaan, M. N., & Farrington, C. P. (2002). Estimation of waning vaccine efficacy. *Journal of the American Statistical Association*, *97*(458), 389–397.

Kohberger, R. C., Jemiolo, D., & Fernando, N. (2008). Prediction of pertussis vaccine efficacy using a correlates of protection model. *Vaccine*, *26*, 35163521.

Mangtani, P., Nguipdop-Djomo, P., Keogh, R. H., Sterne, J. A., Abubakar, I., Smith, P. G., … Rodrigues, L. C. (2018). The duration of protection of school-aged BCG vaccination in England: A population-based case-control study. *International Journal of Epidemiology*, *47*(1), 193–201.

Plotkin, S. A. (2008). Correlates of vaccine-induced immunity. *Clinical Infectious Diseases*, *47*, 401–409.

Ramsay, M. E., Farrington, C. P., & Miller, E. (1993). Age-specific efficacy of pertussis vaccine during epidemic and non-epidemic periods. *Epidemiology and Infection, 111*, 41–48.

Smith, P. G., Rodrigues, L. C., & Fine, P. E. (1984). Assessment of the protective efficacy of vaccines against common diseases using case-control and cohort studies. *International Journal of Epidemiology, 13*(1), 87–93.

Storsaeter, J., Hallander, H. O., Gustaffson, L., & Olin, P. (1998). Levels of anti-pertussis antibodies related to protection after household exposure to Bordetella pertussis. *Vaccine, 16*(20), 1907–1916.

Part IV

Risks associated with vaccination programmes

Chapter 17

Vaccine safety
An introduction

This and the next three chapters are devoted to vaccine safety. The evaluation of vaccine safety includes both the assessment and quantification of adverse events following immunisation, and the accrual of evidence for absence of risk. Risks associated with vaccination include direct risks for a vaccinee due to adverse events. They also include risks associated with vaccination programmes, which have already featured in earlier chapters. Thus, in Chapter 5 we discussed some of the negative impacts that might arise following the introduction of vaccination in a population, resulting from changes in the ecology of the infection: for example, possible changes in the severity profile of cases resulting from a rise in the average age at infection, or post-honeymoon outbreaks resulting from the accumulation of susceptibles. And in Chapter 6, we discussed vaccination programmes from a societal perspective, in which risks as well as benefits shape attitudes to vaccination among the public.

The four chapters in this part of the book on vaccine safety are focused on adverse events following immunisation that affect vaccinated individuals directly. In this brief introductory chapter, we set the scene for subsequent chapters on surveillance and assessment of vaccine safety. In Section 17.1 we describe the different types of adverse events that may arise after vaccination. Then in Section 17.2 we discuss the context in which vaccine safety is assessed.

17.1 Adverse events following immunisation

Individuals who get vaccinated may experience untoward medical events after vaccination. For licensed vaccines, these are very seldom causally related to the vaccination. In order not to limit a priori the set of medical events to be taken into account, vaccine safety evaluations usually consider all adverse events that occur following immunisation (AEFIs). An AEFI is defined as any untoward medical occurrence that follows

DOI: 10.4324/9781315166414-18
This Chapter has been made available under a CC-BY-NC-ND license.

immunisation; it does not necessarily have a causal relationship with the vaccine. The adverse event may be any unfavourable or unintended sign, an abnormal laboratory finding, a symptom or a disease. This definition was proposed by the World Health Organization (WHO), who further classified AEFIs in five different types according to their cause (Box 17.1).

> ### Box 17.1 AEFIs: cause-specific classification
>
> The following classification of AEFIs was proposed by WHO (2018).
>
> 1. *Vaccine product-related reaction*, also called 'side effect', 'adverse vaccine reaction' or 'vaccine-induced reaction': an AEFI caused (or precipitated) by a vaccine due to one or more of the inherent properties of the vaccine product.
> 2. *Vaccine quality defect-related reaction*: an AEFI that is caused (or precipitated) by a vaccine due to one or more quality defects of the vaccine product, including the administration device, as provided by the manufacturer.
> 3. *Immunisation error-related reaction*: an AEFI that is caused by inappropriate vaccine handling, prescribing or administration.
> 4. *Immunisation anxiety-related reaction*: an AEFI arising from anxiety about the immunisation.
> 5. *Coincidental adverse events*: an AEFI that is caused by something other than the vaccine product, immunisation error or immunisation anxiety.

Only the first three types of AEFI in Box 17.1 are directly caused by the vaccine or its administration. When evaluating vaccination programmes, the classification of AEFIs into one of these categories is essential, as it determines the public health intervention needed. This classification may not be straightforward; the assessments required will be discussed in Chapters 18 to 20.

In this section, we describe the mechanisms of how these different types of AEFI can arise and provide examples of each.

17.1.1 Vaccine product-related reactions (side effects)

Vaccines used in current national vaccination programmes are very safe, but no vaccine is free of risks. Side effects of vaccines can be mild, such as transient local reactions at the injection site, malaise and fever. These reactions generally result from the inflammatory response induced by vaccination. In addition, vaccines can cause specific, sometimes severe, side effects. The risk of these for currently used vaccines is extremely low (see Box 17.2).

Box 17.2 Frequencies of some severe vaccine product-related reactions

WHO publishes information sheets detailing the safety evidence for individual vaccines. Table 17.1 provides orders of magnitude for some of the more severe adverse reactions for selected live-attenuated vaccines and killed vaccines. The data are available from www.who.int/vaccine_safety/initiative/tools/vaccinfosheets/en/.

Table 17.1 Frequencies of severe adverse events for selected vaccines

Vaccine	Adverse reaction	Frequency per no. doses
Live-attenuated vaccines		
BCG	Disseminated BCG	1–4 per million*
Measles	Febrile convulsion	3–10 per 10,000
MMR	ITP	1 per 30,000
OPV	Vaccine-associated paralytic polio	1 per million
Killed vaccines		
DTwP	Febrile convulsion	8–60 per 100,000
Influenza	Guillain-Barré syndrome	1 per million**

* In HIV-negative infants.
** In some influenza seasons only.
BCG: Bacille Calmette-Guérin; ITP: idiopathic thrombocytopenic purpura; MMR: measles, mumps and rubella; OPV: oral polio vaccine; DTwP: diphtheria, tetanus and whole-cell pertussis.

As a general principle, the risk of side effects for live-attenuated vaccines is higher for the first dose, while for killed vaccines it is higher for subsequent doses. The explanation for this is that the relatively small dose of live-attenuated organisms in live vaccines is mopped up quickly when adequate immunity is present after a first vaccine dose, while for killed vaccines the host immune response causing side effects gets stronger after subsequent doses due to immune memory.

A side effect specific to some live-attenuated viral vaccines is the occurrence of symptoms resembling a mild form of the viral infection the vaccine is targeted against. These symptoms occur after an incubation period during which the vaccine virus replicates to sufficient amounts to cause vaccine-associated effects. When monitoring a vaccination programme, it is important to distinguish whether the symptoms are caused by the vaccine or result from natural infection. This can be done by genetically characterising the virus in the affected individual, which can provide evidence about the presence of the vaccine or the wild virus.

Oral polio vaccines (OPV), containing live-attenuated polioviruses, have specific safety concerns (see Box 17.3). These concerns are not shared with the inactivated polio vaccines (IPV).

Box 17.3 Side effects of live-attenuated polio vaccines: vaccine-associated paralytic poliomyelitis and vaccine-derived polioviruses

OPV contains live-attenuated polioviruses. This has the advantage that through shedding of vaccine polioviruses by vaccinees, contacts may get immunised. However, OPV does carry the very low risk of causing paralytic poliomyelitis by two different mechanisms.

Vaccine-associated paralytic polio

Vaccine-associated paralytic polio (VAPP) is caused by a genetic reversion of the polio vaccine virus to neurovirulence in the intestine of the OPV recipient (or their immediate contact). The resulting paralysis is clinically indistinguishable from poliomyelitis caused by wild poliovirus. As the virus causing VAPP does not spread, outbreaks of VAPP do not occur. The risk of VAPP is about 2–4 per million birth cohort in countries using OPV.

Vaccine-derived poliovirus

The second mechanism by which OPV can cause paralysis is through mutation of the vaccine virus, causing it to revert to being pathogenic with a capacity for sustained person-to-person transmission. Such mutated viruses are called vaccine-derived polioviruses (VDPVs). VDPVs can arise when there is prolonged replication of a vaccine virus in an individual (usually someone with immunosuppression) or a population (usually when the levels of immunity in the population are inadequate). Adequate immunity against wild poliovirus also protects against VDPVs. VDPVs are defined based on the level of genetic divergence of the mutated virus from the vaccine strain. The level of divergence is related to the duration of circulation of the virus in a population.

WHO has proposed definitions available for further classification of VDPVs. When there is evidence of person-to-person transmission of VDPVs, they are called circulating VDPV (cVDPV). Immunodeficiency-associated VDPVs (iVDPV) are VDPVs found in persons with one of a set of specific immunodeficiency disorders. Ambiguous VDPVs (aVDPVs) are VDPVs that are isolated from a person with no known immunodeficiency or sewage isolates of unknown origin (WHO, 2016).

> To reduce the risk of VAPP and VDPVs in the context of wild poliovirus type 2 being eradicated, a global recommendation was made to use bivalent OPV, containing only type 1 and 3 vaccine strains polioviruses, rather than trivalent OPV (against poliovirus type 1, 2 and 3) from April 2016 onwards (WHO, 2016).

Apart from side effects resulting from the biological action of a vaccine, AEFIs may also occur due to hypersensitivity reactions in the vaccine recipient. These reactions can range from mild local reactions to severe anaphylaxis. The latter is very rare (about one in a million vaccinees) and can be fatal if not treated adequately.

A specific type of side effect is the phenomenon of vaccine-associated enhanced disease (VAED) (see Box 17.4). It is arguable whether it can be classified as a side effect per se, since infection with the pathogen the vaccine intended to protect against is essential for it to occur.

Box 17.4 Vaccine-associated enhanced disease

Vaccine-associated enhanced disease (VAED) is a severe or modified clinical presentation of a known disease, which may occur in someone who is vaccinated against that disease, and subsequently gets infected with the pathogen the vaccine was intended to protect against. VAED has been described for several vaccines, including those against measles and dengue. The immunological mechanism through which it occurs can involve antibodies or T cells. Since there is no definitive (microbiological) diagnostic marker for VAED, the distinction between cases of vaccine failure and of VAED is challenging: all VAEDs are vaccine failures, but not all vaccine failures are cases of VAED. There are laboratory tests that can raise a suspicion of VAED, which together with the clinical manifestation, the time of onset after vaccination and the incidence of the targeted disease around the case can make the diagnosis VAED more or less likely. Systematic surveillance of disease manifestations in vaccinated individuals is important to detect the occurrence of cases of likely VAED.

17.1.2 Vaccine quality defect-related reactions

In the era before the current high safety standards imposed on vaccines, several incidents were documented that were caused by vaccines with quality defects. One of the worst is the 'Cutter' incident (Box 17.5).

> **Box 17.5 The Cutter incident**
>
> In the early years of the polio-vaccination programme in the United States, a vaccine company in California (Cutter Laboratories) produced an inactivated polio vaccine that included, by mistake, incompletely inactivated polioviruses. This vaccine was administered by injection to about 120,000 children, causing an outbreak of polio in spring 1955, including 40,000 children with mild polio, 200 with permanent paralysis and 10 fatal cases. The first polio cases among Cutter vaccinees were reported on 25 and 26 April 1955. A meeting of public health epidemiologists, virologists and others on 26 April suggested the polio cases had been caused by the vaccine, which led to a request on 27 April 1955 to the company to start recalling the vaccine (Nathanson & Langmuir, 1963). This likely prevented many more cases from occurring, highlighting the importance of timely safety surveillance and decision-making.

17.1.3 Immunisation error-related reaction

In this type of AEFI, the vaccine product itself is safe, but an AEFI arises due to prescribing it inadequately or not handling or administering it well. One example of this is the risk of acquisition of a blood-borne infection in the vaccine recipient when needles used for vaccination are reused. To prevent this, single use (auto-disable) needles are recommended. Another example is mixing up vaccine reconstitution products with medicines kept in the same refrigerator, which may cause serious adverse events.

17.1.4 Immunisation anxiety-related reaction

An example of this type of AEFI is fainting due to a vasovagal reaction. Anxiety-related AEFI may occur at higher rates in mass vaccination programmes, when signs of anxiety from one person may increase the levels of anxiety in others.

17.1.5 Coincidental adverse event

Any event occurring after vaccination, when not classified in one of the above categories, falls into this category. For some coincidental AEFIs, there is sufficient evidence that they are not caused by a specific vaccine. Examples of this are autism, which is not linked to measles, mumps and rubella (MMR) vaccination, and Guillain-Barré syndrome, which was demonstrated not to have a causal relation with human papillomavirus (HPV) vaccine. Distinguishing coincidental AEFIs from those causally related to vaccination can be difficult, and typically requires epidemiological studies (see Chapters 19 and 20).

17.2 The context of vaccine safety assessment

Because vaccines are mostly administered to healthy individuals, the acceptability of any adverse reaction caused by the vaccine or its administration (beyond transient pain or mild local or systemic reactions such as a short-lived fever) is much lower for vaccines than for other pharmaceutical products, particularly when compared to those used to treat severe conditions.

Vaccines must therefore meet demanding standards of efficacy and safety before they can be licensed for use in vaccination programmes. Once licensed, their manufacturing for routine use is subject to stringent quality controls. Nevertheless, because vaccination programmes are targeted at large populations, AEFIs even of very low frequency (less than 1 per 100,000 doses, say) may still be expected to occur in significant numbers. All such events are of concern, whatever their frequency.

AEFIs are thoroughly investigated in preclinical studies and in clinical trials prior to licensure. However, such trials are necessarily of limited size and duration, and cannot therefore be expected to identify rare adverse events. This can only be achieved by monitoring the safety of the vaccine in the field once it is in routine use. Studying rare events and seeking to establish whether they are caused by the vaccine is difficult. Statistical difficulties associated with the study of rare events are compounded by the fact that vaccines are complex products, all of whose constituents (preservatives, adjuvants, diluents and other excipients), along with their handling and administration, must undergo close scrutiny in the case of an AEFI that may be causally linked to the vaccine.

The monitoring, evaluation and communication of risks is an essential requirement, both ethical and practical, of every vaccination programme, and a demanding one. It encompasses the quantification of risks of known vaccine reactions; the identification of new or unsuspected risks and their evaluation; accrual of evidence of vaccine safety; and effective communication of information about vaccine risks. Some of the latter issues were discussed in Chapter 6.

The responsibility for these tasks is usually shared between public health bodies operating at subnational, national and international levels, and the vaccine manufacturers. For the reasons given above, the assessment of risks potentially associated with vaccines is a highly specialised subdiscipline of pharmacoepidemiology. WHO, in particular, provides extensive information and advice on vaccine safety, and seeks to strengthen safety monitoring systems worldwide. These activities are described in Box 17.6.

Box 17.6 WHO and global vaccine safety

WHO plays an active role in supporting vaccine safety initiatives worldwide.

The Global Advisory Committee on Vaccine Safety (GACVS) was set up in 1999 to provide independent, authoritative scientific advice to WHO on all vaccine-related safety issues. It reviews scientific data and publications and makes evidence-based recommendations on matters of regional or global concern with the potential to affect national vaccination programmes.

The Global Vaccine Safety Initiative (GVSI) was launched in 2011 to enhance vaccine safety activities worldwide, by building and supporting vaccine pharmacovigilance in all low- and middle-income countries.

> WHO also provides extensive reference documents, including the vaccine information sheets mentioned in Box 17.2. These resources and other information on WHO vaccine safety activities may be found online at www.who.int/teams/regulation-prequalification/regulation-and-safety/pharmacovigilance/vaccine-safety-net.

In the next three chapters, the processes used to evaluate vaccine safety, including the surveillance of AEFIs and their investigation in epidemiological studies, will be described.

Summary

- An AEFI is any untoward medical event occurring after vaccination.
- AEFIs are categorised as vaccine product-related reactions, vaccine quality defect-related reactions, immunisation error-related reactions, immunisation anxiety-related reactions and coincidental adverse events. Only the first three are directly causally related to vaccination.
- The monitoring, evaluation and communication of vaccine safety is an essential requirement of every vaccination programme.

References

Nathanson, N., & Langmuir, A. D. (1963). The Cutter incident: Poliomyelitis following formaldehyde-inactivated poliovirus vaccination in the United States during the spring of 1955. I. Background. *American Journal of Epidemiology*, 78(1), 16–28.

World Health Organization (WHO). (2016). Polio vaccines: WHO position paper – March 2016. *Weekly Epidemiology Record*, 91(12), 145–168.

World Health Organization (WHO). (2018). *Causality assessment of an adverse event following immunization: User manual for the revised WHO classification* (2nd ed.). Geneva, Switzerland: WHO.

Chapter 18

Surveillance of adverse events following immunisation

For the reasons set out in Chapter 17, vaccination programmes should be monitored for safety, even though vaccines are licensed subject to stringent safety criteria. Post-licensure, all vaccine batches are usually tested for safety and potency, and only when the results are satisfactory are these batches released for use. Despite this rigorous process, no vaccine, nor its administration, can be assumed to carry zero risk of an adverse reaction. Thus, surveillance of adverse events following immunisation (AEFIs) is a key component of vaccine programme surveillance.

The present chapter sets out some of the key aspects of vaccine adverse event surveillance. We begin in Section 18.1 with a more detailed description of the rationale and purpose of vaccine safety surveillance. In Sections 18.2 and 18.3 we describe passive and active safety surveillance systems. Finally, in Section 18.4 we discuss the analysis of AEFI surveillance data.

18.1 The rationale for surveillance of adverse events

Pre-licensure, vaccine safety is established in phase 1–3 clinical trials and results are reviewed as part of the licensing process (see Chapter 1, Section 1.5). However, important side effects may only become apparent when the vaccine is used in large-scale vaccination programmes, which is why post-licensure vaccine safety surveillance is an essential aspect of any vaccination programme.

There are several reasons for this. First, a rare side effect may be missed in pre-clinical studies, if the size of the pre-licensure trials were inadequate to detect it. An example is intussusception related to rotavirus vaccination, previously described in Chapter 3. Further details are in Box 18.1.

Box 18.1 Rotavirus vaccine and intussusception in the United States

In pre-licensure studies, the RotaShield anti-rotavirus vaccine was found to be effective and safe and was licensed for use in 1998 with a three-dose vaccination schedule at 2, 4 and 6 months of age.

In 11 pre-licensure trials, intussusception occurred during the first 12 months of life in one of 4,633 placebo recipients (0.022%), compared to five in 10,054 vaccine recipients (0.050%); but only two cases arose in the 8,240 recipients of the vaccine at the dosage proposed for licensure (0.024%). The cases in vaccinees arose between days 6 and 51 after the second or third dose of vaccine. Statistical tests provided no evidence for a difference in the underlying rates of intussusception in vaccinees compared to the placebo group (Rennels et al., 1998).

Subsequent studies, undertaken after the vaccine was licensed, revealed a significantly increased risk of intussusception between 3 and 14 days after the first and second dose of vaccine. However, intussusception is very uncommon, and the risk attributable to the vaccine is low, being of the order of one case per 5,000 to one case per 10,000 children vaccinated (Murphy et al., 2001). Nevertheless, the vaccine was withdrawn, as described in Chapter 3.

The key issue revealed in Box 18.1 is that the pre-licensure clinical trials were too small to detect an effect of the size subsequently revealed in field studies. In statistical terms, the power of the studies – that is, the probability that they would detect a true effect – was too low, and in consequence the effect was missed.

Second, side effects will be missed if they typically occur outside the usually relatively brief period of follow-up of most pre-licensure trials. Third, pre-licensure trials may be undertaken in populations that differ from those in which the vaccine is used, for example because people with certain chronic diseases were excluded from the trials or a different age group from the one in the trial was targeted for vaccination.

Since all types of AEFI (except coincidental adverse events unrelated to vaccination) may require interventions to minimise their occurrence and adequately inform the population, AEFI surveillance is needed throughout the existence of a vaccination programme in order to inform such interventions. The primary aim of post-licensure AEFI surveillance is to identify vaccine side effects that were not detected pre-licensure, to quantify their rate of occurrence and to inform benefit–risks analyses (see Chapter 21). Second, post-licensure AEFI surveillance aims to identify adverse events caused by vaccine quality defects or vaccine administering errors that require interventions to improve the quality of the programme. Finally, post-licensure surveillance is required to build the evidence base underpinning the vaccine's safety profile – even in the absence of any adverse events. Box 18.2 provides some further details.

Box 18.2 Evidence of vaccine safety when no adverse events are observed

While it cannot be proved that a vaccine never causes a given adverse event, evidence of safety can accumulate over time. To this end, the total number of vaccinations followed up should always be specified. A bold statement such as 'no adverse events were observed to be caused by the vaccine' is uninformative about the risk, because it is also consistent with no or little surveillance having taken place. This point is usefully captured by the phrase 'absence of evidence does not constitute evidence of absence'.

Observing 0 events after N vaccinations are given allows both the risk, and the uncertainty associated with it, to be quantified. The risk estimate is 0, and an approximate 95% confidence interval (CI) for the underlying risk is 0 to 3/N.

For example, if no deaths are observed in the month following vaccination in 3,000 children, then the estimated fatality rate for this period is 0, and an approximate 95% CI for the risk is 0 to 1 in 1,000, or (0, 0.001).

Post-licensure vaccine safety surveillance is carried out by public health authorities, regulatory agencies and vaccine manufacturers. Vaccine safety surveillance is based on recording AEFIs, which may come to light by informal reporting in (social) media, by reporting through passive or active surveillance systems or through data-linkage of routine electronic health data.

18.2 Passive surveillance systems for AEFIs

Passive AEFI surveillance is used in almost all countries. Passive surveillance does not involve an active search for AEFIs by health authorities, but relies on spontaneous reporting of AEFIs by medical professionals and sometimes the public. The events reported can include any events that, in the opinion of the reporter, may be associated with vaccination. Some countries use dedicated passive surveillance systems for vaccines (see for example Box 18.3), while in others AEFI reporting is integrated in broader medical products safety monitoring, also called pharmacovigilance.

Box 18.3 Passive AEFI surveillance in the United States: the VAERS system

The US Vaccine Adverse Event Reporting System (VAERS) was launched in 1990 and is jointly organised by the US Centers for Disease Control and Prevention (CDC) and the US Food and Drug Administration (FDA). AEFIs can be submitted to VAERS by health professionals, vaccine manufacturers and also by the public, by filling out a form available on the Internet (https://vaers.hhs.gov). The system and its operation are described in Shimabukuro, Nguyen, Martin, and DeStefano (2015).

> Following the introduction of rotavirus vaccination in the United States in August 1998, VAERS rapidly detected an unusually high number of intussusceptions occurring soon after vaccination. This led to the suspension of the rotavirus vaccination programme in July 1999, as described in Chapter 3 (CDC, 1999).
>
> Other notable signals detected by VAERS include multiple organ system failure (YEL-AVD) after yellow fever vaccine (CDC, 2002), severe adverse events after smallpox vaccine (CDC, 2003) and febrile convulsions in young children after an inactivated influenza vaccine during the 2010–2011 influenza season (Leroy, Broder, Menschik, Shimabukuro, & Martin, 2012).

Passive reporting systems for AEFIs provide data on the number of AEFIs reported, can detect rare AEFIs and may be used to identify changes in the known safety profile of vaccines. In certain countries, it is mandatory for clinicians to report certain AEFIs, which then feed into government compensation schemes.

One of the main strengths of passive surveillance systems based on spontaneous reporting of AEFIs is that they can identify previously unsuspected adverse reactions, by making use of reports from astute clinicians and members of the public. Box 18.4 describes how passive surveillance led to the identification of narcolepsy as an unexpected side effect of one pandemic influenza vaccine.

Box 18.4 Pandemic influenza vaccination and narcolepsy in children and adolescents

In 2009, the H1N1 influenza virus pandemic led to influenza vaccine recommendations for a much wider target group than the usual target groups for seasonal influenza vaccine. Eight different pandemic vaccines were used in Europe, and enhanced passive surveillance of AEFIs was recommended by the European Medicines Agency (EMA).

An apparent excess of narcolepsy, often with catalepsy, was picked up in children and adolescents by clinicians in Finland and in Sweden soon after the introduction of one of these vaccines, Pandemrix. Narcolepsy is a rare neurological sleep disorder, which had never before been reported in association with vaccination; it was not included in the events recommended to be followed by the EMA (Nohynek et al., 2012).

These reports were first made public in August 2010 in a press release from the Swedish Medical Products Agency. In view of the temporal association with narcolepsy, Pandemrix vaccinations were suspended in Finland in August 2010 (Partinen et al., 2012).

Subsequent investigations concluded there was an increased risk of narcolepsy associated with Pandemrix vaccination in children and adolescents aged less than 19 years, and in July 2011 the EMA recommended restrictions on the use of the Pandemrix vaccine in these age groups.

In order to work effectively, passive reporting systems must be accessible and easy to use. Ensuring that this is the case is a public health priority, as is training of a wide range of medical staff about their responsibility for reporting AEFIs.

However, passive AEFI surveillance usually cannot be used to estimate population-based incidence rates of AEFIs, owing to underreporting and lack of data on the number of people who received a particular vaccine. Underreporting is a particularly important weakness of passive reporting systems, and can lead to misplaced optimism regarding the frequency of adverse events. An example is described in Box 18.5.

Box 18.5 Aseptic meningitis after MMR vaccines in the United Kingdom

Aseptic meningitis is a recognised complication of mumps vaccination. In order to assess the risk in the United Kingdom following the introduction of routine measles, mumps and rubella (MMR) vaccination in 1987, a passive surveillance system was initiated. Paediatricians were asked to report all confirmed and suspected cases of aseptic meningitis in 1990–1991. The risk based on confirmed cases was 4 per 1 million doses, all in recipients of MMR vaccines containing the Urabe mumps strain; vaccines with the Jeryl-Lynn mumps strain were also in use. However, investigations based on active case finding found that the true risk was much higher, at 1 per 1,1000 doses in Urabe vaccine recipients; no cases were identified in children who had received MMR vaccines containing the Jeryl-Lynn mumps strain (Miller et al., 1993).

Following this finding, MMR vaccines containing the Urabe mumps strain were replaced in the United Kingdom with vaccines containing the Jeryl-Lynn strain.

In the example in Box 18.5, the true frequency of AEFI was over 20 times higher than that suggested by passive surveillance. Discrepancies of this order of magnitude are typical, rather than the exception.

In addition to underreporting, passive AEFI surveillance is also prone to reporting biases. In particular, media publicity about adverse reactions can distort diagnosis and reporting of such events. An example is described in Box 18.6.

Box 18.6 Increases in vaccine-associated narcolepsy diagnoses after media reports

As described in Box 18.4, narcolepsy was identified as an unexpected side effect of the Pandemrix vaccine during the 2009–2010 influenza pandemic. Confirmation of the signal was complicated by the widespread media attention it received after the Swedish Medical Products Agency issued a press release concerning it on 16 August 2010.

One of the key epidemiological studies on narcolepsy cases collected information on the onset date of excessive daytime sleepiness (EDS) as observed by parents and on the date a physician diagnosed narcolepsy (Nohynek et al., 2012). The data are shown in Figure 18.1.

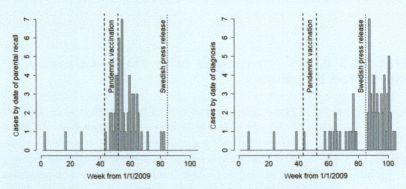

Figure 18.1 **Weekly cases of narcolepsy, Finland, 2009–2010.**

Note: Left: case onset defined by parental reports; Right: case onset defined by physician diagnosis. The central bands denote the period when most persons aged under 19 years were vaccinated. The rightmost vertical dotted lines mark 16 August 2010, when the Swedish press release was issued.

In the left panel of Figure 18.1 the onset of narcolepsy is defined by parental reports of EDS, while in the right panel the onset is defined by the date of physician diagnosis of narcolepsy. The vertical dotted line at 16 August 2010 is when the Swedish Medical Products Agency published the press release on the observation on the association between narcolepsy and Pandemrix vaccination. Whereas parental reports occur shortly after vaccination, the physician diagnoses cluster after 16 August, suggesting a diagnostic bias; the press release having prompted the physicians to diagnose narcolepsy.

Owing to under-reporting, lack of denominator data and potential biases, the interpretation of data from passive surveillance systems, and taking public health decisions on the basis of such data, are complex tasks. These will be touched upon in Section 18.4.

18.3 Active surveillance systems for AEFIs

Unlike passive surveillance, active AEFI surveillance does not rely on spontaneous reports from clinicians or the public, but involves proactively monitoring the occurrence of certain well-defined adverse events.

Active AEFI surveillance has been defined as involving a data collection system that seeks to ascertain as completely as possible the number of AEFIs in a given population via a continuous organised process (Heininger, Holm, Caplanusi, & Bailey, 2017). Active AEFI surveillance requires dedicated health professionals. It can be organised by directly asking vaccinees (or their parents) to provide information on the occurrence of AEFIs; alternatively, it may be based on health records collected systematically in real time. Active AEFI surveillance is also used in phase 4 vaccine trials. These are conducted after licensure of a vaccine with safety as the primary outcome (see Chapter 1). Box 18.7 gives an example of an active surveillance system.

Box 18.7 Active surveillance for AEFIs: the Canadian IMPACT system

In Canada, an active AEFI surveillance scheme has been implemented since 1993 at around 12 paediatric referral centres covering approximately 90% of the country's tertiary care paediatric beds. The system, called Immunization Monitoring Programme, Active (IMPACT) was developed after the existing passive AEFI surveillance system failed to detect an unacceptably high risk of aseptic meningitis associated with mumps-containing vaccines (see Box 18.5). The system is operated by 'nurse monitors' who actively search for recent vaccinees among patients admitted with one out of a list of predefined conditions. Because it is based in tertiary care hospitals, IMPACT is only able to monitor very severe AEFIs (Bettinger, Halperin, Vaudry, Law, & Scheifele, 2014).

Active AEFI surveillance can ensure more complete AEFI ascertainment and allows standardised data collection, but is resource intensive and often limited in scope. In particular, active surveillance systems are unlikely to detect previously unknown vaccine side effects. As with passive AEFI surveillance, descriptive analyses of active AEFI surveillance data do not generally permit causality assessments, which require analytic methods; these are discussed in Chapter 20.

Increasingly, active surveillance systems involve linking databases of routinely recorded clinical events with immunisation records. Such systems do not require a list of conditions to be prespecified, and thus may also be used for analytical studies of vaccine safety. They do, however, need to be validated to ensure that the data are of high quality. An early and influential example is provided in Box 18.8.

Box 18.8 Vaccine safety monitoring through data linkage in the United States: the Vaccine Safety Datalink project

The potential of using large, linked data sources for vaccine safety monitoring was first recognised in the United States in 1990, with the establishment of the Vaccine Safety Datalink (VSD), a collaboration between US CDC and eight health maintenance organisations.

The VSD combines electronic health data on administered vaccines and medical illnesses to assess vaccine safety. The VSD was validated by verifying that it correctly identified known associations between diphtheria, tetanus and pertussis (DTP) and MMR vaccines and febrile convulsions (Chen et al., 1997).

The VSD has since been expanded and its uses have developed over time. It has been used for numerous purposes, including active surveillance of AEFIs, but also analytical studies of vaccine safety, using a multiplicity of study designs (McNeil et al., 2014).

The active surveillance systems described in Boxes 18.7 and 18.8 are permanent, generic systems applicable to all routinely administered vaccines. Active surveillance of AEFIs may take very different forms in different settings, to match local circumstances and needs, and to take advantage of local opportunities. Box 18.9 illustrates this variety.

Box 18.9 Active AEFI surveillance in Ethiopia, Guatemala, Taiwan and Vietnam

In *Ethiopia*, a programme of active surveillance was put in place in 2011–2012 to monitor injection-site reactions to a new presentation of the pneumococcal PCV-10 vaccine as a two-dose vial without preservative. Over 55,000 PCV-10 vaccinations were followed up by home visits. Injection-site reactions to the DTP-HepB-Hib vaccine injection site were used as comparators; frequencies of reactions in first and second aliquot recipients of the PCV-10 vaccine were also compared. No significant differences in risks of injection-site abscess were found (Berhane et al., 2014).

In *Guatemala*, an active surveillance system was set up in 2008–2010 to monitor the safety of a fully liquid combined DTwP-HepB-Hib vaccine. Parents of 3,000 infants vaccinated at two paediatric clinics in the capital were followed up by telephone after each dose and their hospital attendances were monitored for any AEFI. A self-controlled analysis was undertaken; no excess of adverse events was observed (Asturias et al., 2013).

In *Taiwan*, active surveillance was undertaken for the 2009–2010 influenza season to monitor the safety of the influenza vaccine. The system was based on data linkage between medical and vaccination records, with weekly updates on occurrences of Guillain-Barré syndrome, other demyelinating diseases, convulsions, encephalitis, Bell's palsy, anaphylaxis and immune thrombocytopenia within 42 days of vaccination. No excesses of monitored events were identified (Huang et al., 2010).

In *Vietnam*, an active AEFI surveillance database was developed in Khang Hoa province and used to monitor a measles vaccination campaign. All admissions at clinics and hospitals within the study area were recorded and linked via a unique identifier. Visits to local health centres were undertaken to obtain vaccination data. A self-controlled analysis did not identify an excess for any of the events investigated (Ali et al., 2005).

Active surveillance systems based on computerised records operate in real time, or near real time, and are particularly suitable for monitoring newly introduced vaccines, including influenza vaccines and additions to the childhood vaccination schedule. To this end, analyses are repeated at frequent intervals (typically weekly) with the aim of detecting potential safety issues early.

To allow for the multiple statistical tests involved, sequential methods of statistical analysis are employed. These sequential methods ensure that the probability of a false alarm is not inflated by repeatedly interrogating the data as they accumulate; the details of these methods lie outside the scope of this book. An example is described in Box 18.10: this is a development of the VSD surveillance system described in Box 18.8. Some further details of a different application will be given in Box 18.15.

Box 18.10 Rapid cycle analysis in the VSD: febrile convulsions after MMRV vaccine

Rapid cycle analysis (RCA) involves frequent data monitoring using sequential statistical methods. This typically involves comparing observed (after vaccination) and expected (in the absence of vaccination) counts of prespecified events using active surveillance methods in successive time intervals. If an excess is found, additional analyses are undertaken to verify whether it is due to the vaccine. These additional analyses may involve analytical studies (McNeil et al., 2014).

An early success of this system was the detection of a higher risk of febrile convulsions 7–10 days after the combination measles, mumps, rubella, varicella (MMRV) vaccine, compared to MMR and varicella vaccines administered separately, in children aged 12–23 months.

The MMRV vaccine was licensed in the United States in 2005 and recommended for use in 2006. Pre-licensure studies had revealed an increased frequency of fever 1–2 weeks after vaccination with MMRV, but it was not known whether there was an increased risk of febrile convulsions. Weekly active surveillance under the RCA system was undertaken and in August 2007 a preliminary signal of a twofold rise in the risk of febrile convulsions compared to MMR vaccine in the period 7–10 days after vaccination was detected. This was notified to the regulatory authorities in early 2008, resulting in an adjustment to the recommendations for the vaccine. The signal was subsequently confirmed in further investigations on additional data (Klein et al., 2010).

The real-time surveillance methods described so far have made use of medical and administrative databases. The widespread availability of digital platforms and use of social media in some countries provide another avenue for the development of innovative and responsive surveillance systems. One such example is described in Box 18.11.

> ### Box 18.11 Real-time surveillance of influenza vaccine safety in Australia by SMS and email
>
> Reduced confidence resulting from increased rates of febrile reactions in children associated with one influenza vaccine in 2010 prompted the development of this real-time active surveillance system. Children aged 6 months to 4 years receiving seasonal influenza vaccination in 2015 in participating centres were included in this real-time surveillance system; 75% of parents or carers among those invited agreed to participate (Pillsbury et al., 2015).
>
> Participants were contacted within 3 days of vaccination by automated SMS messages or emails and asked to complete an online survey. Demographic and medical data as well as reports of predetermined adverse events were collected and compiled weekly. Cumulative results were periodically made available online. Predetermined alert thresholds were defined: for fever, the expected rate was 6% and the alert threshold was 13%. No alerts were triggered at any time during the surveillance period April to August 2015: fever rates remained below 5% in every week.

18.4 Analysis of AEFI surveillance data

The first step in analysing AEFI reports is the identification of severe events that require an immediate assessment of causality. For example, these can be one or more reports of deaths following receipt of a certain vaccine. Any decisions about interventions, which may involve collecting further data, undertaking further studies and in some cases suspending the vaccination programme, should be made after such an assessment has been completed. Box 18.12 describes an example in which causality could be attributed on the base of individual reports.

> ### Box 18.12 Disseminated BCG in First Nation and Inuit people in Canada
>
> In 1998 a report from the Canadian IMPACT passive surveillance system (see Box 18.7) detailed three deaths associated with vaccination. All three deaths involved Bacille Calmette-Guérin (BCG) administered to First Nation and Inuit (FNI) infants. The case review indicated that the infants were immunocompromised, disseminated BCG being a contributory cause of death. The editorial comment

accompanying this report discussed the benefits and risks of Canada's BCG vaccination programme in FNI populations and outlined the further research required to achieve a better balance between them (Scheifele, Law, & Jadavji, 1998).

The causality assessment of reports of rare and severe AEFI requires both speed and caution. Striking the right balance is difficult: precipitate action at this stage carry the risk of serious negative consequences. Box 18.13 describes such an example.

Box 18.13 An MMR tragedy and a measles disaster in Samoa

On 6 July 2018, two infants in Samoa died within minutes of being given MMR vaccine. In response, the government suspended the MMR immunisation programme. It was restarted in November 2018, but the cause of the tragedy was not made public for months. Two nurses were sentenced to 5 years' imprisonment in July 2019 for inadvertently using a curare-like muscle blocking agent instead of water as a diluent. But it remains unclear why muscle relaxants were kept in immunisation facilities in Samoa.

Lack of transparency about the combination of administrative failures and human error that caused the MMR tragedy resulted in a calamitous drop in immunisation rates and an epidemic of measles. Routine measles vaccination rates fell to 31% by November 2019. The government declared a national emergency and mandated that all 200,000 people on the archipelago should be vaccinated. In spite of this, measles swept through Samoa, causing 4,357 cases with 70 deaths, 61 in children aged less than 5 years, by 9 December 2019 (Isaacs, 2020).

At an individual level, it is usually not possible to conclude definitively whether a certain vaccine caused the reported event except, for example, when it concerns an injection site reaction or an immediate allergic reaction, or in other special circumstances such as those described in Boxes 18.12 and 18.13. The aim of the causality assessment is rather to assess the level of confidence that a particular vaccination caused an AEFI. The World Health Organization (WHO) has produced a guide for such assessments, described in Box 18.14.

Box 18.14 WHO approach to causality assessment for individual AEFI

When clinicians or public health staff receive a report of an individual with a severe AEFI, it is important to assess the likelihood of a causal relation between the AEFI and the vaccine that was administered. The 2018 WHO guide for this

> describes the types of AEFI for which a causality assessment is recommended (excluding, for example, events that are listed on the product label) (WHO, 2018).
>
> The assessment, which can also be done using an online tool (http://gvsi-aefi-tools.org), consists of several steps, which result in the classification of the AEFI into one of four categories: 'consistent with causal association to immunisation', 'indeterminate', 'inconsistent with causal association with immunisation' and 'adequate information not available'. Actions subsequent to the assessment should be outlined in protocols established by national immunisation programmes.
>
> Events classified as 'consistent with causal association to immunisation' or 'indeterminate' (which might apply to new vaccines for which definitive evidence is not available) may be regarded as signals to be investigated further.
>
> WHO defines a signal as follows:
>
>> Information (from one or multiple sources) which suggests a new and potentially causal association, or a new aspect of a known association, between an intervention and an event or set of related events, either adverse or beneficial, that is judged to be of sufficient likelihood to justify verificatory action.
>>
>> (WHO, 2018, p. viii)

As set out in Box 18.14, a signal indicates that an unproven association with immunisation is plausibly causal and merits further investigation. In addition to qualitative assessments, quantitative methods may also be used to identify AEFI signals.

The design of the AEFI surveillance system can help in facilitating the evaluation of signals. Standardised case definitions for AEFIs greatly facilitate the interpretation of results from AEFI surveillance, and indeed epidemiologic studies of AEFIs more widely. The Brighton Collaboration has been instrumental in establishing such standard definitions; details are available from www.brightoncollaboration.org (Bonhoeffer et al., 2002).

Data from passive surveillance systems typically do not feature any denominator data. Furthermore, spontaneous reports are usually made when a clinician or member of the public suspects there may be a causal association. These features greatly complicate the quantitative analysis of data from passive surveillance systems. However, some standard tools of pharmacovigilance, such as disproportionality analyses, may be used to help identify signals. Some of these methods, as applied to vaccines, are described in Shimabukuro et al. (2015). An application, using the proportional reporting ratio or *PRR*, will be described in Box 18.16.

Active surveillance systems, on the other hand, often do include denominator data, so that rates can be calculated, approximately at least. These rates may then be compared, between vaccinated individuals and historical baselines, or between vaccines. Alternatively, provided events are documented independently of their temporal relationship with vaccination, self-controlled methods of analysis (to be described in Chapter 20) may be used. Thus, rough quantitative measures of association may be obtained, potential signals being generated when such measures exceed a given statistical threshold; an example is discussed in Box 18.15.

SURVEILLANCE OF ADVERSE EVENTS

After review by trained epidemiologists, some signals may be set aside (e.g., if they are obviously the result of reporting artefacts), while others may be selected for further investigation. This process may be described as one of hypothesis generation: the surveillance data suggests that a causal link between a vaccine and an adverse event is possible, but does not provide conclusive evidence that such a link exists. Further investigations are then required to determine whether the signal is most likely due to artefacts or data quality issues (e.g., reporting delays or incompletely confirmed cases), to confounding effects or other biases, or whether it could represent a genuine effect. These processes are illustrated in Box 18.15.

Box 18.15 Bell's palsy and monovalent inactivated pandemic influenza vaccine in the United States

As part of comprehensive surveillance of AEFIs and influenza vaccines, the rapid cycle analysis prospective active surveillance system described in Box 18.10 was deployed during the 2009–2010 influenza season to monitor Bell's palsy after the pandemic H1N1 monovalent inactivated vaccine (MIV) (Lee et al., 2011).

Weekly sequential surveillance began in November 2009 and ended in June 2010. A signal was detected for MIV and Bell's palsy in adults aged 25 years or older. Figure 18.2 summarises the progress of several surveillance indicators over the period.

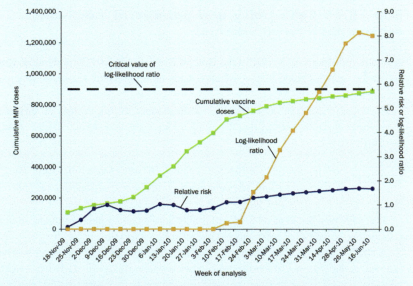

Figure 18.2 Surveillance indicators for Bell's palsy and MIV in adults: cumulative MIV doses administered (left scale), relative risk and log-likelihood ratio (right scale).

Note: The horizontal dashed line is the signalling threshold.
Source: Reproduced with permission from Lee et al. (2011).

> The signalling indicator is the log-likelihood ratio, a probabilistic measure, which is tracked over time. A potential signal is declared when it crosses the signalling threshold: this occurred on 31 March 2010. The relative risk on 1 May 2010 was 1.67 for the association between MIV and Bell's palsy, by which time some 900,000 MIV doses had been administered within the catchment of the surveillance system to persons aged 25 years or older.
>
> Subsequent review of the data, and further analyses, suggested that the effect picked up in sequential monitoring was most likely an artefact induced by seasonality of Bell's palsy. Thus, this potential signal was discounted.

In the example described in Box 18.15, the sequential surveillance system identified a potential signal, which was then reviewed and, in this case, set aside.

One of the problems confronting active surveillance systems based on large databases is that the best data available are scanned for signals, and thus are used to generate hypotheses. But a hypothesis cannot validly be tested on the same data that led to the generation of that hypothesis. It follows that such verification may require waiting till more data have accumulated, as was done in the example described in Box 18.10. Alternatively, hypothesis-testing analyses can be undertaken independently with other data or in other populations. An example is described in Box 18.16.

Box 18.16 Bell's palsy and parenteral inactivated seasonal influenza vaccines

A review of reports to VAERS (see Box 18.3) from 1991 to 2001 flagged up a signal for an association between Bell's palsy and parenteral seasonal influenza vaccines (Zhou et al., 2004).

Among the multiple considerations underpinning the signal was an analysis using the proportional reporting ratio (*PRR*). This is defined as follows (BP stands for Bell's palsy):

$$PRR = \frac{BP\ reports\ after\ influenza\ vaccine}{All\ reports\ after\ influenza\ vaccine} \bigg/ \frac{BP\ reports\ after\ other\ vaccines}{All\ reports\ after\ other\ vaccines}$$

The *PRR* was found to be 3.78 and highly statistically significant, indicating a relative excess of Bell's palsy cases after influenza vaccines.

A similar signal having been obtained from the UK passive reporting system (known as the Yellow Card system), a separate epidemiological study was undertaken in the United Kingdom to test the hypothesis of an association (Stowe, Andrews, Wise, & Miller, 2006).

This study, undertaken in the UK Clinical Practice Research Datalink, a large database of clinical data, found no evidence of an increased risk of Bell's palsy in the three months after vaccination with the parenteral inactivated influenza vaccine, in any age group, or in association with pneumococcal vaccine.

> Thus, it appears that the original signals from VAERS (US) and the Yellow Card (UK) systems were most likely have been false positives, due to chance, bias or confounding.

In Box 18.16, hypothesis testing based on epidemiological studies was undertaken independently from the hypothesis generation process based on signals from surveillance systems. This separation between signal generation and hypothesis testing is of fundamental importance from a methodological point of view. The terms 'signal refinement' and 'signal strengthening' have been used to describe more analytical approaches to signal detection, including, for example, the sequential methods described in Section 18.3. However, such processes still lie within the domain of hypothesis generation. The analytical epidemiological studies required for causality assessment at a population level are discussed in Chapters 19 and 20.

Summary

- Monitoring AEFIs is an essential component of surveillance for vaccine-preventable diseases to detect safety problems and maintain public trust.
- The purpose of AEFI surveillance systems is to detect safety signals and generate hypotheses about changes in the occurrence of AEFIs, which can subsequently be studied in analytical epidemiologic or other studies.
- Passive AEFI surveillance schemes may identify previously unknown vaccine reactions. Training of a wide range of medical staff about their responsibility for early warning is an important role for public health.
- Active surveillance schemes are less prone to under-reporting than passive schemes, and can take many different forms according to local circumstances.
- Electronic health record linkage is increasingly used in AEFI surveillance, including prospective real-time surveillance.
- A first priority in the analyses of AEFI reports is to identify severe events that require an immediate assessment of causality, preferably by using the dedicated WHO guide for this.
- AEFI signals are vaccine-event pairs where causality is plausible but as yet unproven, and merit further investigation.
- AEFI signals are hypotheses, which must then be tested in independent epidemiological studies.

References

Ali, M., Do, C. G., Clemens, J. D., Park, J. -K., von Seidlein, L., Truong, M. T., … Dang, T. D. (2005). The use of a computerized database to monitor vaccine safety in Viet Nam. *Bulletin of the WHO*, *83*, 604–610.

Asturias, E. J., Contreras-Roldan, I. L., Ram, M., Garcia-Melgar, A. J., Morales-Oquendo, V., Hartman, K., … Halsey, N. A. (2013). Post-authorization safety surveillance of a liquid pentavalent vaccine in Guatemalan children. *Vaccine*, *31*, 5909–5914.

Berhane, Y., Worku, A., Demissie, M., Tesfaye, N., Asefa, N., Aniemaw, W., … Ayele, G. (2014). Children who received PCV-10 vaccine from a 2-dose vial without preservative are not more likely to develop injection site abscess compared with those who received pentavalent (DTP-HepB-Hib) vaccine: A longitudinal multi-site study. *PLoS-ONE, 9*(3), e97376.

Bettinger, J. A., Halperin, S. A., Vaudry, W., Law, B. J., & Scheifele, D. W. (2014). The Canadian Immunization Monitoring Program, ACTive (IMPACT): Active surveillance for vaccine adverse events and vaccine-preventable diseases. *Canada Communicable Disease Report, 40*(Suppl. 3), 41–43.

Bonhoeffer, J., Kohl, K., Chen, R., Duclos, P., Heijbel, H., Heininger, U., ... Loupi, E. (2002). The Brighton Collaboration: Addressing the need for standardized case definitions of adverse events following immunization (AEFI). *Vaccine, 21*, 298–302.

Centers for Disease Control and Prevention (CDC). (1999). Intussusception among recipients of rotavirus vaccine, United States, 1998–1999. *Morbidity and Mortality Weekly Report, 48*(27), 577–581.

Centers for Disease Control and Prevention (CDC). (2002). Adverse events associated with 17D-derived yellow fever vaccination, United States, 2001–2002. *Morbidity and Mortality Weekly Report, 51*(44), 989–993.

Centers for Disease Control and Prevention (CDC). (2003). Smallpox vaccine adverse events among civilians, United States, February 25–March 3, 2003. *Morbidity and Mortality Weekly Report, 52*(9), 180–191.

Chen, R. T., Glasser, J. W., Rhodes, P. H., Davis, R. L., Barlow, W. E., Thompson, R. S., ... Hadler, S. C. (1997). Vaccine Safety Datalink Project: A new tool for improving vaccine safety monitoring in the United States. *Pediatrics, 99*, 765–773.

Heininger, U., Holm, K., Caplanusi, I., & Bailey, S. R. (2017). Guide to active vaccine safety surveillance: report of CIOMS working group on vaccine safety: Executive summary. *Vaccine, 35*(32), 3917–3921.

Huang, W. -T., Chen, W. -W., Yang, H. -W., Chen, W. -C., Chao, Y. -N., Huang, Y. -W., ... Kuo, H. -S. (2010). Design of a robust infrastructure to monitor the safety of the pandemic A(H1N1) 2009 vaccination program in Taiwan. *Vaccine, 28*, 7161–7166.

Isaacs, D. (2020). Lessons from the tragic measles outbreak in Samoa. *Journal of Paediatrics and Child Health, 56*, 175.

Klein, N. P., Fireman, B., Yih, W. K., Lewis, E., Kulldorff, M., Ray, P., ... Weintraub, E. (2010). Measles-mumps-rubella-varicella combination vaccine and the risk of febrile seizures. *Pediatrics, 126*, e1–e8.

Lee, G. M., Greene, S. K., Weintraub, E. S., Baggs, J., Kulldorff, M., Fireman, B. H., ... Lieu, T. A. (2011). H1N1 and seasonal influenza vaccine safety in the Vaccine Safety Datalink project. *American Journal of Preventive Medicine, 41*(2), 121–128.

Leroy, Z., Broder, K., Menschik, D., Shimabukuro, T., & Martin, D. (2012). Febrile seizures after 2010–2011 influenza vaccine in young children, United States: A vaccine safety signal from the vaccine adverse event reporting system. *Vaccine, 30*, 2020–2023.

McNeil, M. M., Gee, J., Weintraub, E. S., Belongia, E. A., Lee, G. M., Glanz, J. M., ... DeStefano, F. (2014). The Vaccine Safety Datalink: Successes and challenges monitoring vaccine safety. *Vaccine, 32*, 5390–5398.

Miller, E., Goldacre, M., Pugh, S., Colville, A., Farrington, P., Flower, A., ... Tettmar, R. (1993). Risk of aseptic meningitis after measles, mumps and rubella vaccine in the UK. *Lancet, 341*, 979–982.

Murphy, T. V., Gargiullo, P. M., Massoudi, M. S., Nelson, D. B., Jumaan, A. O., Okoro, C. A., ... Livingood, J. R. (2001). Intussusception among infants given an oral rotavirus vaccine. *New England Journal of Medicine, 344*, 564–572.

Nohynek, H., Jokinen, J., Partinen, M., Vaarala, M., Kirjavainen, T., Sundman, J., ... Kilpi, T. (2012). AS03 adjuvanted AH1N1 vaccine associated with an abrupt increase in the incidence of childhood narcolepsy in Finland. *PLoS One, 7*(3), e33536.

Partinen, M., Seerenpaa-Heikkila, O., Ilveskoski, I., Hublin, C., Linna, M., Olsen, P., ... Kirjavainen, T. (2012). Increased incidence and clinical picture of childhood narcolepsy following the 2009 H1N1 pandemic vaccination campaign in Finland. *PLoS One, 7*(3), e33723.

Pillsbury, A., Cashman, P., Leeb, A., Regab, A., Westphal, D., Snelling, T., ... Macartney, K. (2015). Real-time safety surveillance of seasonal influenza vaccines in children, Australia, 2015. *Eurosurveillance, 20*(43), pii=30050.

Rennels, M. B., Parashar, U. D., Holman, R. C., Le, C. T., Chang, H., & Glass, R. (1998). Lack of an apparent association between intussusception and wild or vaccine rotavirus infection. *Pediatric Infectious Disease Journal, 17*(10), 924–925.

Scheifele, D., Law, B., & Jadavji, T. (1998). Disseminated Bacille Calmette-Guérin infection: Three recent Canadian cases. *Canada Communicable Disease Report, 24*(9), 69–75.

Shimabukuro, T. T., Nguyen, M., Martin, D., & DeStefano, F. (2015). Safety monitoring in the Vaccine Adverse Event Reporting System (VAERS). *Vaccine, 33*(36), 4398–4405.

Stowe, J., Andrews, N., Wise, L., & Miller, E. (2006). Bell's palsy and parenteral inactivated influenza vaccine. *Human Vaccines, 2*(3), 110–112.

World Health Organization (WHO). (2018). *Causality assessment of an adverse event following immunization (AEFI): User manual for the revised WHO classification* (2nd ed.). Geneva: WHO.

Zhou, W., Pool, V., DeStefano, F., Iskander, J. K., Haber, P., & Chen, R. T. (2004). A potential signal of Bell's palsy after parenteral inactivated influenza vaccines: Reports to the Vaccine Adverse Event Reporting System (VAERS) – United States, 1991–2001. *Pharmacoepidemiology and Drug Safety, 13*, 505–510.

Chapter 19

Estimating vaccination risks
General methodological principles

This chapter is the first of two about the methods that are used to estimate risks of adverse events following immunisation (AEFI), using epidemiological data obtained in field studies (as distinct from the pre-licensure studies of vaccines undertaken in randomised controlled clinical trials). In the present chapter, we focus on methodological issues specific to epidemiological studies of vaccine safety. In the next chapter, we shall describe the most commonly used methods.

Some methodological issues arise specifically in studies of AEFI, and are less relevant for safety studies of other pharmaceutical products. For example, many of the AEFIs of greatest concern are acute, and are likely to be causally related to vaccination only in a limited time frame. Thus, it makes sense to focus on adverse events occurring during this period, known as the risk period. Accordingly, in Section 19.1 we discuss risk periods, and how to select them.

In studies of AEFI, both relative and absolute measures of risk are relevant: relative measures to quantify the association with vaccination, and absolute measures to weigh the risks and the benefits of vaccination. These measures will be described in Section 19.2.

Vaccines are often administered in several doses, which may have different risk profiles (see also Chapter 17, Section 17.1). Information on dose-specific risks is important from a public health perspective in order to mitigate such risks. Thus, in Section 19.3 we address matters relating to multiple doses, timing of events and recurrent events.

In Section 19.4 we discuss issues of bias and confounding in field studies of vaccine safety. Finally, in Section 19.5 we make some remarks about the use of patient databases and data networks, as they relate to vaccine safety studies.

DOI: 10.4324/9781315166414-20
This Chapter has been made available under a CC-BY-NC-ND license.

19.1 Risk periods

The risk period following vaccination is the time period during which adverse events caused by the vaccine are most likely to arise. More generally, the term 'risk period' may be used to denote any time period of special interest, or during which a causal vaccine effect is hypothesised. Because many AEFI are acute, the risk period is often brief. The risk period may be subdivided into several shorter intervals to capture temporal changes in risk over time since vaccination, or to allow for uncertainty in the specification of the risk period. Examples of risk periods are given in Box 19.1.

Box 19.1 Risk periods for MMR and DTP safety studies in England

A study of adverse events including febrile convulsions after diphtheria, tetanus and pertussis (DTP) and measles, mumps and rubella (MMR) vaccines was undertaken in England over the period 1988 to 1993 in children aged under 2 years (Farrington et al., 1995).

For the DTP vaccine, which included a whole-cell pertussis component, the risk periods of interest were 0–3, 4–7 and 8–14 days after vaccination with any of the three vaccine doses. Day 0 represents the day of vaccination. This choice of risk periods was based on prior evidence from an earlier case-control study of neurological reactions to the DTP vaccine. The risk periods are shown diagrammatically in Figure 19.1.

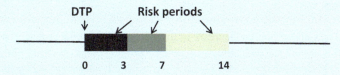

Figure 19.1 Risk periods for febrile convulsions after each dose of DTP vaccine. The numbers represent days since the last DTP dose (day 0).

For the MMR vaccines, the risk periods of interest were 6–11 days and 15–35 days after vaccination. These periods were also chosen based on prior evidence that vaccine-related neurological events might be most likely to occur at these times. Specifically, the 6–11-day period corresponds to a potentially increased risk from the measles component of the vaccine, while the 15–35-day period corresponds to a potentially increased risk from the mumps component of the vaccine, for those MMR vaccines containing the Urabe mumps strain. These risk periods are illustrated in Figure 19.2.

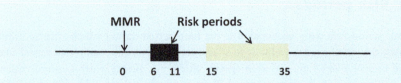

Figure 19.2 Risk periods for febrile convulsions after MMR vaccine. The numbers represent days since MMR vaccination (day 0).

Vaccinated individuals were not considered to be at higher risk from febrile convulsions outside these risk periods (both before and after them).

The key feature of the risk periods described in Box 19.1 is that they cover only a relatively brief period of days or weeks after vaccination. This is because, when studying rare adverse events, it helps to be as precise as possible about the likely time frame over which the events may occur in relation to vaccination. Sometimes, it is not possible to be as precise as for MMR vaccines in Box 19.1: in this case it is usual to use a small number of adjacent risk intervals after vaccination, as was done for DTP vaccines in Box 19.1.

Sometimes, there is no information about the relative timing of the adverse event in relation to vaccination. In this case, the risk period may include all post-vaccination time. An example of such an indefinite risk period is described in Box 19.2.

Box 19.2 Risk periods for MMR vaccine and autism studies

A study was undertaken in Denmark to investigate the hypothesis that MMR vaccination is associated with autism spectrum disorders (Madsen et al., 2002). The timing of the hypothesised MMR-associated autism in relation to vaccination was not clearly specified.

The Danish study therefore assumed that the risk of autism might be elevated at any time after MMR vaccination. All times post-MMR were therefore included in the risk period. Additional analyses were undertaken in which the time since vaccination was split into separate but adjacent risk periods: under 6 months, 6 to 11 months, then yearly intervals up to 59 months after vaccination and a final period 60 months or more since vaccination. The risk periods are shown diagrammatically in Figure 19.3.

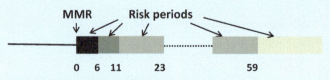

Figure 19.3 Risk periods for autism after MMR vaccine. The numbers represent months since MMR vaccination (day 0).

ESTIMATING VACCINATION RISKS

> Thus, vaccinated individuals were considered as being potentially at higher risk of autism at any time after receipt of the MMR vaccine. In the study, no association was identified, overall or in any individual risk period.

The choice of risk period should be based on prior hypotheses, documented evidence or an understanding of the biological mechanisms involved (see Chapter 17). Whatever risk periods are used, it is important that they should be chosen prior to data collection. This is because clustering of events may be expected to occur by chance, so that data-dependent choices of risk periods will tend to yield spurious results. Results based on data-driven risk periods can only ever be regarded as hypothesis-generating rather than hypothesis-testing.

As previously indicated, the term 'risk period' may be used to denote any time period of special interest. For example, an adverse event that would have occurred anyway might be precipitated by vaccination, that is, brought forward in time. This gives rise to a positive association during an initial risk period combined with an apparently protective effect in a second risk period immediately following it; when the two risk periods are combined there is no association. This phenomenon is sometimes referred to as a harvesting effect.

Periods of time that are not presumed to be potentially at higher or lower risk of the adverse event of interest, or are not otherwise of special interest, are reference periods. Reference periods include all times contributed by unvaccinated individuals, as well as times outside risk periods for vaccinated individuals.

19.2 Measures of risk

Risks associated with vaccination are evaluated using the same measures as those used to evaluate the safety of pharmaceutical drugs. The main measures used can be classified as relative quantities (such as the relative incidence or odds ratio), and absolute quantities (such as the attributable fraction or attributable risk). Relative measures are used to quantify the strength of the association with vaccination, whereas absolute measures are used to quantify the burden of adverse events attributable to vaccination.

The distinction between risk-based and rate-based measures is not particularly relevant for vaccine-related risks, because these risks are usually low (under 10%). The most convenient measures are rate-based, because they allow for risk periods and reference periods of different durations. For potentially recurrent adverse events (such as febrile convulsions), a commonly used measure is the relative incidence RI, or incidence rate ratio:

$$RI = \frac{incidence\ of\ adverse\ events\ during\ the\ risk\ period}{incidence\ of\ adverse\ events\ during\ the\ reference\ period}.$$

In this expression, the incidences are event rates per unit time. For non-recurrent adverse events (e.g., first febrile convulsion), the hazard ratio HR is used rather than the relative incidence, though when the adverse event of interest is rare, as is usually the case, the distinction is immaterial. For this reason, either measure is commonly referred to simply as the relative risk RR. In case-control studies, the odds ratio OR is used; this will be discussed in more detail in Section 20.2. Confidence intervals for relative risks and odds ratios are obtained in a similar way as described for vaccine effectiveness; in practice, they are usually adjusted for potential confounders.

The attributable fraction AF is the proportion of adverse events arising within a risk period that are attributable to the vaccine. This notion only makes sense if there is evidence that vaccination is causally and positively associated with the event, implying that the relative risk and its lower 95% confidence limit are both greater than 1. There is a simple relationship between the relative risk and the attributable fraction:

$$AF = \frac{RR-1}{RR}. \tag{19.1}$$

A 95% confidence interval (CI) (AF^-, AF^+) for AF may be obtained from the 95% CI (RR^-, RR^+) for the relative risk as follows:

$$AF^- = \frac{RR^- - 1}{RR^-}, \quad AF^+ = \frac{RR^+ - 1}{RR^+}.$$

The attributable risk, or risk difference, is the quantity

$$AR = p_v - p_u = p_v \times AF = p_u \times (RR - 1), \tag{19.2}$$

where p_v is the risk of an adverse event in the risk period and p_u is the risk of an adverse event in a comparable period in the absence of vaccination. The attributable risk is sometimes presented in the form 1 event per N doses of vaccine, or 1 event per N persons vaccinated.

Relative and absolute measures of risk convey quite different types of information. This is illustrated in Box 19.3.

Box 19.3 Intussusception and rotavirus vaccination with the RotaShield vaccine

After licensure of the RotaShield vaccine (see Chapter 18), an epidemiological study was undertaken to assess the relative and absolute risks of intussusception associated with this vaccine (Murphy et al., 2001).

In one analysis, the relative risk of intussusception in the 3–14-day risk period after the first dose was $RR = 29.4$ with 95% CI (16.1, 53.6). On the other hand, the attributable risk was estimated to be of the order of 1 per 10,000 to 1 per 5,000 children vaccinated.

Thus, while the relative risks indicate a very strong positive association between intussusception and vaccination, the attributable risk remained low. The decision was taken to withdraw the vaccine; since then, safer rotavirus vaccines have been developed.

As illustrated in Box 19.3, the attributable risk can be very low even when the relative risk is high: the relative risk is a measure of association, whereas the attributable risk is an absolute measure. Both measures are relevant to vaccine risk assessments.

The relative risk and attributable fraction may be estimated from field studies, to be described in the present chapter and the next. The attributable risk, on the other hand, requires an estimate of the absolute risk either during the risk period after vaccination (p_v in Equation 19.2) or in an equivalent period in the absence of vaccination (p_u in Equation 19.2), or both. Often, such estimates may be available only indirectly from field data, and so are likely to be approximate. For this reason, it is common for attributable risks to be presented as orders of magnitude, or as a range of values obtained in different populations, rather than as precise estimates with 95% confidence intervals. This contrast is illustrated in Box 19.4.

Box 19.4 Relative and attributable risks of febrile convulsions after MMR vaccine in England

The study of febrile convulsions after MMR vaccine described in Box 19.1 found an increased risk of febrile convulsions for the 6–11-day risk period after MMR vaccination. The relative risk (in this case, a relative incidence) was $RR = 3.04$, with 95% CI (2.27, 4.07).

Thus, the attributable fraction, obtained using Equation 19.1, is:

$$AF = \frac{3.04 - 1}{3.04} = 0.67.$$

This signifies that 67% of febrile convulsions in the 6–11-day risk period after MMR vaccination are attributable to the vaccine; the remaining 33% are background events unrelated to the vaccine. The 95% CI is (56%, 75%).

In this study, 49 febrile convulsions were observed within the 6–11-day post-vaccination period. These cases were obtained from hospital records. It was estimated that 97,300 doses of MMR vaccine had been administered in the catchment areas of these hospitals during the study period. From these data, an estimate of the absolute risk following vaccination may be obtained:

$$p_v = \frac{49}{97,300} = 50.4 \text{ per } 100,000.$$

Then, applying Equation 19.2, we obtain

$$AR = p_v \times AF = 50.4 \times 0.67 = 33.8,$$

so the attributable risk is about 34 per 100,000 MMR doses. Equivalently, this may be quoted as one attributable febrile convulsion per 3,000 MMR doses.

Note that while a precise estimate, with 95% CI, is obtained in Box 19.4 for the relative risk and the attributable fraction, the attributable risk is approximate and is aimed at conveying an order of magnitude.

Approximate absolute risk estimates are typical when derived from studies other than cohort studies (as in Box 19.4), since detailed information on the vaccinated population is usually not available. However, such approximate estimates are still useful: the attributable risk is used to convey the likely magnitude of such risk in absolute terms, and a correct order of magnitude is usually sufficient. In contrast, a precise estimation of the relative risk, adjusted for possible confounding variables, is essential to determine whether vaccination is causally associated with the adverse event of interest.

Both relative risks and absolute risks may vary between populations, and so it is always of interest to compare results obtained in different contexts. This is illustrated in Box 19.5.

Box 19.5 Relative and attributable risks of febrile convulsions after MMR vaccine in the United States

A large cohort study of febrile and non-febrile convulsions after childhood vaccinations was undertaken in the United States using administrative data from four large health maintenance organisations (HMOs) (Barlow et al., 2001). For MMR vaccine, the risk periods investigated were day of vaccination (day 0) and 1–7 days, 8–14 and 15–30 days post-vaccination.

A significantly increased risk was observed only for first febrile convulsions in the 8–14-day period after MMR vaccine. The adjusted relative risk (more precisely, the hazard ratio) was $RR = 2.83$ with 95% CI (1.44, 5.55).

From this estimate, the attributable fraction may be obtained: $AF = 65\%$, signifying that 65% of first febrile convulsions observed between 8 and 14 days after receipt of the MMR vaccine are attributable to the vaccine. The 95% CI for AF is (31%, 82%).

To calculate attributable risks, the authors used background rates of convulsions in the second year of life in two of the participating HMOs. The resulting attributable risk estimates were 25.0 and 34.2 additional febrile convulsions per 100,000 vaccinated children.

The estimates, both relative and absolute, obtained in the US cohort study described in Box 19.5 are similar to those obtained in England (see Box 19.4), even though the studies used slightly different post-vaccination risk periods and very different statistical methods.

19.3 Multiple doses, concomitant vaccines, timing of events and recurrences

Many vaccines are administered in multi-dose schedules. Unlike the estimation of vaccine effectiveness, where emphasis in post-licensure studies focuses on the protection afforded by a complete course of vaccination, the study of AEFIs should be dose-specific: as indicated in Chapter 17, Section 17.1, the association may differ between doses. Dose effects should, if possible, be estimated separately from age effects; this is feasible provided, as is usually the case, there is variation between individuals in the ages at which each dose is administered. Clearly, if a similar effect is found at different doses then this may be summarised by a global estimate of the relative risk after any dose. Box 19.6 describes an example where the dose effect was important, independently of age.

Box 19.6 RotaShield vaccine and intussusception: dose effect

This example, relating to intussusception and the RotaShield vaccine against rotavirus infection, was described in Box 19.3. The vaccine was administered in a three-dose schedule at 2, 4 and 6 months of age. In one analysis, the relative risk for the 3–14 days post-vaccination risk period was $RR = 29.4$, 95% CI (16.1, 53.6) and $RR = 6.8$, 95% CI (2.8, 16.3) after the second dose. For the third dose, there were too few events to obtain reliable estimates (Murphy et al., 2001).

The occurrence of intussusceptions in vaccinated cases in relation to the timing of the three vaccine doses is shown in Figure 19.4.

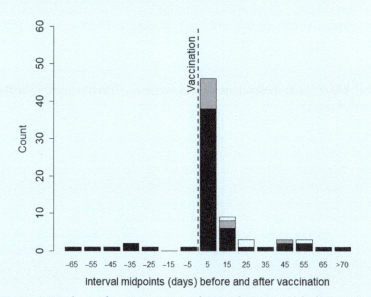

Figure 19.4 Numbers of intussusceptions by 10-day interval before and after each vaccine dose.

Note: Black bars: cases occurring before dose 1, or after dose 1 but not after subsequent doses. Grey bars: cases occurring after dose 2 but not after dose 3. White bars: cases occurring after dose 3. The dashed vertical line represents time of vaccination for all three doses.

> Figure 19.4 shows a clear clustering of intussusception onsets soon after the first dose, and to a lesser extent after the second dose of vaccine. After the third dose the occurrences of intussusceptions are very sparse, as indeed they are prior to the first dose.

A graph showing the time lags between event onsets and vaccination, like that presented in Figure 19.4, can be a useful aid to visualising dose effects, though it does not take account of age effects and thus cannot replace a full statistical analysis.

One issue that arises when dealing with multi-dose vaccines is that observation periods may overlap. For example, if doses 1 and 2 are separated by 28 days but the risk period of interest is 0–42 days, then the risk periods for the two doses will overlap. A commonly used procedure is to give precedence to the most recent dose: in this case this means truncating the risk period after dose 1 at 28 days. Other choices are possible and results can be compared in sensitivity analyses.

With combined vaccines, such as MMR vaccine or DTP vaccine, it is not generally possible to separate the effects of the different vaccine components, unless prior information is available suggesting that they might occur in different risk periods. An example for MMR vaccine was described in Box 19.1. Similarly, if the vaccine of interest is usually administered concomitantly with another, it may be difficult to separate their effects. Generally, this is only possible if some infants receive the vaccines at different times. Then, a global analysis of all the vaccines involved, with each as a risk factor, is required to separate their effects. An example is described in Box 19.7.

Box 19.7 Hib booster vaccination, MMR and febrile convulsions

In the United Kingdom, a *Haemophilus influenzae* type b (Hib) vaccine booster dose is administered in the second year of life, often at the same time or in close temporal proximity to MMR. To investigate the association, if any, between Hib booster vaccine and convulsions, it is essential to allow for the effect of MMR. Thus, both exposures must be studied simultaneously in a joint analysis.

Analyses of vaccines administered concomitantly may be undertaken with all study designs to be described in Chapter 20. Examples using the self-controlled case series (SCCS) method may be found in Farrington, Whitaker, and Ghebremichael Weldeselassie (2018, pp. 66 ff).

An important issue, which arises more commonly with vaccines than other pharmaceutical products, is the timing of events. This is important particularly when the risk periods to be investigated are brief. Accurate data on the timing of events is then very important. If timing is inaccurate, for example because it is subject to delays or measurement errors, exposure status is likely to be misclassified. Thus, events that occur within the risk period may be counted as arising outside the risk period, and vice versa. This will generally bias the relative risk towards unity.

Assigning event dates should be based on objective criteria, for example date of consultation or date of hospital admission. Dating event onsets should as far as possible be done with vaccination status concealed. If media publicity about a link with vaccination may have influenced the dating (as was the case in the narcolepsy example presented in Chapter 18), then the study should be restricted to cases ascertained prior to the publicity, to avoid bias.

For some types of events it may be difficult to define onsets accurately, or diagnosis may be delayed. This is likely to be an issue for non-acute events. In this case, analyses using very short risk periods are inappropriate, as the extent of misclassification is likely to be severe. An example in which this issue arose is described in Box 19.8.

Box 19.8 MMR vaccine and autism

An early epidemiological study of the alleged link between MMR vaccination and autism was that undertaken by Taylor et al. (1999). The hypothesis of a link, published in a 1998 study that has since been retracted, was based on a series of 12 cases, of whom 8 had received MMR. Of these, 7 were deemed to present symptoms of behavioural regression within 24 hours to 2 weeks after vaccination.

Setting aside any considerations of biological plausibility, the hypothesis suggested by the study was that the onset of regressive autism may be associated with MMR vaccination, with a risk period of up to a few weeks. However, the diagnosis of autism is only made many months later, and the retrospective dating of behavioural regression may be inaccurate. For this reason, risk periods longer than the 2 weeks post-MMR suggested by the original data were employed. One set of analyses, based on 105 cases of regressive autism, produced the results in Table 19.1.

Owing to the uncertainty about which risk period was most appropriate, the three risk periods displayed in Table 19.1 were used. None was associated with a significant excess of regressive autism. Subsequently, other analyses were undertaken, not limited to cases of regressive autism, and using an indefinite post-vaccination risk period; the results were similar (see Box 19.2).

Table 19.1 Relative risk (95% CI) of regressive autism after MMR vaccination

Risk period	Relative risk	95% CI
0–2 months	0.92	(0.38–2.21)
0–4 months	1.00	(0.52–1.95)
0–6 months	0.85	(0.45–1.60)

Some AEFIs may be potentially recurrent. The analysis may then be restricted to first occurrences. In some applications (e.g., when recurrences are believed to be independent), it may be desirable to undertake analyses in which all events, both incident and recurrent, are included. Then it becomes important to avoid double counting events that are part of the same episode. Criteria for doing this need to be set out in advance. An example is described in Box 19.9.

Box 19.9 Febrile convulsions and DTP vaccine

A study to investigate febrile convulsions in relation to DTP vaccine was described in Box 19.1. Events were hospital admissions for febrile convulsion in infants and children aged between 29 and 365 days, with a discharge diagnosis of febrile convulsion. The event date was the date of admission. To distinguish incident admissions from repeat admissions that were part of the same episode, readmissions within 72 hours with the same diagnosis were excluded: only the first admission within each episode was retained. The DTP analysis included 491 admissions (corresponding to distinct episodes) in 443 children aged 1–12 months (Farrington et al., 1995).

The data described in Box 19.9 include repeat events (occurring in distinct episodes). For potentially recurrent events, it is usually advisable to undertake separate analyses for first events, and for all episodes.

19.4 Bias and confounding in studies of vaccine safety

Studies of vaccine safety may be subject to bias and confounding, just as are studies of other pharmaceutical products. Vaccines are not administered randomly in the population: they may be given preferentially to groups at higher risk, or at lower risk, of adverse events in relation to environmental factors, socio-economic indicators or individual predisposition. These factors may in turn confound the association between vaccination and adverse events. Selection bias may arise in the choice of individuals for study, and information bias may arise in the collection of data on these individuals. Thus, studies of AEFIs must confront the same problems as other pharmaco-epidemiological investigations; and broadly, the methods available for controlling these biases are largely the same.

There are, however, some differences of emphasis between studies of vaccine safety and safety studies of other pharmaceutical drugs. In this section, we will focus specifically on these issues.

The first is the issue of age. Vaccines are often administered to infants and young children, for whom the age-related variation in the background incidence of adverse events can be extremely large, on short time scales (of days or weeks). For this reason, careful control of age in study design and analysis is particularly important, all the more so because vaccines, unlike most other pharmaceutical products, are often administered according to tight age-dependent vaccination schedules. Nevertheless, in practice there is usually sufficient variation in ages at vaccination between individuals to separate the effect of age from the effect of vaccination, and estimate both. Sometimes, seasonal effects are also important, particularly for vaccines administered according to a seasonal schedule, for the same reason. An illustration is provided in Box 19.10.

Box 19.10 Intussusception and oral polio vaccine in Cuba

Following the withdrawal of the RotaShield rotavirus vaccine in the United States, concerns arose as to whether other oral vaccines, in particular the oral polio vaccine (OPV), might cause similar reactions. A study was undertaken in Cuba to investigate this issue (Galindo Sardinas et al., 2001).

Some 297 first cases of intussusception in infants arising in 1995–2000 were documented in the study. Intussusception in Cuba is very strongly age-dependent and seasonal, as shown in Figure 19.5.

Intussusception incidence peaks at age 4 months and in spring and winter. Furthermore, in Cuba OPV is administered to infants in biannual campaigns, which typically occur in February and April. Thus, both age and time of year could confound the association between vaccination and intussusception, and must therefore be taken into account in the analysis.

No statistically significant effects were found in the 0–14-, 15–28- and 29–42-day risk periods after each of two doses. The relative risk in the 0–42-day risk period, both doses combined, was $RR = 1.11$, 95% CI (0.74, 1.67).

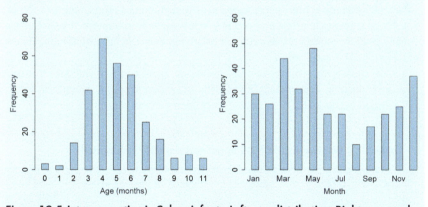

Figure 19.5 Intussusception in Cuban infants. Left: age distribution. Right: seasonal distribution.
Source: Reproduced with permission from Galindo Sardinas et al. (2001).

When strong age or seasonal effects are present, it is advisable to check that the results obtained are not unduly sensitive to the particular age or time categorisation chosen in the analysis – for example, by using a finer age stratification and comparing results.

When discussing the estimation of vaccine effectiveness in Chapter 13, Section 13.3, we emphasised the importance of two types of confounding bias that may arise: the healthy vaccinee bias and bias by indication. These biases are also potentially an issue when investigating vaccine safety.

The healthy vaccinee effect arises when individuals who access vaccines are at a lower risk of adverse events than those who don't. Socio-economic indicators, for example, may come into play, and need to be taken into account in the analysis. But in addition, a more subtle effect may be present, related to the timing of vaccination. If an individual is unwell, vaccination is likely to be delayed until they recover. Thus, a healthy vaccinee effect may be present that is related to the timing of vaccination. The timing of vaccination may, in turn, influence the propensity for adverse events to occur. This confounding mechanism is discussed in Box 19.11.

Box 19.11 DTP vaccination, the healthy vaccinee effect and sudden infant death syndrome

This example is based on a review of the literature on serious AEFI and their possible association with whole-cell pertussis vaccines, with a focus on potential confounding factors (Fine & Chen, 1992). We consider the potential association between pertussis vaccines and sudden infant death syndrome (SIDS).

The authors identified several factors that were associated both with avoidance or delay of vaccination, and with increased risk of SIDS. These included low parental education, high parity/large family size, ethnic origin, age of mother, maternal smoking in pregnancy and low birth weight. Furthermore, they noted that many studies reported relative risks of SIDS less than 1 in the period immediately following DTP vaccination.

One such study, which we shall use as an exemplar, was undertaken using record linkage in Tennessee, USA (Griffin, Ray, Livengood, & Schaffner, 1988). The relative risks of SIDS in infants were as shown in Table 19.2.

Table 19.2 Relative risk of SIDS in defined post-DTP risk periods

Days since DTP	0–3	4–7	8–14	15–30	≥ 31 (reference)
RR	0.18	0.17	0.75	1.00	1
95% CI	0.04–0.8	0.04–0.7	0.4–1.5	0.6–1.6	-

> These results are adjusted for age; further adjustments for sex, ethnic origin, calendar year, birth weight and Medicaid enrolment produced similar results. Table 19.2 shows an apparently protective effect of DTP vaccination against SIDS in the first week after vaccination. The authors argue that the most plausible explanation for this unexpected observation is that children may be immunised when they are in better health, and that this healthier state is associated with a lower risk of SIDS. Further investigations by Fine and Chen (1992) tended to reinforce this interpretation.

The example in Box 19.11 suggests that delaying vaccination until a child is well may introduce confounding, at least for some adverse events. Like the effect of age, this is a time-varying confounder. It is distinct from the effect of time-invariant potential confounders, such as those also described in Box 19.11. It will tend to bias the relative risk towards zero.

Indication bias arises when the indication for the vaccine is associated with potential adverse events. The potential for indication bias is often a major issue in non-vaccine pharmacoepidemiology. Generally, it is less of an issue for studies of AEFIs in relation to universally administered vaccines. However, indication bias may arise for studies of vaccines used in selective vaccination programmes, if those individuals targeted for vaccination are also those at higher (or lower) risk of adverse events.

The methods available for adjusting for time-invariant confounders, including confounding by indication, include those used in general pharmacoepidemiology. Commonly used methods are confounder adjustment by regression techniques or propensity score methods, matching in case-control studies followed by a matched analysis and self-controlled methods. Some of the latter (to be discussed in Chapter 20) were developed specifically to investigate vaccine safety, though they are now used more generally. Regression and propensity score methods are generic statistical techniques, the details of which lie outside the scope of this book. Box 19.12 describes one application where bias by indication was particularly important.

Box 19.12 Asthma exacerbations after influenza vaccination

This study was undertaken within the Vaccine Safety Datalink (see Chapter 18), to investigate whether influenza vaccination of children with asthma precipitated asthma exacerbations (Kramarz et al., 2000). The children were aged between 1 and 6 years; those with asthma were identified by the medications prescribed. Asthma exacerbations were defined as hospitalisations or emergency department visits for asthma. The main analysis used a 2-week risk interval after influenza vaccination. The results for the three influenza seasons studied are in Table 19.3.

Table 19.3 Relative risk (95% CI) of asthma exacerbation in the 2 weeks following influenza vaccination, by analysis method, in the 1993–1994, 1994–1995 and 1995–1996 influenza seasons

Model	1993–1994	1994–1995	1995–1996
Unadjusted	2.51 (1.51–3.88)	2.22 (1.38–3.35)	3.29 (2.55–4.15)
Adjusted	1.00 (0.60–1.56)	1.09 (0.67–1.67)	1.39 (1.08–1.77)
Self-controlled	0.58 (0.36–0.95)	0.74 (0.47–1.17)	0.98 (0.76–1.27)

In the absence of any adjustment for confounders, there is a strong positive association between asthma exacerbations and influenza vaccination. This is most likely due to indication bias: children with more severe underlying asthma are more likely to be vaccinated against influenza.

Adjusting for covariates including several predictors of asthma severity (use of asthma medication and hospitalisations for asthma outside the influenza seasons) and several other variables (sex, age, health maintenance organisation and calendar time) reduced the relative risk to $RR = 1$ during the 1993–1994 influenza season and to $RR = 1.09$ during the 1994–1995 season. For the 1995–1996 season, the relative risk $RR = 1.39$ is reduced but still significantly above 1, as shown by the 95% CI (1.08, 1.77).

The self-controlled model reported in Table 19.3 adjusts automatically for all time-invariant confounders, whether measured or not, and also for calendar time. Using this model, the influenza vaccine was found to be significantly protective against asthma exacerbations during the 1993–1994 influenza season. There was no association during the other seasons.

The example in Box 19.12 demonstrates the importance of allowing for potential confounders in epidemiological studies of adverse events following vaccination.

We end this section by mentioning some further time-varying covariates that may require adjustment. Concomitant vaccinations associated with the same AEFI of interest were discussed in Section 19.3. Similarly, infections (which may be the same infection as that against which the vaccine is targeted, or different infections) may also cause the same adverse event of interest. In this case, it may be desirable to adjust for them. An example is described in Box 19.13.

Box 19.13 Influenza vaccine, influenza-like illness and Guillain-Barré syndrome

In 1976 the national swine influenza vaccination programme in the United States was suspended owing to an increased risk of Guillain-Barré syndrome (GBS). The present study was undertaken to investigate and quantify the association between seasonal influenza vaccine and GBS in the United Kingdom. There is also strong evidence to suggest that influenza is associated with GBS: thus, the risk associated with influenza-like illness (ILI) and GBS was also quantified, in the same study (Stowe, Andrews, Wise, & Miller, 2009).

The study was undertaken in the UK General Practice Research Database (since renamed Clinical Practice Research Datalink), using data recorded in 1990–2005. Repeat GBS diagnoses within 6 months were counted as part of the same episode. The risk periods were 0–90 days from vaccination and 0–90 days after consultation for ILI. Age was controlled in broad age groups, and season was controlled by calendar month. The analysis was self-controlled using the SCCS method (see Chapter 20).

No association was found with influenza vaccination: $RI = 0.76$ with 95% CI (0.41, 1.40). For ILI, however, an elevated risk was found: $RI = 7.35$ with 95% CI (4.36, 12.4). The association was particularly strong within the first 30 days after a consultation for ILI: $RI = 16.6$, 95% CI (9.37, 29.5).

The study described in Box 19.13 provides an opportunity to contrast directly the vaccine-associated risk with the infection-associated risk in the same population. Such comparisons are relevant to benefit–risk evaluations of vaccination programmes (see Chapter 21).

19.5 Use of electronic databases and data networks for vaccine studies

Most studies of vaccine safety today are undertaken wholly or partly within clinical or administrative databases of electronic patient records, linked to or including information on vaccination. The epidemiological study designs to be described in Chapter 20 may all be, and often are, undertaken retrospectively within electronic databases. These databases are very diverse, ranging from population registers, health insurance databases, general practitioner records, linked hospital admissions and vaccination registers. The use of health databases for vaccine safety research has been reviewed by Verstraeten, DeStefano, Chen, and Miller (2003).

In spite of the size and versatility of clinical databases, single database studies of vaccine safety may still be underpowered for rare adverse events, especially for recently introduced vaccines. Thus, more robust assessments of vaccine safety from several data sources are often required, whether through analyses of pooled data or meta-analyses. However, differences in definitions of safety outcomes, variability of observation time and poor reporting of safety in the published literature, impair the ability to conduct high-quality meta-analyses and systematic reviews (Dimova, Egelebo, & Izurieta, 2020). Such issues may be resolved by international collaborations based on common data models. Moves to develop such global vaccine data networks has gained added impetus by the unprecedented rate of vaccine development in response to the COVID-19 pandemic (Petousis-Harris & Dodd, 2020).

We end with some notes of caution. Different databases have different strengths and weaknesses, and may be prone to different sources of bias. It is essential to understand these idiosyncrasies when applied to studies on vaccines, as they may generate spurious associations. A striking example is presented in Box 19.14.

> **Box 19.14 Influenza vaccination, asthma and chronic obstructive pulmonary disorder in the General Practice Research Database**
>
> A study was undertaken within the UK General Practice Research Database (GPRD) to investigate potential associations between influenza vaccination and consultation for asthma in 2,552 vaccinated patients with asthma, and between influenza vaccination and consultations for chronic obstructive pulmonary disorder (COPD) in 2,100 vaccinated patients with COPD (Tata et al., 2003). The results for the 1991–1992 influenza year are shown in Table 19.4 for three risk periods: the day of vaccination (day 0), and days 1–2 and 3–14 after influenza vaccination.
>
> Table 19.4 does not suggest a positive association between influenza vaccination and consultations for asthma or COPD in the period 1–14 days post-vaccination. For the day of vaccination, however, the relative risks for both events are very high, with 95% confidence intervals located well above 1. Similar results were obtained for influenza years 1992–1993 and 1993–1994.
>
> These results are suggestive of biased ascertainment on the day of vaccination; this bias is apparent in Figure 19.6 (a similar graph is obtained for COPD).
>
> *Table 19.4* Relative risk of consultation for asthma and COPD, with 95% CI
>
> | Event | Risk period (days post-vaccination) | | |
> |---|---|---|---|
> | | 0 (day of vaccination) | 1–2 days | 3–14 days |
> | Asthma | 14.9 (11.8, 18.9) | 0.76 (0.39, 1.47) | 0.88 (0.67, 1.14) |
> | COPD | 11.4 (8.02, 16.3) | 0.31 (0.08, 1.24) | 0.61 (0.40, 0.93) |
>
>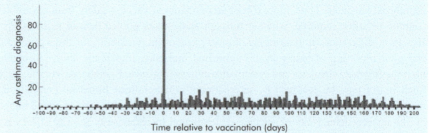
>
> *Figure 19.6* Days between asthma diagnosis and influenza vaccination.
> Source: Reproduced with permission from Tata et al. (2003).

> The authors concluded that the apparent association at day 0 is an artefact resulting from how events are coded in the GPRD: histories of chronic events, including asthma and COPD, are taken on the day of vaccination, and are coded to that day when in fact they occurred in the past.

The undoubted benefit of clinical databases is that they enable large studies to be done relatively rapidly and cheaply. A disadvantage, however, is that detailed information on potential confounding variables may not be available, and that recording of some data may be suboptimal. For example, a prescription database may indicate that a vaccine has been prescribed, but not whether – or exactly when – it has been administered. A hospital admissions database will indicate date of admission, but not necessarily date of onset. Contrasting studies undertaken across different databases can help to shed light on their differences, and any inherent biases they may possess.

Summary

- Studies of adverse events after vaccination often require one or more risk intervals to be specified. A risk interval is the time period after vaccination during which the risk of an adverse event may be increased.
- The relative risk, relative incidence or odds ratio are commonly used to measure the strength of association between vaccination and AEFIs. Attributable risks are used to quantify absolute risks.
- Dose-specific analyses should be undertaken, separating out dose and age effects.
- Care is required in defining event dates, in order to avoid misclassifying events in or out of risk periods. Event dates should where possible be determined objectively and independently of vaccination.
- Recurrent events may be included in some analyses, provided that they relate to distinct episodes.
- It is essential to adjust for age when vaccinations are administered according to age-dependent schedules. Adjustment for season may also be required, especially for seasonal vaccines.
- Indication bias may arise, particularly for selective vaccination programmes.
- Electronic databases are a key resource for vaccine safety studies. They enable large studies to be undertaken rapidly, but may provide limited information on potential confounders.
- International collaborations and global vaccine data networks using common data models can contribute to robust, high-quality meta-analyses.

References

Barlow, W. E., Davis, R. L., Glasser, J. W., Rhodes, P. H., Thompson, R. S., Mullooly, J. P., ... Chen, R. T. (2001). The risk of seizures after receipt of whole-cell pertussis or measles, mumps and rubella vaccine. *New England Journal of Medicine*, 345, 656–661.

Dimova, R. B., Egelebo, C. C., & Izurieta, H. S. (2020). Systematic review of published meta-analyses of vaccine safety. *Statistics in Biopharmaceutical Research*, 12(3), 293–302.

Farrington, P., Pugh, S., Colville, A., Flower, A., Nash, J., Morgan-Capner, P., ... Miller, E. (1995). A new method for active surveillance of adverse events from diphtheria tetanus pertussis and measles mumps rubella vaccines. *Lancet, 345*, 567–569.

Farrington, P., Whitaker, H., & Ghebremichael Weldeselassie, Y. (2018). *Self-controlled case series studies: A modelling guide with R.* Boca Raton, FL: CRC Press.

Fine, P. E., & Chen, R. T. (1992). Confounding in studies of adverse reactions to vaccines. *American Journal of Epidemiology, 136*, 121–135.

Galindo Sardinas, M. A., Zambrano Cardenas, A., Coutin Marie, G., Santin Pena, M., Alino Santiago, M., Valcardel Sanchez, M., & Farrington, C. P. (2001). Lack of association between intussusception and oral polio vaccine in Cuban children. *European Journal of Epidemiology, 17*, 783–787.

Griffin, M. R., Ray, W. A., Livengood, J. R., & Schaffner, W. (1988). Risk of sudden infant death syndrome after immunization with the diphtheria-tetanus-pertussis vaccine. *New England Journal of Medicine, 319*, 618–623.

Kramarz, P., DeStefano, F., Garguillo, P. M., Davis, R. L., Chen, R. T., Mulooly, J. P., ... Marcy, M. S. (2000). Does influenza vaccination exacerbate asthma? *Archives of Family Medicine, 9*, 617–623.

Madsen, K. M., Hviid, A., Vestergaard, M., Schendel, D., Wohlfahrt, J., Thorsen, P., ... Melbye, M. (2002). A population-based study of measles, mumps and rubella vaccination and autism. *New England Journal of Medicine, 347*, 1477–1482.

Murphy, T. V., Gargiullo, P. M., Massoudi, M. S., Nelson, D. B., Jumaan, A. O., Okoro, C. A., ... Livingood, J. R. (2001). Intussusception among infants given an oral rotavirus vaccine. *New England Journal of Medicine, 344*, 564–572.

Petousis-Harris, H., & Dodd, C. N. (2020). Progress towards a global vaccine data network. *Pediatric Infectious Disease Journal, 39*(11), 1023–1025.

Stowe, J., Andrews, N., Wise, L., & Miller, E. (2009). Investigation of the temporal association of Guillain-Barré syndrome with influenza vaccine and influenza-like illness using the United Kingdom General Practice Research Database. *American Journal of Epidemiology, 169*, 382–388.

Tata, L. J., West, J., Harrison, T., Farrington, P., Smith, C., & Hubbard, R. (2003). Does influenza vaccination increase consultations, corticosteroid prescriptions, or exacerbations in subjects with asthma or chronic obstructive pulmonary disease? *Thorax, 58*, 835–839.

Taylor, B., Miller, E., Farrington, C. P., Petropoulos, M. -C., Favot-Mayaud, I., Li, J., & Waight, P. A. (1999). Autism and measles, mumps and rubella vaccines: No epidemiological evidence for a causal association. *Lancet, 353*, 2026–2029.

Verstraeten, T., DeStefano, F., Chen, R. T., & Miller, E. (2003). Vaccine safety surveillance using large linked databases: Opportunities, hazards and proposed guidelines. *Expert Review of Vaccines, 2*(1), 21–29.

Chapter 20

Epidemiological study designs for evaluating vaccine safety

In this chapter we describe the main study designs used to evaluate vaccine safety after the vaccine has been licensed and is in routine use. These field studies are confirmatory: they seek to address pre-existing hypotheses, which may have emerged from surveillance systems such as those described in Chapter 18, from other clinical or epidemiological studies or from the media.

The study designs may be grouped in three categories: cohort studies, case-control studies and self-controlled studies. Cohort and case-control studies share many of the features of those described in Chapters 14 and 15 for estimating vaccine effectiveness. In contrast, the self-controlled designs apply primarily to vaccine safety evaluation. We shall not attempt an exhaustive description of all the variants of cohort and case-control designs, which would largely mirror the material in these earlier chapters, but will seek simply to illustrate the most common types of studies used. For self-controlled studies, on the other hand, we will provide a more complete description.

In Sections 20.1 and 20.2 we describe cohort studies and case-control studies, respectively. In Sections 20.3 and 20.4 we describe the self-controlled case series method and variants of it. In Section 20.5 we describe the case-crossover method. These various methods differ according to their properties and data requirements. The chapter ends with a table in which some of these features are summarised.

20.1 Cohort studies of vaccine safety

Most cohort studies of vaccine safety are grouped or individual time-to-event studies, often undertaken retrospectively within electronic databases (see Chapter 19, Section

19.5), with vaccinations (or more precisely, the risk periods following vaccination) as time-varying exposures. They may be analysed by Poisson or related regression methods, or by survival methods including the Cox proportional hazards model. Follow-up is usually determined by age and time constraints, together with presence within the database. When non-recurrent or first recurrent events are to be studied, follow-up should end at the earliest of: the age and time constraint applied, time at which the individual leaves the database (or dies) and time of event. For recurrent events, this final constraint (time of event) is not applied, individuals remaining at risk of recurrence after each event.

Subject to these constraints, a typical individual may enter the study unvaccinated and thus, at first, contribute unexposed person-time. If this person is vaccinated at some point, they then contribute exposed person-time during the risk periods, and unexposed person-time outside the risk periods. Finally, if the risk period is not indefinite, they may again contribute unexposed person-time.

If Poisson regression (as described in Chapter 14, Section 14.2.1) is employed, events and person-time are aggregated in discrete categories cross-classified by exposure status (i.e., risk period and perhaps dose), age group and/or season and stratified by other covariates (e.g., sex). An example is described in Box 20.1.

Box 20.1 Febrile convulsions after DTaP vaccine in the United States

Receipt of whole-cell pertussis vaccines is associated with an increased risk of convulsions immediately after vaccination. This study was undertaken to evaluate the corresponding risk for acellular pertussis vaccines (Huang et al., 2010).

The study was a cohort study within the Vaccine Safety Datalink (VSD; see Chapter 18). In the United States, the primary course of diphtheria, tetanus, acellular pertussis (DTaP) vaccine is administered in four primary doses at recommended ages 2, 4, 6 and 15–18 months, with a booster dose at 4–6 years. This study included children aged 6 weeks to 23 months and enrolled within 6 weeks of birth in the participating VSD care organisation between 1 January 1997 and December 2006. Some further restrictions were applied: children receiving diphtheria, tetanus and pertussis (DTP) vaccines with a whole-cell pertussis component were excluded, as were some of those who received two successive DTaP doses less than the recommended minimum interval apart. The risk period of interest was 0–3 days after each dose. All convulsions, including recurrences, were included in the analysis.

The study cohort included 433,654 children. There were 7,191 convulsions in 5,205 children. Table 20.1 contains a summary of the results; as there were no substantial differences between doses, the data for the four primary doses are combined.

Table 20.1 **Numbers of convulsions and total follow-up time in exposed and unexposed groups**

Risk period	Events	Person-years	Rate
0–3 days	112	14,708	761.5 × 10⁻⁵
Control	7,079	588,390	1,203.1 × 10⁻⁵

The rates in Table 20.1 are the numbers of events divided by the person-years. The unadjusted relative rate for the 0–3-day post-vaccination risk period was thus

$$RR = \frac{761.5 \times 10^{-5}}{1,203.1 \times 10^{-5}} = 0.63.$$

The following variables were adjusted in the analysis: gender, participating care organisation, grouped calendar year, season, age (in 3-month intervals), and receipt of measles, mumps and rubella (MMR) vaccines within 8 to 14 days. After adjustment in a Poisson generalised linear model, the relative rate was $RR = 0.87$ with 95% confidence interval (CI) (0.72, 1.05). Thus, there is no evidence of an increased risk of convulsions in the 0–3-day risk period following DTaP vaccination.

In field studies of vaccine safety such as that described in Box 20.1, it is important to adjust for potential confounders, notably the effect of age and possibly season, which can be particularly important as described in Chapter 19, Section 19.4. A second, contrasting example is described in Box 20.2.

Box 20.2 Autism and MMR vaccine in Denmark

This study was undertaken within six linked registers in Denmark to evaluate the risk of autism in relation to vaccination with the MMR vaccine (Madsen et al., 2002).

The study cohort included all children born in Denmark between 1 January 1991 and 31 December 1998, identified through the Danish civil registration system. Vaccination data on MMR was obtained from general practitioners. Information on autism diagnoses was obtained from a central psychiatric register. Information on birth weight and gestational age was obtained from a medical registry of births and from hospital records. Data on potential confounders, such as the household's socio-economic status and mother's education, was obtained from Statistics Denmark. All these databases are linked by a unique personal identification number that is allocated at birth. Follow-up of these children began on their first birthday and continued until the earliest of autism diagnosis (or diagnosis of an associated condition), emigration, death or 31 December 1999. The risk period included all time after MMR vaccination, subdivided in successive adjacent periods (see Chapter 19). The analysis was by Poisson generalised linear modelling.

A total of 537,303 children were included. There were 316 cases of autism and 422 of other autistic spectrum disorders. As the events are non-recurrent, follow-up time for the cases was curtailed at time of event. The relative rate did not vary significantly in different post-vaccination time intervals. The results, with all risk intervals combined, are in Table 20.2.

Table 20.2 Cases of autism and autism spectrum disorders, and person-time in exposed and unexposed groups

Risk period	Autism disorders	Other autistic spectrum disorders	Person-years
Post MMR	263	345	1,647,504
Unexposed	53	77	482,360

Based on the data in Table 20.2, the unadjusted relative rates, for autism disorders and other autistic spectrum disorders (ASD), are:

$$RR_{Autism} = \frac{263/1647,504}{53/482,360} = 1.45; \quad RR_{Other\ ASD} = \frac{345/1647,504}{77/482,360} = 1.31.$$

However, it is essential to adjust for the confounding effect of age, since much unexposed time is accrued at young ages prior to MMR vaccination, when autism or ASD diagnoses are uncommon. After adjustment for age and other potential confounders, the relative rates and 95% confidence intervals are as follows:

$$RR_{Autism} = 0.92, 95\%\ CI\ (0.68, 1.24); \quad RR_{Other\ ASD} = 0.83, 95\%\ CI\ (0.65, 1.07).$$

Thus, the study does not support the hypothesis of an association between MMR vaccination and autism, or other autistic spectrum disorders.

Both the examples described so far exploited the availability of computerised databases or population registers, and thus were able to include very large samples of children. Such databases are invaluable for investigating rare potential adverse reactions to vaccination.

However, informative cohort studies of vaccine safety need not require vast databases, as demonstrated by the example in Box 20.3.

Box 20.3 Hepatitis B vaccination in children and risk of relapse of inflammatory demyelination

Vaccination of children and adolescents against infection with the hepatitis B virus (HBV) fell to a low level in France following persistent concerns about a possible link with multiple sclerosis (MS). Furthermore, it was widely believed that HBV vaccination should be avoided in children who had had an episode of acute central nervous system (CNS) inflammatory demyelination. This cohort study was undertaken to quantify the risk of relapse and its potential association with HBV in such children (Mikaeloff, Caridade, Assi, Tardieu, & Suissa, 2007).

The study was undertaken within a neuropaediatric cohort, and included patients who had experienced a first demyelinating event before the age of 16 years between 1 January 1994 and 31 December 2003. Patients were followed up until December 2005. Documented vaccination histories were obtained. The adverse event of interest was a second episode of neurological symptoms, indicating a conversion to MS. Several risk periods were investigated: any time after vaccination, and defined risk periods of 3, 6, 12 and 36 months after vaccination. The analysis used a Cox proportional hazards model.

A total of 356 patients were enrolled. There were 136 relapses among the 323 patients who did not receive HBV vaccine after their first demyelinating event, and 10 among the 33 patients who did. The hazard ratio for relapse at any time post-vaccination was 1.09, 95% CI (0.53, 2.24). This was adjusted for several covariates, including age and time of onset, sex, socio-economic status and familial history of MS.

The hazard ratio was not elevated in any of the shorter risk periods investigated. Thus, this study does not support the hypothesis that HBV vaccination increases the risk of relapse and conversion to MS, within 3 years or at any time since vaccination, in patients with a first episode of CNS inflammatory demyelination in childhood.

Cohort studies enable direct and accurate estimation of absolute risks in the population studied, as well as relative risks. However, as was noted in Chapter 19, it may be difficult to control completely for potential confounding factors, especially when data are obtained from administrative databases.

20.2 Case-control studies of vaccine safety and their variants

Many case-control studies of vaccine safety are individually matched on potential confounders, such as age, and analysed using conditional logistic regression. These methods were previously described in the context of vaccine effectiveness studies in Chapter 14. In the case of vaccine safety studies, nested case-control studies undertaken within clinical or other databases are particularly common.

Within a matched set comprising one case and one or more controls, the event time of the case determines the index time of the case-control set; this may be based on age or calendar time depending on context. The index times are then used to determine the exposure status of each case and each control, using previously specified risk periods. The procedure is described in more detail in Box 20.4.

Box 20.4 Oral polio vaccine and intussusception in the United Kingdom

This study was undertaken to investigate a potential association between the oral polio vaccine (OPV) and intussusception in infants, using data from a UK clinical database that has since been renamed the Clinical Practice Research Datalink or CPRD (Jick, Vasilakis-Scaramozza, & Jick, 2001).

The study identified all infants under 1 year of age and born between 1 January 1988 and 31 October 1998 with confirmed intussusception, and without prior disease predisposing to intussusception.

Each case was matched with up to four control infants without intussusception, selected randomly from the same database. The matching variables were month of birth, sex and age of the mother (within 1 year). The calendar time of diagnosis of the case was used as the index date for the matched case-control set.

The risk period of interest comprised the first 42 days after any dose of OPV, subdivided into six 7-day periods. Cases and controls were classified as unexposed if they had not received a dose of OPV on one of the 42 days prior to the index date. The time from the last OPV dose to the index date was used to classify the exposure into the six exposure periods; all infants had received OPV.

There were 133 cases and 515 controls. The odds ratios were estimated by conditional logistic regression. The results are in Table 20.3.

Table 20.3 Cases and controls with odds ratio (OR) and 95% CI

Days since last OPV dose	No. of cases	No. of controls	OR (95% CI)
1–7	12	47	0.9 (0.4–2.0)
8–14	7	34	0.8 (0.3–2.1)
15–21	12	45	1.0 (0.4–2.3)
22–28	12	46	0.9 (0.4–2.0)
29–35	5	26	0.7 (0.2–2.1)
36–42	8	32	0.9 (0.2–2.1)
> 42 (unexposed)	77	285	–

> The odds ratios are not statistically significantly higher (or lower) than 1 for any risk period. In consequence, this study provides no evidence that OPV is associated with intussusception in this population.

The study described in Box 20.4 is analysed using conditional logistic regression. In other contexts, it may be required to investigate whether there is a dose effect, or to correct for other potential confounders not included in the matching variables.

In Box 20.3 we described a cohort study of hepatitis B vaccination and relapses of demyelinating episodes in children who had experienced a first such attack. The possibility of a link between hepatitis B vaccination and MS led to the temporary suspension of the school-based HBV vaccination programme in France in October 1998. The study described in Box 20.5 was undertaken to investigate this hypothesis.

Box 20.5 HBV vaccination and MS in the United States

A nested case-control study was undertaken within two large cohorts of nurses in the United States. These cohorts were chosen because the uptake of vaccination against HBV is high in healthcare workers, and because reliable vaccination records are available for a large proportion (Ascherio et al., 2001).

The case notes of MS cases in these cohorts were reviewed to classify the diagnosis as definite or probable and to determine the date of onset. Each case was matched with five controls chosen randomly from the same database among women with no history of MS or breast cancer (healthy controls). Each case was also matched with one woman with breast cancer (breast cancer control). Matching was on year of birth, study cohort and, for the breast cancer control, date of diagnosis. The index date for each matched case-control set was the date of diagnosis of the case. Two exposure definitions were used in the primary analyses: receipt of at least one dose of hepatitis B vaccine at any time before the index date, and receipt of the first dose of the vaccine within 2 years before the index date. Exposure status was determined from vaccination certificates. Further adjustments were made using conditional logistic regression for the potential confounding effects of latitude of residence at birth, pack-years of smoking, past history of infections and ancestry. The results are in Table 20.4.

Table 20.4 Odds ratio of MS according to exposure definition and control type

Vaccination interval prior to index date	190 MS cases and 534 healthy controls OR	95% CI	111 MS cases and 111 breast cancer controls OR	95% CI	192 MS cases and pooled controls OR	95% CI
≤2 years	0.7	0.3–1.7	1.3	0.3–6.1	0.7	0.3–1.8
Any time	0.8	0.5–1.5	1.3	0.5–3.7	0.9	0.5–1.6

From Table 20.4, none of the primary analyses suggest an association between HBV vaccination and MS. Secondary analyses included number of vaccine doses received and several sensitivity analyses, which did not alter the results. The authors concluded that the study suggests no association between HBV vaccination and MS.

The advantage of a nested case-control study is that it reduces the potential for selection bias, since cases and controls are sampled from the same cohort. Using both healthy and breast cancer controls in Box 20.5 also provided some protection against information biases relating to the diagnosis of a severe disease. An important feature of the study described in Box 20.5 was the use of contemporaneously recorded vaccination histories: the authors showed that using self-reported vaccination histories would have introduced recall bias, which would have increased the odds ratio.

Case-cohort methods (described in Chapter 14 in the context of vaccine effectiveness estimation) and other variants of the case-control method may also be used in vaccine safety studies, but are less common.

If individual data are available, they should be used to adjust for confounding. However, in some circumstances, it may be unclear how to select individual controls. When the post-vaccination risk periods are indefinite and good vaccine coverage data are available, the case-coverage method may then be appropriate. This method, which is akin to the screening method for vaccine effectiveness, is illustrated in Box 20.6. Each case is matched to the vaccine coverage of the population segment (typically including time and age group) from which the case arises. The model is fitted exactly as the screening model using logistic regression, with the exposure status of the case as the response variable and the log odds of vaccination coverage as an offset.

In the application described in Box 20.6, cases were selected nationally from a multiplicity of different types of sources, which makes selection of individual controls difficult. However, the case-coverage method shares the weaknesses of the screening method, notably limited opportunities for adjusting for potential confounders, this being achieved by stratification. More information on the case-coverage method may be found in Farrington (2004).

Box 20.6 Narcolepsy and pandemic influenza vaccination in England

A possible link between narcolepsy in adolescents and the pandemic influenza A (H1N1) Pandemrix vaccine was discussed in Chapter 18. The present study was undertaken retrospectively in England. Cases in children and adolescents aged 4–18 years at onset of narcolepsy were identified from sleep centres and paediatric neurology centres, as well as hospital databases (Miller et al., 2013).

The 2009–2010 pandemic vaccination programme was targeted initially at people at high risk, and later extended to all children aged less than 5 years. One of the analyses presented used the case-coverage method. For each case, the vaccine coverage was calculated for the population comprising children of the same age as the case, and within the same risk group as the case, on the date of symptoms onset of the case. The risk interval in this analysis includes all time after vaccination. In an attempt to reduce ascertainment bias, cases were restricted to those diagnosed prior to July 2011, when the European Medicines Agency (EMA) announced restrictions on the use of Pandemrix.

Out of 17 cases of narcolepsy eligible for vaccination prior to disease onset, 10 were vaccinated. The average coverage in the matched populations was 16%. The relative risk of narcolepsy associated with vaccination was $RR = 14.4$, with 95% CI (4.3 to 48.5).

Other case-coverage analyses (with different risk intervals, different matching criteria and different event onset definitions) produced different relative risks, yet all statistically significantly raised. The study is consistent with a causal association between Pandemrix vaccine and narcolepsy.

The study described in Box 20.6 illustrates how difficult it can be to assess causality in situations where the onset of the adverse of event of interest is difficult to determine, and where bias due to unmeasured confounding may be an issue. In particular, bias by indication could affect the results in view of the relatively low vaccine coverage and the targeted nature of the vaccination programme.

Finally, we describe a case-control method called case-centred analysis. This method is used within databases, using stratification by time period to adjust for temporal effects. The method shares some features with nested case-control studies and with the case-coverage method, and has been shown to be equivalent to a stratified Cox model (Fireman et al., 2009).

In a case-centred analysis, each case is matched to all individuals within the database who are at risk at the time the case occurred, and who lie within the same stratum as the case (the strata are determined by possible confounders). The proportion of this risk set who are exposed is then contrasted, within a logistic regression model, with the exposure status of the case. The analysis proceeds as in the case-coverage method, the log odds of the proportion exposed within the risk set being included as an offset in the model. Thus, as with the case-coverage method, confounders are controlled by stratification. An application of the method is described in Box 20.7.

> **Box 20.7 Bell's palsy and vaccinations in US children**
>
> This case-centred analysis was undertaken to study the association between vaccination and Bell's palsy in children aged up to 18 years (Rowhani-Rahbar et al., 2012). The study was undertaken in a health maintenance organisation (HMO) database, with cases ascertained over the period 2001–2006. Three analyses were undertaken: for inactivated trivalent influenza vaccine (TIV), HBV and any vaccine.
>
> Cases and matched risk sets were restricted to those who received the vaccine of interest (or any vaccine) in the year prior to onset of Bell's palsy in the case. The risk set for each case comprised all children who were matched to the case on age group and sex. Exposure was determined using three risk periods: 1–14, 1–28 and 29–56 days after vaccination. For each case, the proportion exposed within the matched risk set was obtained.
>
> The analysis uses only the exposure status of the cases, the proportions exposed in the risk sets and the stratum variables. No evidence of an association was found for TIV, HBV or any vaccine. For example, for the 1–28-day risk period, the odds ratio (OR) was 0.7 for TIV, 95% CI (0.2, 2.8); for HBV, OR = 0.8, 95% CI (0.2, 2.4); and for any vaccine, OR = 0.9, 95% CI (0.6, 1.4).

The merit of the case-centred method is that the analysis is simple. A disadvantage is the need to adjust covariates by stratification. The number of variables than can be adjusted in this way is usually limited, and the role of the potential confounders is perhaps less transparent than when analysed with regression methods that make use of the individual data available.

20.3 The self-controlled case series method

The self-controlled case series (or SCCS) method was developed specifically for the purposes of vaccine safety evaluation, though it has since been used in other areas of pharmacoepidemiology. Unlike cohort and case-control methods, control is achieved not through comparisons between exposed and unexposed individuals, but by contrasting risk periods and unexposed control periods within cases, that is, individuals who have experienced the event of interest. The parameter estimated is the relative incidence, or incidence rate ratio described in Chapter 19, Section 19.2. However, absolute rates are not estimated or compared: estimation is direct via the likelihood function (this is a standard statistical technique, but lies beyond the scope of this book). The SCCS model is fitted using conditional Poisson regression. The technical details of the method are set out, along with many vaccine examples, in Farrington, Whitaker, and Ghebremichael Weldeselassie (2018). The assumptions needed for the SCCS method will be discussed in Section 20.4.

Two key features of the SCCS method are, first, that it uses only cases, that is, individuals who have experienced the event of interest (whether or not it occurred after vaccination); and, second, that the method automatically adjusts for all time-invariant confounding factors, whether these are known or not. These may include sex, birth weight, genetic factors and, over limited time-spans, socio-economic status, location and underlying state of health. The fact that only cases are used greatly simplifies the application of the method; the fact that time-invariant confounders are automatically adjusted removes any concern about confounding from such variables, notably confounding by indication. (Strictly speaking, only confounders acting multiplicatively on the baseline incidence are controlled, but the distinction is largely theoretical.) Control of confounding makes the method particularly attractive for use with administrative databases, in which information on confounders is often very limited and not within the control of the investigator.

On the other hand, confounding by variables that vary over time, notably age and season, is not automatically adjusted. However, this is readily handled by inclusion of suitable age and season variables in the model, usually in the form of age groups and calendar time periods through which individuals progress.

In addition to the risk periods described in Chapter 19, Section 19.1, the SCCS method requires the specification of the observation period for each case. This is the period of time over which an individual is observed, and during which the event of interest might occur. The observation period is specified using age and calendar time constraints, or in terms of vaccination; it is not censored at the time of event, even if events are non-recurrent.

Further details will be given after the example in Box 20.8, which illustrates the application of the method in a concrete example.

Box 20.8 ITP and MMR vaccines

Idiopathic thrombocytopenic purpura (ITP) is a rare, potentially recurrent blood clotting disorder that has been linked to MMR vaccines, with risk period 15–35 days post-vaccination. This SCCS study was undertaken to quantify the strength of association more accurately than had hitherto been possible (Miller et al., 2001).

ITP cases were identified from hospital admissions of children during their second year of life in the regions and time periods in which the data were collected. Vaccination records were obtained by data linkage. The observation period for each case stretches from the latest of age 365 days and start of case ascertainment in that hospital, to the earliest of age 730 days and end of case ascertainment in the hospital.

There were 35 ITP cases with 44 distinct episodes of ITP. A 6-week risk period 0–42 days after MMR was used. Figure 20.1 shows the time interval from MMR vaccine to ITP for those episodes for which the interval is less than a year.

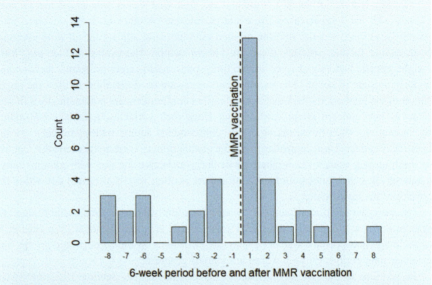

Figure 20.1 ITP cases by interval (in 6-week periods) between MMR and ITP. The timing of MMR vaccination is indicated by the vertical dashed line.

Figure 20.1 suggests that ITP clusters within the 6 weeks after receipt of MMR vaccine. The SCCS analysis, adjusted for age in six groups of roughly 2 months, found a relative incidence $RI = 3.27$ with 95% CI (1.49 to 7.16) for the 0–42-day risk period. When the risk period was subdivided into three 2-week periods, the strongest association was found for the 15–28-day period with $RI = 5.80$, 95% CI (2.30 to 14.6).

In the study described in Box 20.8, only events arising in the second year of life were included. This was because the recommended age for MMR vaccination is within the second year of life. Generally, it is sensible to define the observation period with reference to the actual and recommended ages at vaccination in this way. Note also that all events, including recurrences, were included. An assumption of the method is that the event is either potentially recurrent, or uncommon and non-recurrent. Thus, since ITP is an uncommon condition (by which we mean the risk is less than 10% over the observation period), the analysis could be repeated including only first ITPs (which by definition are non-recurrent). Finally, in this analysis all 35 cases had received MMR vaccine. The reason for excluding ITP cases without an MMR history in this particular study was that it could not be guaranteed that lack of a match with the vaccine database genuinely indicated absence of MMR.

However, inclusion of unvaccinated cases in other contexts can help to estimate the temporal effects (age or season). This can be particularly important when longer risk periods are used, as illustrated in Box 20.9.

Box 20.9 MMR vaccine and autism

This SCCS analysis of UK autism and MMR vaccine data used an indefinite post-vaccination risk period (Farrington, Miller, & Taylor, 2001). The study included 357 cases with a diagnosis of autism in children up to age 16 years who were born between 1979 and 1998. The observation period for each case was time from birth to age 191 months or August 1998, whichever was earlier. Some 64 cases did not receive any MMR vaccine; in 30 cases autism was diagnosed before MMR. The oldest age at autism diagnosis was 15 years. Owing to the MMR catch-up programme, the ages at vaccination were very spread out, with median 57 months and maximum 165 months.

The SCCS analysis adjusted for age in 17 distinct age groups, and for temporal effects. The relative incidence was $RI = 1.06$ with 95% CI (0.49 to 2.30).

The use of an indefinite post-vaccination risk period in the autism example of Box 20.9 poses special challenges, as then age and time since vaccination are substantially confounded. The inclusion of unvaccinated cases removes this source of confounding. However, the SCCS method is most powerful when used with a short risk period.

In the examples presented so far, the observation periods have spanned the age range over which the vaccine is administered. Typically, this range could include many months or even years. The age effects (and seasonal effect, if relevant) must then be accounted for in the model, which can be achieved in a variety of ways: by explicitly specifying age groups as in the examples above, or by fitting a semi-parametric model in which age groups need not be specified in advance (Farrington et al., 2018).

The self-controlled risk interval (SCRI) design is a special case of the SCCS design with a short observation period, defined in terms of the time of vaccination. As for some SCCS studies, only vaccinated cases are included. The key difference with other SCCS studies lies in the selection of control period: in the SCRI design, short control intervals are chosen before or after, or both before and after, the risk period. The brief observation periods (risk and control periods combined) of the SCRI design make it especially suitable for use in sequential monitoring systems, where analyses are updated at frequent intervals; the Bell's palsy example in Chapter 18, Section 18.4, was of this type.

The SCRI design has also been used for substantive evaluations of vaccine safety; one such example is described in Box 20.10.

Box 20.10 Adverse events following varicella vaccine in Taiwan

This study was undertaken using linked vaccination and health insurance databases, within a cohort of children aged between 12 and 35 months during the January 2004 to September 2014 study period. The prespecified events of interest were pneumonia, ITP, meningitis, encephalitis and ischemic stroke. Fracture was also included as a negative control. The risk period included days 1–42 after receipt of the varicella vaccine, and the control period included days 43–84. Age was controlled in eight 3-month periods, and season in four 3-month periods (Liu, Yeh, Huang, Chie, & Chan, 2020). The results are in Table 20.5

None of the prespecified events are significantly positively associated with varicella vaccination in the adjusted SCRI analysis.

Table 20.5 Total number and relative incidence (RI) of selected adverse events after varicella vaccine

Event	Total events in 1–84-day period	Unadjusted analysis RI	95% CI	Analysis adjusted for age and season RI	95% CI
Pneumonia	10,614	0.94	0.90–0.97	0.97	0.93–1.01
ITP	248	1.07	0.83–1.36	1.00	0.76–1.33
Meningitis	29	1.55	0.72–3.30	1.21	0.49–2.95
Encephalitis	92	1.00	0.66–1.51	1.00	0.62–1.60
Stroke	15	2.00	0.68–5.85	1.24	0.31–4.95
Fracture	240	1.18	0.92–1.53	1.06	0.79–1.41

SCRI studies are sometimes analysed without adjusting for temporal effects (age, season or both), this being justified by the short observation period used. However, the study described in Box 20.10 shows that, even with relatively brief 12-week observation periods, confounding by time and season can alter the relative incidences and their statistical significance. Especially when there are few cases, better control of age or season effects may be achieved by using the longer observation periods available in the more general SCCS method. We recommend that age (or season, if relevant) are controlled with narrow age bands in confirmatory SCCS studies of adverse events following immunisation (AEFIs) in childhood, because event rates may be very age-dependent.

The SCRI method is particularly well-suited for sequential surveillance purposes. However, for substantive evaluations of vaccine safety, the SCRI method requires reliable a priori information about the risk period. This is because the results are likely to be more sensitive to misspecification of the risk period than a standard SCCS design. For example, no effect may be identified if the true risk period overlaps with the control period used in the SCRI analysis, or vice versa.

The SCRI method has the advantage of great simplicity. However, longer observation periods enable a more complete characterisation of the risk profile of the vaccine: the SCRI method only allows a short-term risk gradient in vaccinees to be determined.

SCCS analyses also provide a more flexible framework for studying age and dose effects, and for studying several vaccines concurrently, as required when two or more vaccines may be administered concomitantly (see Chapter 19).

20.4 SCCS analyses for event-dependent vaccinations

The SCCS method requires two major assumptions: occurrence of an event should not affect subsequent vaccination and occurrence of an event should not affect the observation period. The second is seldom an issue for SCCS studies of vaccines: it typically arises when the event of interest substantially increases the short-term risk of death. However, most AEFIs of interest are not of that nature.

The first assumption, however, can be problematic in some vaccine studies. Most commonly, the assumption is violated because the event may delay or preclude subsequent vaccination. Left uncorrected, the SCCS method will then produce a relative incidence *RI* that is too high. The fact that the direction of bias is known can help: for example, if no association is found, then because the true *RI* is lower than that estimated, inferences are robust to failure of the assumption.

One of several adjustments to the SCCS method can be made to remove this bias. Suppose first that the occurrence of an adverse event may cause a delay in vaccination. In consequence, few adverse events would be observed shortly before vaccination. A simple way in which to adjust the SCCS analysis in this particular case is to include an additional risk period immediately prior to vaccination. Then, if events do delay vaccination, this should be revealed by an $RI < 1$ for this pre-exposure risk period (if, on the other hand, the event precipitates vaccination, $RI > 1$ would be observed). An example is in Box 20.11.

Box 20.11 Influenza vaccination and Bell's palsy

Concern over a possible link between parenteral inactivated influenza vaccine and Bell's palsy led to this study in the UK Clinical Practice Research Datalink (Stowe, Andrews, Wise, & Miller, 2006). Consultations for Bell's palsy were ascertained between 1 July 1992 and 30 June 2005; consultations less than 6 months apart were regarded as part of the same episode. The observation period for each case started at the latest of 1 June 1992 and registration in the database; it ended at the earliest of 30 June 2005, death and the date when the patient left the practice. The analysis was limited to cases with at least one influenza vaccination. Age was adjusted in 5-year age bands, season and year were adjusted by year and quarter. The risk period included days 1 to 91 after any influenza vaccine. Opportunistic recording of episodes on the day of vaccination is a known feature of this database, so the day of vaccination (day 0) was given its own risk period. A pre-vaccination period of 2 weeks from day −14 to day −1 was included to correct for delays in vaccination caused by Bell's palsy.

There were 2,263 episodes in 1,156 females and 972 males. The results are in Table 20.6.

Table 20.6 Bell's palsy episodes, relative incidence (*RI*) and 95% CI by risk period

Risk period	Episodes	RI	95% CI
Control	2015	–	–
−14 to −1 days	25	0.72	0.48, 1.07
day 0	11	4.38	2.47, 7.79
1 to 91 days	212	0.92	0.78, 1.27

The value $RI = 0.72$ for the 2-week pre-exposure period is suggestive of deficit of events just prior to vaccination (thought the effect is not statistically significant). The relative incidence in the 1–91-day risk period is 0.92 with 95% CI (0.78, 1.27), indicating no association between influenza vaccination and Bell's palsy. The results were confirmed in further analyses, in which the risk period was split into three 30-day periods.

Note that in Box 20.11, the day 0 (vaccination day) effect is spurious, as explained in Chapter 19, Section 19.5. By using separate risk periods for the immediate pre-vaccination period and the day of vaccination, these spurious effects are made explicit, and removed from influencing the effect of primary interest that pertains to the 1–91-day risk period.

In a more extreme scenario, occurrence of an event may discourage or even (if it is a contraindication to vaccination) preclude subsequent vaccination. This also constitutes a violation of the assumptions of the SCCS method. In this more extreme scenario, two approaches are possible. The first, which works when the vaccine is administered in a single dose, is to begin every observation period with the day of vaccination, since subsequent events can no longer affect future vaccinations (since there are none). This is illustrated in Box 20.12.

Box 20.12 Influenza vaccination and Guillain-Barré syndrome in France

Many studies of seasonal and pandemic influenza vaccines have since studied a possible association between Guillain-Barré syndrome (GBS) and influenza vaccination, yielding contrasting results. The present study included data from four influenza seasons (September to March of 2010–2014) and was undertaken within the French national health data system (Grave et al., 2020).

The study used a SCCS design with risk period 1–42 days post-vaccination. In France, a history of GBS is considered to be a contraindication to vaccination by some patients and some physicians. Accordingly, only vaccinated cases were included in the study, with observation starting on day of vaccination. The control period extended from day 43 post-vaccination until 31 March of the same influenza season. The temporal confounders adjusted included season (by calendar month) and acute respiratory and gastrointestinal infections, each with a post-infection risk period of 42 days, as these infections could also cause GBS (see also Chapter 19, Section 19.4).

The study included 463 vaccinated GBS cases. The relative incidence was $RI = 1.10$ with 95% CI (0.89, 1.37), thus not significantly raised for the 42-day post-vaccination risk period. Subgroup analyses suggested a possible association during the 2012–2013 season ($RI = 1.60$, 95% CI (1.05 to 2.44)) and for the 1–28-day post-vaccination risk period ($RI = 1.27$, 95% CI (1.00 to 1.60)). In contrast, the relative incidences of GBS associated with infections were very significantly raised: $RI = 3.64$, 95% CI (3.10 to 4.40) for acute gastrointestinal infections, and $RI = 3.89$, 95% CI (3.52 to 4.30) for acute respiratory tract infections.

Using only post-vaccination times is possible in Box 20.12 because influenza vaccines are given in single doses. Note also that, in this example, infections that could cause GBS are also adjusted as time-varying covariates.

A different SCCS model, based on a pseudolikelihood method (the details of which lie beyond the scope of this book), has been developed that applies for all vaccines, including multi-dose vaccines, with finite risk periods, in situations where the event of interest is a contraindication to vaccination. The details of the method may be found in Farrington et al. (2018). An example is provided in Box 20.13.

Box 20.13 Rotavirus vaccination and intussusception in sub-Saharan Africa

This SCCS study was undertaken by the African Intussusception Network, using data contributed by hospital patients in Ethiopia, Ghana, Kenya, Malawi, Tanzania, Zambia and Zimbabwe, where the monovalent Rotarix vaccine is in use, with a two-dose vaccination schedule (Tate et al., 2018).

Cases of intussusception in infants younger than 12 months of age who met the Brighton Collaboration criteria were enrolled. Vaccination status was determined using vaccination cards. The two risk periods 1–7 and 8–21 days after any dose of vaccine were used. The observation period stretched from age 28 to age 245 days; age was adjusted in 14 age groups.

In total, 717 intussusception cases with confirmed vaccination were included in the analysis. The results, obtained using the pseudolikelihood SCCS method, are shown in Table 20.7.

Table 20.7 Number of events, relative incidence (RI) and 95% CI by dose

Risk period (days)	Dose 1 Events	RI	95% CI	Dose 2 Events	RI	95% CI
1–7	1	0.25	0.00–1.16	5	0.76	0.16–1.87
8–21	6	1.01	0.26–2.24	16	0.74	0.39–1.20
1–21	7	0.85	0.35–1.73	21	0.81	0.49–1.22

The study did not find any evidence of an increased risk of intussusception after either dose of monovalent rotavirus vaccine.

20.5 The case-crossover method

In this section we describe the case-crossover method. This method, like SCCS, uses only cases and is self-controlled, and thus adjusts for all time-invariant confounders. However, while the SCCS method is akin to a cohort method, the case-crossover method is akin to a case-control method.

Briefly, a case interval is assigned to each case prior to the event time, corresponding to the risk period as in a case-control study (see, for example, Box 20.4). One or more control times are defined at predetermined times prior to the event time, and control intervals are assigned to these control times. For each case, the case interval and control intervals constitute a matched set. The data are then analysed exactly as in a matched case-control study, with vaccination during the case and control intervals determining exposure status. For further details of the case-crossover method, see Maclure (1991).

Unlike the SCCS method, the case-crossover method does not make use of post-event time, and so it may be used whether or not events influence subsequent vaccinations. However, it requires a major assumption not shared with the SCCS method: the risk of vaccination must be constant over time. In fact, a slightly stronger assumption is required: exposures in the matched set must be exchangeable. This mirrors the tacit assumption in matched case-control studies that the controls matched to each case are interchangeable.

Such an assumption is untenable for many vaccines because they are administered according to a strongly temporal schedule. However, in some circumstances the assumption may not be unreasonable. An example is given in Box 20.14.

Box 20.14 Vaccinations and the risk of relapse in MS in Europe

This study was undertaken to determine whether vaccination of patients with MS precipitates a relapse (Confavreux, Suissa, Saddier, Bourdes, & Vukusic, 2001). Patients with a definite or probable diagnosis of MS and with at least one relapse were identified from a European database. The index relapse was the first occurring in 1993–1997 with the previous 12 months relapse-free. The risk period included the 2 months after vaccination. Thus, the 2-month period prior to time of relapse is the case interval. Four control times were chosen 2, 4, 6 and 8 months prior to the time of the relapse. The four 2-month periods prior to these control times were used as control intervals. Figure 20.2 illustrates the design of the study.

The majority of vaccinations were confirmed. A total 643 index relapses were included in the study. None of the vaccines studied were associated with a significant increase in relapses. For all vaccines combined, $OR = 0.71$ with 95% CI (0.40 to 1.26). For hepatitis B vaccine, $OR = 0.67$ with 95% CI (0.20 to 2.17) and for influenza vaccine, $OR = 1.08$ with 95% CI (0.37 to 3.10).

The results remained stable when the duration of the risk and control periods were varied. The authors remarked that the proportion of patients vaccinated was stable over the 12 months preceding the relapse.

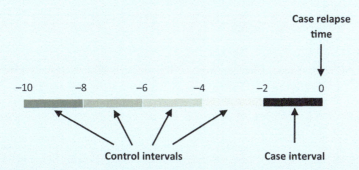

Figure 20.2 Case interval and control intervals for MS relapse study. The control times are at −2, −4, −6 and −8 months relative to the case relapse time at time 0. The control and case intervals are the two-month periods prior to these times.

Case-crossover methods that allow for trends in exposures over time have been proposed, notably the case-time-control method (Suissa, 1995). However, vaccinations are often administered according to more complex schedules than can be adequately described by linear trends.

Summary

- Standard cohort and case-control methods may be used to study vaccine safety, with predetermined risk periods.
- These methods are often applied retrospectively using data from administrative, clinical or linked databases; however, information on potential confounders may be limited.
- Self-controlled methods use cases as their own controls and adjust automatically for time-invariant confounders.
- The SCCS method, and its variant the SCRI method, are widely used in vaccine safety studies.
- The SCCS method requires an assumption that events do not influence subsequent vaccinations. Several SCCS methods are available to circumvent this assumption.
- The case-crossover method is a different self-controlled method. It requires the assumption that the chance of vaccination does not vary over time.
- Some of the key properties of these various methods are summarised in the Table 20.8.

Table 20.8 **Summary table**

Method	What is estimable	Time-invariant confounder adjustment	Time-varying confounder adjustment	Risk period durations	Data required
Cohort	RI, absolute risks	Explicit	Explicit	Any	Full cohort
Case-control	OR	Explicit or matching	Explicit or matching	Any	Cases and controls
Case coverage	RI	Stratification	Stratification	Indefinite	Cases and coverage
Case-centred	RI	Stratification	Stratification	Any	Cases and risk set coverage
SCCS	RI	Automatic	Explicit	Any	Cases
SCRI	RI	Automatic	Explicit	Short	Cases
SCCS for EDE*	RI	Automatic	Explicit	Short	Cases
Case-crossover	OR	Automatic	Exposures must be exchangeable	Short	Cases

* Event-dependent exposures.

References

Ascherio, A., Zhang, S. M., Hernan, M. A., Olek, M. J., Coplan, P. M., Brodovicz, K., & Walker, A. M. (2001). Hepatitis B vaccination and the risk of multiple sclerosis. *New England Journal of Medicine*, *344*(5), 327–332.

Confavreux, C., Suissa, S., Saddier, P., Bourdes, V., & Vukusic, S. (2001). Vaccinations and the risk of relapse in multiple sclerosis. *New England Journal of Medicine*, *344*(5), 319–326.

Farrington, C. P. (2004). Control without separate controls: Evaluation of vaccine safety using case-only methods. *Vaccine*, *22*, 2064–2070.

Farrington, C. P., Miller, E., & Taylor, B. (2001). MMR and autism: Further evidence against a causal association. *Vaccine*, *19*, 3632–3635.

Farrington, P., Whitaker, H., & Ghebremichael Weldeselassie, Y. (2018). *Self-controlled case series studies: A modelling guide with R*. Boca Raton, FL: Chapman & Hall/CRC Press.

Fireman, B., Lee, J., Lewis, N., Bembom, O., van der Laan, M., & Baxter, R. (2009). Influenza vaccination and mortality: Differentiating vaccine effects from bias. *American Journal of Epidemiology*, *170*, 650–656.

Grave, C., Boucheron, P., Rudant, J., Mikaeloff, Y., Tubert-Bitter, P., Escolano, S., ... Weill, A. (2020). Seasonal influenza vaccine and Guillain-Barré syndrome: A self-controlled case series study. *Neurology*, *94*(20), e2168–e2179.

Huang, W. -T., Garguillo, P. M., Broder, K. R., Weintraub, E. S., Iskander, J. K., Klein, N. P., & Baggs, J. M. (2010). Lack of association between acellular pertussis vaccine and seizures in early childhood. *Pediatrics*, *126*(2), e263–e269.

Jick, H., Vasilakis-Scaramozza, C., & Jick, S. S. (2001). Live attenuated polio vaccine and the risk of intussusception. *British Journal of Clinical Pharmacology*, *52*, 451–453.

Liu, C. -H., Yeh, Y. -C., Huang, W. -T., Chie, W. -C., & Chan, K. A. (2020). Assessment of pre-specified adverse events following varicella vaccine: A population-based self-controlled risk interval study. *Vaccine*, *38*(11), 2495–2502.

Maclure, M. (1991). The case-crossover design: a method for stydying transient effects on the risk of acute events. *American Journal of Epidemiology*, *133*, 144–153.

Madsen, K. M., Hviid, A., Vestergaard, M., Schendel, D., Wohlfahrt, J., Thorsen, P., ... Melbye, M. (2002). A population-based study of measles, mumps and rubella vaccination and autism. *New England Journal of Medicine*, *347*, 1477–1482.

Mikaeloff, Y., Caridade, G., Assi, S., Tardieu, M., & Suissa, S. (2007). Hepatitis B vaccine and risk of relapse after a first childhood episode of CNS inflammatory demyelination. *Brain*, *130*, 1105–1110.

Miller, E., Andrews, N., Stellitano, L., Stowe, J., Winstone, A. M., Shneerson, J., & Verity, C. (2013). Risk of narcolepsy in children and ypoung people receiving AS03 adjuvanted pandemic A/H1N1 2009 influenza vaccine: Retrospective analysis. *British Medical Journal*, *346*, f794.

Miller, E., Waight, P., Farrington, P., Andrews, N., Stowe, J., & Taylor, B. (2001). Idiopathic thrombocytopenic purpura and MMR vaccine. *Archives of Disease in Childhood*, *84*, 227–229.

Rowhani-Rahbar, A., Klein, N. P., Lewis, N., Fireman, B., Ray, P., Rasgon, B., ... Baxter, R. (2012). Immunization and Bell's palsy in children: A case-centered analysis. *American Journal of Epidemiology*, *175*(9), 878–885.

Stowe, J., Andrews, N., Wise, L., & Miller, E. (2006). Bell's palsy and parenteral inactivated influenza vaccine. *Human Vaccines*, *2*(3), 110–112.

Suissa, S. (1995). The case-time-control design. *Epidemiology*, *6*, 248–253.

Tate, J. E., Mwenda, J. M., Armah, G., Jani, B., Omore, R., Ademe, A., … Parashar, U. D. (2018). Evaluation of intussusception after monovalent rotavirus vaccination in Africa. *New England Journal of Medicine*, *378*, 1521–1528.

Part V

Benefit–risk assessment of vaccination programmes

Chapter 21

Benefit–risk assessment of vaccination programmes

A well-implemented vaccination programme using an effective vaccine reduces the burden of disease and death due to the infection it targets. Vaccination programmes have generally been very successful in achieving this. However, no vaccine is completely safe, despite rigorous safety assessment of vaccines pre-licensure. An overview of vaccine safety and its assessment is provided in Chapter 17, explaining why some risks associated with vaccination may become apparent only after implementation of a vaccination programme. Therefore, post-implementation decision-making regarding vaccination programmes ideally should be informed by an integrated evaluation of benefits and risks. Benefit–risk assessments show many similarities with cost-effectiveness analyses in terms of methodology used. However, cost-effectiveness analyses are out of scope of the current book, since they are mostly used prior to the implementation of vaccination programmes while the current book focuses on the evaluation of existing vaccination programmes.

While benefits and risks of vaccination programmes are usually monitored routinely, integrated and explicit benefit–risk assessments are often lacking. This involves the integration of data and information from different sources, typically associated with different levels of uncertainty, on both benefits and risks. In addition, new evidence on the benefits and risks of a vaccination programme might become available over time, which implies that the initial benefit–risk assessment needs to be updated in the light of the new evidence.

Benefit–risk assessment methodology is frequently used pre-licensure and for therapeutic drugs. However, benefit–risk assessment for decision-making about vaccination programmes is still in its infancy (Arlegui, Bollaerts et al., 2020). Benefit–risk methodologies aim to provide transparency to the process of assessing benefit–risk profiles by

DOI: 10.4324/9781315166414-22
This Chapter has been made available under a CC-BY-NC-ND license.

structuring the approach and making a clear distinction between evidence (prevented and induced disease) and value judgements (relative importance of the different health outcomes). Thus, integrated benefit–risk analyses are a systematic way of collating and presenting the evidence on benefits and risks, facilitating decision-making on the continuation, modification or cessation of vaccination programmes. These decisions should ideally be based on a scientific approach, taking into account not only an integrated, comprehensive and rigorous assessment of benefits and risks, but also of other relevant evidence and associated uncertainty, as well as contextual information and ethical aspects.

When serious adverse events following immunisation (AEFIs) are detected, urgent causality assessment precedes any benefit–risk assessment, as outlined in Chapter 18, Section 18.4. When this is inconclusive, or has not led to decisions to modify the programme, benefit–risk analyses are an important next step. In the present chapter we start with some examples illustrating why conducting benefit–risk assessments of vaccination programmes is important. We then describe benefit–risk frameworks, integrated benefit–risk measures and population health metrics.

21.1 The need for benefit–risk assessment of vaccination programmes

Vaccination programmes may need to be modified or extended, for example to target new populations, adjust vaccination schedules, introduce booster doses or to switch vaccines. Such adaptations may be necessary to respond to emerging concerns over vaccine safety. These adjustments and responses should be evidence-based. Concerns about vaccine safety have a negative impact on the uptake of the vaccine for which concerns exist, and may affect uptake of other vaccines. Hence, such vaccine safety concerns need to be addressed with urgency but also with care. In particular, it is important to place adverse events and their frequency of occurrence in the context of the benefits provided by the vaccine. Yet all too often, such assessments are undertaken in crisis management mode, without careful consideration for the implications of different courses of action. In this section we provide several examples to illustrate the importance of benefit–risk assessments to support public health decision-making. Box 21.1 describes benefit–risk assessments used for rotavirus vaccination.

Box 21.1 Rotavirus vaccination and intussusception

Nine months after an oral rhesus-human reassortant rotavirus tetravalent vaccine (RotaShield) was licensed in the United States in October 1998, the immunisation programme was suspended because of a temporal association between rotavirus vaccination and intussusception (IS), a condition in which one segment of the intestine telescopes inside another. If left untreated, IS can be fatal. The estimated relative risk (RR) of IS during the 3–7 days after RotaShield administration was

58.9 (95% confidence interval (CI), 31.7–109.6) after dose 1 and 11.0 (95% CI, 4.1–29.5) after dose 2. These increased risks resulted in the withdrawal of the RotaShield vaccine recommendation in the United States. This decision made it impossible for the vaccine to be used elsewhere, including regions for which the rotavirus burden is much higher compared to the United States.

Since 2006, two live-attenuated rotavirus vaccines have been licensed in more than 100 countries: Rotarix, a two-dose schedule oral human rotavirus vaccine, and RotaTeq, a three-dose schedule oral human–bovine reassortant rotavirus vaccine. A meta-analysis reported an overall estimate of RR for IS following Rotarix of 5.4 (95% CI, 3.9–7.4) after dose 1 and of 1.8 (95% CI, 1.3–2.5) after dose 2. For RotaTeq, the estimates were 5.5 (95% CI, 3.3–9.3) after dose 1 and 1.7 (95% CI, 1.1–2.6) after dose 2.

It is important to evaluate the increased risk of IS associated with rotavirus immunisation in relation to the benefits of vaccination in reducing hospitalisations and deaths related to rotavirus gastroenteritis (RVGE). The baseline incidences of hospitalisations or deaths for RVGE and IS in the absence of vaccination are country-specific and are higher in low- and middle-income countries. Several studies have been conducted in different geographical settings to investigate the benefit–risk profile of rotavirus vaccination. A systematic review by Arlegui, Nachbaur, Praet, and Begaud (2020) found that, depending on the benefit–risk model used, vaccination with Rotarix or RotaTeq according to the national or World Health Organization (WHO) recommended vaccination schedule would prevent 190 to 1,624 RVGE-related hospitalisations for every IS-related hospitalisation induced and 71 to 743 RVGE-related deaths for every IS-related death induced. All studies concluded that the benefits outweigh the risks.

The example of rotavirus vaccination illustrates the importance of considering a confirmed risk in relation to the benefits conferred by vaccination. Even when the risks are not yet confirmed or the benefits not well established, a benefit–risk assessment might help decision-making. This is illustrated in Box 21.2, describing contrasting responses to the controversy in the early 1990s surrounding hepatitis B vaccination in France and Italy.

Box 21.2 Hepatitis B vaccination in France and Italy

Since the early 1990s, several cases of multiple sclerosis (MS) were reported in France among people who had received hepatitis B vaccine. Because of this and the growing public concern, the Health Ministry of France decided to suspend the school-based hepatitis B vaccination campaign. The decision was based on spontaneous reports of MS cases in hepatitis B vaccinees, a pilot case-control study and two case-control studies. The studies all showed odds ratios suggesting an

(continued)

increased risk, though the individual odds ratios were not statistically significant (pilot study: 1.7, 95% CI: 0.5–6.3; French case-control study: 1.4. 95% CI: 0.4–4.5 and UK case-control study: 1.4, 95% CI: 0.8–2.4). The overall evidence was assessed as indicating a true causal relationship between hepatitis B vaccination and MS. The decision was taken to suspend the hepatitis B vaccination campaign despite an endorsement of the efficacy of the vaccine by the French government. This decision was strongly criticised by WHO for the potentially negative consequences on the acceptance and vaccination uptake of hepatitis B and other vaccines (Jefferson & Traversa, 2002).

At the same time, modifications to the hepatitis B vaccination policy in Italy were under discussion. To support decision-making, a simulation study was carried out for Italy assuming that there was a true causal association between hepatitis B vaccination and MS. The study showed that vaccinating 100,000 adolescents would incur 0.7 cases of MS but also prevent 1,099 cases of hepatitis B, including 58 cases with chronic progression. The Italian government decided not to change the vaccination strategy adopted in Italy (Jefferson & Traversa, 2002).

A third example illustrating the importance of benefit–risk assessments is the human papillomavirus (HPV) vaccination controversy that started in Japan in 2013. After a cluster of adverse events suspected to be linked to HPV vaccination were reported in the Japanese media, the Japanese government decided to suspend the HPV vaccine recommendations. Box 21.3 describes these events and their consequences.

Box 21.3 HPV vaccine controversy in Japan

In Japan, free HPV vaccination started in 2010 followed by its inclusion in the national immunisation programme in April 2013 for girls aged 12 to 16 years. Soon after the implementation of routine HPV vaccination, several adverse events suspected to be linked to HPV, such as chronic pain after HPV vaccination, were reported. The concerns spread widely via the Japanese mass media, and the Japanese government decided to suspend the recommendations for the HPV vaccine. As a consequence, the HPV vaccine coverage in Japan has dropped from more than 70% to less than 1% since 2013. The adverse events have since been found to be unrelated to HPV vaccination (Ikeda et al., 2019).

In 2020, HPV vaccine coverage was still very low in Japan, despite the vaccine being freely available but not being proactively recommended. Given the long latency period between HPV infection and diagnosis of invasive cancer, the long-term consequences of the low HPV vaccine coverage in terms of morbidity and mortality due to cervical cancer and other HPV-related cancers will not be seen for many years. To assess the impact, a mathematical simulation model was developed. This model suggested that the suspension of the HPV vaccination recommendation in Japan would result in an additional 24,600–27,300 cases and 5,000–5,700 deaths due to cervical cancer compared with what would occur had the coverage remained at around 70% (Simms, Hanley, Smith, Keane, & Canfell, 2020).

21.2 Benefit–risk assessment frameworks

For a benefit–risk assessment to be comprehensive and useful, it should start with clearly framing the benefit–risk question. To this end, benefit–risk assessment frameworks have been developed listing a certain number of generic steps to perform the assessment. These frameworks are useful to ensure that all elements important to the benefit–risk assessment have been considered and are rendered explicit, thereby aiming to improve transparency and to facilitate communication.

The PrOACT-URL and Benefit Risk Action Team (BRAT) frameworks are both frequently used within pharmaceutical and regulatory science to describe the benefit–risk assessment of pharmaceutical products, including vaccines. The two frameworks are similar, with the European Medicines Agency (EMA) referring to the effects table of the PrOACT-URL framework in its documentation while the US Food and Drug Administration (FDA) refers to the BRAT framework. Both descriptive frameworks are standardised, yet flexible, and allow for the inclusion of quantitative methods. Both frameworks are generally suited for the evaluation of vaccination programmes. The main difference is that, unlike the BRAT framework, the PrOACT-URL framework explicitly considers wider issues of risk attitudes and consistency with similar past decisions, which are both important considerations for vaccination programmes. Box 21.4 gives a description of the PrOACT-URL framework, which derived its name from the eight steps described there.

Box 21.4 PrOACT-URL framework

The PrOACT-URL framework is an eight-step decision-analysis framework (Hammond, Keeney, & Raiffa, 1999). It is not specific to the benefit–risk assessment of vaccines, which explains its generic terminology (such as 'criteria', 'alternatives' and 'consequences'). It is slightly adapted here for use with vaccines (Table 21.1).

Table 21.1 The eight steps of the PrOACT-URL framework

1. Problem	To determine the nature of the problem, its context and to frame the benefit–risk question. This includes a description of the vaccine-preventable disease epidemiology, the unmet medical need, the vaccine product, the vaccination schedule (number of doses and age at vaccination) and the target population(s).

(continued)

Table 21.1 Cont.

2. Objective	To establish the objectives that indicate the overall purposes of the benefit–risk assessment (e.g., informing vaccine introduction or cessation, changing the vaccination schedule or updating after a safety signal) and identify the relevant criteria related to the benefits and risks of the vaccination programme. These are usually health outcomes, but could also include others (e.g., the risk of over-burdening the health system during winter months). Hereby, conservative choices can be made by, for instance including possible, not confirmed risks. It is important to also specify the time period over which the benefits and risks are measured (the analytic horizon) and the perspective (individual or societal). An individual perspective means that only the benefits and risks to the vaccinated individuals are considered. A societal perspective means that the benefits and risks of vaccination to the whole society are considered (including the indirect effects). The benefits and risks are often summarised hierarchically using a value tree (see Box 21.6).
3. Alternatives	To identify relevant alternatives (or comparators) to the intervention for which the benefit–risk assessment is initiated. A common alternative is absence of vaccination. Other potential alternatives include withdrawal of the vaccine, the use of an alternative vaccine or alternative vaccination schedule (e.g., changes to the number of doses or age at vaccination).
4. Consequences	To describe how the intervention of interest and its alternative(s) perform on the different benefit and risk criteria. These include measures of vaccine effectiveness and impact (benefits), vaccine safety (risks) but might also include other measures such as the expected number of cases, hospitalisations and deaths prevented and induced. The effects are summarised using benefit–risk tables.
5. Trade-offs	To assess the balance between benefits and risks. This assessment is often based on qualitative clinical judgement. Sometimes a quantitative approach is taken by eliciting preference weights using standardised preference elicitation methods. The weights then reflect the relative importance of the different benefit and risk criteria and allow the calculation of overall benefit–risk scores. The question of which weights to use for vaccines is challenging. For therapeutic drugs, it is the patient who is benefiting from the drugs but is also taking the risks, so patient preferences are informative. For vaccination programmes with major implications for the wider community, the preferences of health authorities, the general, non-patient public and healthcare providers may be most informative.
6. Uncertainty	To describe qualitatively the uncertainty regarding the performance of the intervention of interest and its alternative(s) in terms of benefit and risk criteria. For instance, there might be substantial uncertainty regarding the long-term benefits of vaccination or additional safety studies may be needed to estimate more accurately the vaccine risk.

7. Risk tolerance	To evaluate the relative importance of the decision maker's tolerance towards the risks (adverse reactions in case of vaccine-related decisions) associated with the decision and how this affects the benefit-risk balance reported in step 5. In general, the tolerance towards adverse reactions is lower for vaccines given to healthy people – especially healthy infants and toddlers – to prevent certain conditions than towards other pharmaceutical products used to treat people with an illness. The risk tolerance might be further affected by whether vaccination is recommended or mandated.
8. Linked decisions	To consider the consistency of this decision with similar past decisions, and assess whether this decision could impact on future decisions. This is particularly important as the decision on a particular vaccine might have consequences on the public acceptance of other vaccines.

The PrOACT-URL framework is illustrated for HPV vaccination in boys in Box 21.5. This benefit–risk assessment is meant for illustration only and is not intended to be comprehensive: a rigorous assessment would stretch to many pages. The studies and epidemiological evidence are selected from recent guidance from the European Centre for Disease Prevention and Control (ECDC) on HPV vaccination (ECDC, 2020).

Box 21.5 PrOACT-URL framework applied to HPV vaccination in boys

HPV is a common sexually transmitted infection causing cervical cancer, other less common genital and non-genital cancers, as well as genital warts. HPV vaccination for girls is generally recommended in Europe. Recently, some European countries recommended the use of HPV vaccination in boys. The benefit–risk assessment presented in Table 21.2 is meant for illustration only.

Table 21.2 A benefit–risk assessment of HPV vaccination in boys

1. Problem	In Europe, 14,700 annual cases of anogenital cancers other than cervical are attributable to HPV, with 5,400 cases diagnosed in men (about half in the anus and half in the penis). It is estimated that 1,097 cases of anal intraepithelial neoplasia stages 2/3 (AIN2/3) in men are diagnosed each year. Head and neck cancers also constitute a heavy burden, with an estimated 11,000 cases diagnosed annually in males. No organised screening for HPV-related cancers is currently available for men. Currently, three HPV vaccines are licensed in Europe; a bivalent, a quadrivalent and a nonavalent vaccine.

(*continued*)

Table 21.2 Cont.

2. Objective	To assess the benefit–risk of HPV vaccination in young males (16–26 years old). The benefits are the prevention of 6-month persistent infection, anal intraepithelial neoplasia, penile intraepithelial neoplasia and genital warts. The risks are syncope and anaphylaxis. A value tree is given in Box 21.6. The analytic horizon is as long as possible, within the limits of data availability. The perspective is societal, allowing for data on vaccination impact when available. The age at vaccination and the number of doses are as reported.
3. Alternatives	The assessment compares HPV vaccination to 'no vaccination' as there is currently no other prevention strategy (no organised screening for HPV-related cancer in men).
4. Consequences	As HPV vaccination for boys has only recently been introduced in a limited number of countries, the evidence on the benefits of vaccinating boys currently comes from randomised clinical trials. There is no evidence on clinical outcomes in boys for the bivalent HPV vaccine. For safety, evidence on HPV vaccine safety in girls can be used. The evidence on HPV vaccine safety has been recently reviewed by the Global Advisory Committee for Vaccine Safety (GACVS) of WHO. The evidence is summarised in the benefit–risk table provided in Box 21.7.
5. Trade-offs	Given the long-standing use of HPV vaccination in girls and the excellent safety profiles of the three HPV vaccines, the benefit–risk of HPV vaccination in boys is considered positive.
6. Uncertainty	The uncertainty of the evidence has been assessed. The uncertainty of the efficacy against penile intraepithelial neoplasia is high due to its wide confidence intervals.
7. Risk tolerance	For countries with high HPV vaccine coverage in girls, the tolerance towards potential adverse reactions to HPV vaccines is considered high.
8. Linked decisions	Recommending gender-neutral HPV vaccination is consistent with the current recommendations for HPV vaccination in girls.

A value tree (also called an attribute tree or outcome tree) is sometimes used in conjunction with specific steps within the benefit–risk assessment frameworks. A value tree is a visual, hierarchical display of key benefit and risk outcomes relevant to the benefit–risk assessment. An example of a value tree related to HPV vaccination in boys is given in Box 21.6.

Box 21.6 A value tree applied to HPV vaccination in boys

Figure 21.1 gives an example of a value tree related to HPV vaccination in boys. For illustration, only the main benefits and risks in boys are represented in this tree, although vaccinating boys also induces benefits for girls.

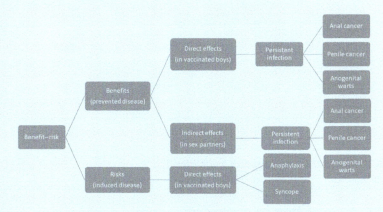

Figure 21.1 Example of a value tree related to HPV vaccination in boys, showing the benefits for boys only.

The tabular summaries then take as their starting columns the terminal nodes of the value tree and minimally include the effect measures for the vaccination programme under evaluation (and its comparator when the comparator is different from 'no vaccination'), the sources and the associated uncertainty. Box 21.7 provides a benefit–risk table for HPV vaccination in boys.

Box 21.7 Benefit–risk table applied to HPV vaccination in boys

Table 21.3 contains the benefit–risk table for HPV vaccines. The row headings correspond to the terminal nodes of the value tree in Box 21.6. The uncertainty is a judgement about the reliability of the estimate, based here on the width of the confidence intervals.

(continued)

Table 21.3 Benefit–risk assessment of HPV vaccination in boys and young men (16–26 years)

Benefits*		Vaccine efficacy (95% CI)	Uncertainty	Source
	6MPI	85.6% (73.4–92.9)	Low	Giuliano et al. (2011)
	AIN2/3	89.6% (57.2–98.8)	Low	Goldstone et al. (2013)
	PeIN2/3	100.0% (–425.5–100)	high	Goldstone et al. (2013)
	Anogenital warts	90.4% (69.2–98.1)	Low	Giuliano et al. (2011)
Risks (severe adverse events)		Vaccine-associated risk		
	Anaphylaxis	1.7 (0.04–9.3) cases per million doses	Low	Gee et al. (2011)
	Syncope	Common anxiety reaction to injection	Low	Bernard, Cooper Robbins, McCaffery, Scott, and Skinner (2011)

Note: 6MPI: 6-month persistent infection; AIN2/3: anal intraepithelial neoplasia grade 2 and 3 (precursor of anal cancer); CI: confidence interval; PeIN2/3: penile intraepithelial neoplasia grade 2 and 3 (precursor of penile cancer).
* Vaccine efficacy based on the per-protocol analysis against the four HPV genotypes of the quadrivalent vaccine. The same efficacy is assumed for the nonavalent vaccine.

To be able to take a decision on a positive or negative benefit–risk balance of a certain health intervention, it is often sufficient to set out the benefits and risks systematically and in context as described in this section, without combining them into an integrated benefit–risk measure. This is the case when the benefits far outweigh the risks, or, alternatively, when the risks are more frequent than the benefits. When the benefit–risk balance is not obvious, when multiple benefit and risk outcomes are involved or when a summary measure for communication to the general public is required, integrated benefit–risk measures might be helpful. These are discussed in the following section.

21.3 Integrated measures of benefit and risk

These measures seek to combine quantitative evaluations of benefits and risks in a single numerical summary. Several options are commonly used, which are described in the following subsections. Very often in benefit–risk assessments, simulation models are used to predict the expected benefits and risks based on input parameters related to the vaccine-preventable disease burden, vaccine coverage, vaccine effectiveness, impact and safety. These input parameters are obtained from a range of sources such as surveillance or epidemiological studies.

Like all numerical summaries, benefit–risk measures are subject to uncertainty. This uncertainty may be statistical as represented by a 95% confidence interval (95% CI), but it may also be derived from the simulation model. In this case, the uncertainty is represented by a 95% uncertainty interval (95% UI), which represents the typical variation obtained in such simulations. Sensitivity analyses, undertaken by varying the assumptions upon which the calculations are based, may also help to determine the robustness of the results.

21.3.1 Ratio of benefit and risk

The benefit–risk ratio is intended as a programmatic or policy-oriented benefit–risk measure, which can encompass the direct and indirect effects of a vaccination programme or the consequences of a certain policy decision regarding the programme. The benefit–risk ratio, denoted BRR, is the ratio of a specified benefit and a specified risk, expressed in terms of numbers of cases averted (the benefit) or caused (the risk) by the vaccine under a particular course of action. The BRR is defined as:

$$BRR = \frac{Number\ of\ cases\ of\ disease\ averted}{Number\ of\ cases\ of\ harm\ caused}.$$

In this definition, the number of cases averted need not all be in vaccinees: it may include cases averted through indirect effects. The number of cases of harm, on the other hand, may include adverse reactions to vaccination, or the wider adverse consequences of a given policy. The interpretation of the BRR is the number of disease events prevented by the programme or policy for every adverse event caused. The BRR can be used to assess the benefit–risk associated with the introduction of a vaccination programme or a modification to a vaccination programme, or its suspension: the numerator and denominator in the BRR then correspond to the numbers of cases averted or caused by that modification. The BRR, however, does not account for potential differences in severity between vaccine-prevented and vaccine-induced events; these are addressed in Section 21.4. An example is provided in Box 21.8 showing a benefit–risk analysis of suspending routine childhood immunisation during the COVID-19 pandemic in Africa. Several of the mathematical models used to predict the benefit of sustained routine childhood immunisation accounted for the indirect effects of vaccination.

Box 21.8 Benefit–risk of suspending routine childhood immunisation during the COVID-19 pandemic in Africa

Abbas et al. (2020) compared the health benefits of sustaining routine childhood immunisation as part of the Expanded Programme on Immunization (EPI) to the risk of acquiring severe acute respiratory syndrome coronavirus 2 (SARS-CoV-2) infection through visiting routine vaccination service delivery points in Africa.

The benefits of sustained routine childhood immunisation were predicted using various pathogen-specific mathematical models, several of them accounting for the indirect effects of vaccination. An additional mathematical model was developed to predict the excess risk of COVID-19 disease during immunisation visits. The scenario of sustained immunisation was compared to a scenario where routine vaccination was suspended for 6 months without catch-up. The benefits from immunisation relate to children up to 5 years of age while the additional SARS-CoV-2 risks were modelled for the vaccinated child, their carer and household members. The results are presented in terms of prevented and excess deaths. The results for diphtheria, tetanus, pertussis and measles are given in Table 21.4.

Table 21.4 Vaccine-specific benefits and risks of sustaining routine childhood immunisation in Africa during the COVID-19 pandemic

Vaccine	Vaccination schedule	Deaths averted by vaccination (95% UI)	Excess COVID-19 deaths (95% UI)	Benefit–risk ratio (95% UI)
Diphtheria	6, 10, 14 weeks	12,944 (10,180–16,539)	5,674 (846–16,830)	2 (0.4–7)
Tetanus	6, 10, 14 weeks	69,254 (54,268–87,343)	5,674 (846–16,830)	12 (2–39)
Pertussis	6, 10, 14 weeks	271,422 (207,238–344,147)	5,674 (846–16,830)	48 (8–155)
Measles	9 months	194,388 (181,469–209,379)	1,896 (228–5,778)	103 (16–332)

Note: UI: uncertainty interval.

Benefit–risk ratios favourable for sustained routine childhood immunisation were found for all vaccines covered by the EPI. The authors recommended that routine childhood immunisation should be sustained in Africa as much as possible during the COVID-19 pandemic.

The quantification of the *BRR* illustrated in Box 21.8 is widely applicable, and particularly useful when the benefits and risks relate to directly comparable outcomes.

Estimates of vaccine effectiveness and vaccine-associated risks, obtained in epidemiological studies, are typically used to derive estimates of the *BRR*. In some circumstances the benefits may only relate to the direct effects of vaccination, often leading to an underestimation of the *BRR*. An example is provided in Box 21.9.

Box 21.9 Benefit–risk ratio of rotavirus vaccination in Latin America

Routine rotavirus vaccination was introduced in 2006 in Brazil and in 2007 in Mexico. Patel et al. (2011) performed a benefit–risk analysis using epidemiological data to assess the likely benefits and risks associated with the rotavirus vaccination programme as compared to no programme in Mexico and Brazil. For their calculations, they assumed that the entire birth cohort would be vaccinated and was followed for 5 years.

The benefits of the rotavirus vaccination programme were calculated as the estimated number of rotavirus-associated deaths and hospitalisations prevented by the age of 5 years, on the basis of published estimates of vaccine effectiveness and the baseline rotavirus disease burden in the region. The risk of the rotavirus vaccination programme was calculated as the excess number of vaccine-associated deaths and hospitalisations due to IS, which was obtained as the product of the baseline incidence of IS and the country-specific risk of IS associated with rotavirus vaccination.

The results for Mexico (see Table 21.5) indicated a *BRR* of 331.5 rotavirus-related deaths prevented for every IS-related death induced. The *BRR* ratio for hospitalisations was 281.7 rotavirus-related hospitalisations prevented for every IS-related hospitalisation induced. The authors concluded that the real-world benefits of the rotavirus vaccination programme far outweigh the potential short-term risk of IS associated with the vaccine.

Table 21.5 Effect of rotavirus vaccination programme as compared with no rotavirus vaccination programme, on deaths and hospitalisations associated with diarrhoea and intussusception in Mexico

	Without vaccination programme	With vaccination programme	Number of events averted or caused	Benefit–risk ratio
Deaths				
Rotavirus diarrhoea	923	260	663 averted	331.5
Intussusception	61	63	2 caused	

(continued)

Table 21.5 Cont.

Hospitalisations				
Rotavirus diarrhoea	16,086	4,535	11,551 averted	281.7
Intussusception	1,215	1,256	41 caused	

Source: Patel et al. (2011).

Often, conclusive *BRR* estimates can be obtained without accounting for indirect effects. Allowing for indirect effects increases the *BRR* compared to its value based on direct effects only. However, the likely indirect effects may be difficult to estimate during the early days of a vaccination programme, as only a small proportion of the population is vaccinated. For this reason, mathematical models are sometimes used to allow for them. An example will be presented in Box 21.13.

21.3.2 Numbers needed to vaccinate and to harm

When the *BRR* is restricted to direct effects, the numerator is the number of cases of disease directly averted by vaccination. In this case, the *BRR* can be written as

$$BRR = \frac{P_u - P_v}{Q_v - Q_u},$$

where P_u and P_v are the risks of the vaccine-preventable disease in unvaccinated and vaccinated individuals and Q_v and Q_u are the adverse event risks.

In this special case when only direct effects are considered, the *BRR* is also equal to the ratio of number needed to harm (*NNH*) to the number needed to vaccinate (*NNV*), or

$$BRR = \frac{P_u - P_v}{Q_v - Q_u} = \frac{1/NNV}{1/NNH} = \frac{NNH}{NNV}.$$

The *NNV* indicates the average number of patients who have to be vaccinated to prevent one adverse outcome of the disease within a specific period of time. Thus, the *NNV* is the reciprocal of the absolute risk reduction or

$$NNV = \frac{1}{P_u - P_v},$$

where P_u and P_v is the risk of the vaccine-preventable disease in unvaccinated and vaccinated individuals, respectively, during a specified period of follow-up (typically some years after vaccination). Note that the *NNV* is only defined when $P_u > P_v$, otherwise its value is negative or infinite. Similarly, the *NNH* is

$$NNH = \frac{1}{Q_v - Q_u},$$

where Q_u and Q_v are the adverse event risks in unvaccinated and vaccinated individuals at any time during follow-up. The *NNH* is then to be interpreted as the average number of patients who need to be vaccinated to induce one adverse event during follow-up (for acute adverse events, this may be a few days or weeks after vaccination). Similarly to the *NNV*, the *NNH* is only defined when $Q_v > Q_u$.

Then, to evaluate the direct benefit–risk of vaccination in individuals, *NNV* and *NNH* can be simply compared, with *NNV* < *NNH* indicating a positive benefit–risk balance. However, such a comparison is only valid when the *NNV* and *NNH* calculations are calculated for the same population and when equal importance can be attached to the benefit and risk outcome. An example is given in Box 21.10.

Box 21.10 *NNV* and *NNH* for a specific influenza vaccine

In 2010, Australian and New Zealand health authorities identified a trivalent inactivated seasonal influenza vaccine as the probable cause of increased febrile convulsions in children <5 years of age within 24 hours of vaccination and recommended against its use in this age group. A benefit–risk assessment based on *NNV* and *NNH* was subsequently carried out (Kelly, Carcione, Dowse, & Effler, 2010). The comparator was no vaccination.

Based on the estimated influenza hospitalisation risk in unvaccinated children of 90/100,000 children < 5 years and an assumed vaccine effectiveness of 60% the *NNV* was calculated as

$$NNV = \frac{1}{90/100,000 \times 0.6} = 1,852,$$

meaning that 1,852 children need to be vaccinated to prevent one influenza-related hospitalisation that season.

The risk of febrile convulsions following vaccination with the influenza vaccine of concern was estimated to be 0.39%. It was further estimated that 34% of children with febrile convulsions require hospitalisation. When no vaccine was given (the comparator), the risk of febrile convulsions was set to 0%. Based on these numbers the *NNH* was calculated as

$$NNH = \frac{1}{0.0039 \times 0.34 - 0} = 754,$$

meaning that for every 754 vaccinated children one child is expected to be hospitalised for febrile convulsions. As the *NNV* was substantially larger than the *NNH*, it was concluded that the benefit–risk balance of that specific influenza

(continued)

> vaccine was not favourable for children < 5 years of age. The Ministry of Health in New Zealand recommended specifically against the use of the influenza vaccine of concern in children < 5 years but recommended the continued use of other influenza vaccines licensed for children in this age group.

The example in Box 21.10 illustrates how a benefit–risk analysis can help to identify a negative benefit–risk balance, resulting in immediate action by the health authorities. It may be less clear to determine the policy implications of a positive benefit–risk balance. The policy implications will depend on the severity of the health outcomes involved: a vaccination programme that might induce some vaccine-related deaths needs a decidedly more positive *BRR* compared to a vaccination programme without vaccine-related deaths. The uncertainty associated with the *BRR* should also be acceptably low before policy decisions can be taken. In some circumstances, a *BRR* only marginally greater than 1 may not be sufficiently beneficial to alter an existing vaccination programme.

The *BRR* as well as the *NNV–NNH* comparison cannot handle multiple benefits and risks. However, they have the advantage of the straightforward interpretation of the number of disease events prevented for every adverse event incurred. Sometimes, the risk–benefit ratio (*RBR*) is used instead. The *RBR* is simply the reciprocal of the *BRR* and gives the number of adverse events incurred for every disease event prevented.

21.3.3 Difference in benefit and risk

The benefit–risk difference is the difference in benefits and risks where both benefits and risks are expressed using the same type of health outcome. The benefit–risk difference is also called the net health benefit, denoted *NHB*. The *NHB* for a single benefit and single risk outcome is calculated as

$$NHB = E - R,$$

where E refers to the benefit (number of cases prevented or averted potentially including indirect effects) and R to the risk (number of cases induced or incurred) of the vaccination programme with both E and R expressed using the same type of health outcome. An example is given in Box 21.11.

> **Box 21.11 Benefit–risk difference of rotavirus vaccination in Japan**
>
> Ledent et al. (2016) evaluated the benefits and risks of rotavirus vaccination in Japanese children. Using a simulation model, events of RVGE and IS were generated for a birth cohort of 1 million Japanese children followed for a period of 5-year post-vaccination. Data from disease surveillance, efficacy/effectiveness and safety studies were used to inform the parameters of the simulation model.

The simulation model has the advantage of translating vaccine effectiveness and relative risk estimates into numbers of disease prevented and induced, which can then be used to obtain a benefit–risk difference. To account for the uncertainty in the parameters of the simulation model, Monte Carlo simulation was used to generate 95% uncertainty intervals.

The benefit–risk difference shows that 17,855 hospitalisations and 6.3 deaths could be averted in a birth cohort of 1 million Japanese children followed for 5 years after rotavirus vaccination (Table 21.6).

Table 21.6 Benefit–risk of rotavirus vaccination in a birth cohort of 1 million Japanese children followed for 5 years post-vaccination (with 95% UI)

	Benefits	Risks	Benefit–risk difference
	Prevented RVGE	Excess IS	Prevented RVGE minus excess IS
Hospitalisations	17,925 (11,715–23,276)	50 (7.2–237)	17,855 (11,643–23,213)
Deaths	6.3 (4.1–8.2)	0.017 (0.0020–0.097)	6.3 (4.1–8.2)

IS: intussusception; RVGE: rotavirus gastroenteritis.

A second example is provided in Box 21.12. In this example, the benefits and risks of rotavirus vaccination with and without age restrictions are compared.

Box 21.12 Benefits and risks of removing the age restrictions for rotavirus vaccination

A simulation model was used to predict the number of deaths prevented by rotavirus vaccination and the number of IS deaths caused by rotavirus vaccination when administered on the previously recommended, restricted schedule (initiate by 15 weeks and complete by 32 weeks) versus a schedule allowing vaccination up to 3 years of age (Patel, Clarke, Sanderson, Tate, & Parashar, 2012).

The simulated cohort included children < 5 y of age in 158 low- and middle-income countries with a birth cohort of 123.6 million where 99.9% of the global rotavirus mortality occurs. Inputs to the simulation model were estimates of rotavirus mortality, IS mortality and predicted vaccination rates by week of age, vaccine effectiveness and vaccine-associated IS risk.

The model predicted that removing the age restrictions would avert an additional 47,200 rotavirus deaths (5th–95th centiles: 18,700–63,000) and cause an

(*continued*)

additional 294 (5th–95th centiles: 161–471) IS deaths. It was concluded that, in low- and middle-income countries, the additional lives saved by removing age restrictions for rotavirus vaccination would by far outnumber the excess vaccine-associated IS deaths, the benefit–risk difference being of the order of 47,000 deaths (Table 21.7).

Table 21.7 Rotavirus deaths averted versus excess IS deaths caused under age-restricted and age-unrestricted rotavirus vaccination strategies

	Rotavirus deaths averted Median (5th–95th centile)	IS deaths caused Median (5th–95th centile)
Vaccination strategy		
(A) Age restriction	155,800 (83,300–217,700)	253 (76–689)
(B) No age restriction	203,000 (102,000–281,500)	547 (237–1,160)
Comparison of vaccination strategies		
Difference (strategy B minus strategy A)	47,200 (18,700–63,700)	294 (161–471)

Source: Patel et al. (2012).

Whether to use benefit–risk differences or benefit–risk ratios depends in part on context. One advantage of the ratio measure is that it is invariant to scaling of benefits and risks by the same constant. This may be an advantage if only a proportion of events included in the benefit and risk calculations are ascertained, or if simulation models are used with approximate scaling. On the other hand, the benefit–risk difference is more clearly a measure of impact, and may be preferable when indirect effects are allowed for. This issue is brought to the fore in the example in Box 21.13, also on rotavirus vaccination. This example accounts for the indirect effects of vaccination, and compares the relationship between benefit–risk ratios and benefit–risk differences in this context.

Box 21.13 Benefit–risk ratio of rotavirus vaccination in France

Escolano, Mueller, and Tubert-Bitter (2020) developed a simulation model to quantify the benefits and risks of rotavirus vaccination in France. Key parameters were epidemiological and demographic data (number of children eligible for vaccination, vaccine coverage), the relative risk of IS in the 3 weeks following administration and the vaccine effectiveness, including direct and indirect effects. The direct effects are in vaccinated individuals only and correspond to the vaccine efficacy estimated in clinical trials, with decreasing protection during the first 3 years after vaccination. The indirect effects relate to the reduction of disease incidence in vaccinated and non-vaccinated individuals from herd immunity and were quantified approximately using a formula involving vaccine coverage, the basic reproduction number and the vaccine efficacy. The results for both benefit–risk ratios and benefit–risk differences and for different vaccine coverages are summarised in Table 21.8.

Table 21.8 Estimated annual benefit–risk ratio and difference of hospitalisations due to rotavirus vaccination in France, assuming various vaccine coverages, with and without accounting for the indirect effects of vaccination

	Vaccine coverage		
	10%	50%	90%
Direct effects only (95% UI)			
Rotavirus diarrhoea hospitalisations prevented	998.4 (756.1–1,280)	4,990 (3,800–6,420)	8,970 (6,830–11,540)
IS hospitalisations induced	6.1 (3.9–9.3)	30.3 (19.3–46.3)	54.6 (35.0–83.8)
Benefit–risk ratio	164.4	164.4	164.4
Benefit–risk difference	992.3	4,959.7	8,915.4
Direct and indirect effects (95% UI)			
Rotavirus diarrhoea hospitalisations prevented	1,696 (1,274–2,173)	7,120 (5,416–9,170)	10,500 (8,050–13,420)
IS hospitalisations induced	6.1 (3.9–9.3)	30.3 (19.3–46.3)	54.6 (35.0–83.8)
Benefit–risk ratio	278.0	234.9	192.3
Benefit–risk difference	1,689.9	7,089.7	10,445.4

Source: Escolano et al. (2020).

For each of the assumed levels of vaccine coverage, the benefit–risk ratios and benefit–risk differences are higher when accounting for indirect effects compared to not accounting for indirect effects. This is explained because the additional indirect benefits arise without any additional vaccination risk. When only accounting for direct effects, the benefit–risk ratio is not affected by the vaccine coverage: both the benefits and risk are proportional to coverage. When also accounting for indirect effects, both the benefit–risk difference and the benefit–risk ratio are affected by the vaccine coverage.

Box 21.13 shows that benefit–risk differences increase with vaccine coverage (for coverages below the critical threshold), whether or not indirect effects are allowed for. However, this may not be true for the benefit–risk ratio: indeed, in Box 21.13, the highest value of the *BRR* is obtained at low vaccine coverage. This reflects the fact that the marginal benefit from indirect effects is greatest at low coverages. This observation suggests that the *BRR* should not generally be used to identify optimal vaccination policies incorporating indirect effects: benefit–risk differences are likely to be more useful measures of global impact for such purposes.

21.4 Population health metrics

The benefit–risk examples provided so far were for a comparison of a single benefit to a single risk or for a comparison of benefits and risks of the same type, such as hospitalisations induced to hospitalisations prevented or deaths induced to deaths prevented. However, evaluating the benefit–risk balance is more complicated when several benefit and risk outcomes of varying severity are to be considered. In this case, population health metrics can be used. Population health metrics typically combine data on the frequency of disease occurrence and the severity of disease.

The most commonly used population health metrics are quality-adjusted life years (QALYs) and disability-adjusted life years (DALYs). Both the DALY and QALY measures can be viewed as complements of each other and are often used interchangeably (Sassi, 2006). QALYs were initially developed to perform cost-effectiveness analysis while DALYs were developed to quantify and regionally compare burden of disease.

21.4.1 Quality-adjusted life years

Today, quality-adjusted life years or QALYs are used in most health economic evaluations to assess the value of medical interventions, typically in terms of QALYs gained from the intervention (Sassi, 2006). QALY is a health expectancy measure. It is used to correct someone's life expectancy based on the levels of health-related quality of life they are predicted to experience throughout the course of their life, or part of it. The QALY metric is thus a function of length of life and quality of life and is calculated (for a given health state) as

$$QALY = years\ of\ life\ spent\ in\ health\ state \times utitlity\ value,$$

where the utility value reflects the quality of life and ranges from 1 (perfect health) to 0 (comparable to death). Health states worse than death have negative values. The QALYs for each health state are then summed to give the overall QALY. An illustration of how to calculate QALYs is provided in Box 21.14.

Box 21.14 Calculating QALYs

HPV infection is a sexually transmitted infection that can be prevented by vaccination and is the main and necessary cause of cervical cancer. Consider calculating the number of QALYs lived by a woman in a period of 20 years, in which 10 years are lived in perfect health (assigned utility weight: 1), after which cervical cancer was diagnosed and treated for a period of 1 year (assigned utility weight: 0.617) while the remaining 9 years are lived with cured cervical cancer (assigned utility weight: 0.95). For this event history, the QALYs are:

$$10 \times 1 + 1 \times 0.617 + 9 \times 0.95 = 19.167 \, QALYs.$$

The utility values needed to calculate QALYs reflect the preference or value that a person or society gives to a particular health state. Broadly, techniques to measure utility values may be categorised in two groups: direct and indirect methods. Direct methods are based on mapping preferences directly on to the utility scale, often done by means of trade-off methods such as standard gamble or time trade-off. Indirect methods are based on mapping preferences on to the utility scale indirectly via a generic health-related quality-of-life questionnaire. For a more in-depth discussion on health utility estimation, see Torrance, Furlong, and Feeny (2002).

The benefit–risk balance is then evaluated as described above, using ratios or differences of QALYs. Box 21.15 illustrates how QALYs were used to quantify the benefits and risks of HPV vaccination of 12-year-old Japanese girls compared to no vaccination. The risk–benefit ratio (RBR) was calculated to obtain an integrated benefit–risk measure.

Box 21.15 Quantifying benefits and risks of HPV vaccination based on QALYs, Japan

Kitano (2020) evaluated the benefits and risks of HPV vaccination in Japan. A cohort of 12-year-old children was followed lifelong in a simulation model. The benefits were: prevented cervical cancer, cervical intraepithelial neoplasm stage 3 (CIN3) and genital warts. The risks were: acute reactions, chronic reactions requiring assistance and chronic reactions not requiring assistance. A conservative approach was adopted by assuming that all adverse events were caused by the vaccine, despite the paucity of data on which to base causality assessments. A literature search was conducted to identify data on utility weights for the outcomes of interest.

The model results, shown in Table 21.9, indicated that the benefits of the HPV vaccine in terms of QALYs gained were 749.00 per 100,000 persons while the estimated QALY loss due to adverse events was 11.71 per 100,000 persons. The risk–benefit ratio in QALY change was 0.0156.

(continued)

Table 21.9 Risks and benefits of the HPV vaccine in terms of QALY change

Benefits	QALY gain/100,000 persons
Cervical cancer	98.17
Cervical cancer-related death	605.55
CIN 3	14.45
Genital warts	30.83
Total benefit	749.00

Risks	QALY loss/100,000 persons
Acute reactions	0.07
Chronic reactions without assistance needs	5.83
Chronic reactions with assistance needs	5.82
Total risk	11.71
Risk–benefit ratio in QALY change	0.0156

CIN: cervical intraepithelial neoplasm; QALY: quality-adjusted life year.

The author concluded that the benefits are much greater than the risks, even if it is assumed that all reported adverse events were due to vaccination, and urged the Japanese government to resume its active recommendation of HPV vaccination in girls.

A second example is given in Box 21.16, illustrating how QALYs were used to evaluate vaccination with a meningococcal conjugate vaccine. In this example, a simulation model was used to predict the number of cases of meningococcal disease and of Guillain-Barré syndrome (GBS) in the presence and absence of a vaccination programme. GBS is a possible but not yet proven side effect of meningococcal conjugate vaccination. The benefit–risk difference was calculated to obtain an integrated benefit–risk measure.

Box 21.16 Net health benefit of meningococcal vaccination based on QALYs

Cho et al. (2010) evaluated the benefits of meningococcal conjugate vaccine (MCV4) against the burden of vaccine-associated GBS. A cohort of 11-year-old children was followed over an 8-year period in a simulation model. Data from disease surveillance, efficacy and safety studies were used to inform the parameters of the simulation model. The utility weights were taken from published sources. A conservative approach was taken and the simulation model was built assuming a causal association between MCV4 vaccination and GBS.

To account for the uncertainty in the parameters of the simulation model, Monte Carlo simulation was used, based on which 95% uncertainty intervals were obtained. The uncertainty intervals reflect both the statistical and parameter uncertainty.

The model results, shown in Table 21.10, indicated that MCV4 vaccination would prevent 3,053 QALYs while vaccine-associated GBS could induce 12 QALYs. Based on these numbers the net health benefit would be 3,053 QALYs − 12 QALYs = 3,041 QALYs saved by the vaccination programme compared to no vaccination. The authors concluded that MCV4 vaccination was strongly favoured against no vaccination despite the possible vaccine-associated GBS risk.

Table 21.10 Projected number of cases, deaths and QALYs lost due to Guillain-Barré syndrome and meningococcal disease

Guillain-Barré syndrome

	Cases[†]	Deaths	QALYs lost[†]	QALYs induced[†]
Vaccination	504 (492–532)		533 (245–977)	
No vaccination	494 (491–497)		522 (241–945)	
Vaccination minus no vaccination				12 (0–45)

Meningococcal disease

	Cases[†]	Deaths[†]	QALYs lost[†]	QALY prevented[†]
Vaccination	29 (12–51)	3 (1–5)	335 (124–639)	
No vaccination	388 (388–388)	40 (28–48)	3,389 (2,271–5,094)	
Vaccination minus no vaccination				3,053 (2,031–4,645)

[†] Mean (95% uncertainty interval). QALY: quality adjusted life year.

21.4.2 Disability-adjusted life years

Disability-adjusted life years or DALYs are a summary measure of public health widely used to quantify the burden of disease. The DALY concept was specifically developed as a burden of disease measure for the WHO Global Burden of Disease (GBD) study in the 1990s. The GBD study is a worldwide observational study describing mortality and morbidity from major diseases, injuries and their risk factors at global, national and regional levels (Murray, Lopez, & Jamison, 1994). It is updated at regular intervals.

DALY is a health gap measure. It is assumed that every person is born with a certain number of life years potentially lived in optimal health. Egalitarian principles are explicitly built into the DALY metric by using the same 'ideal' life expectancy for all population subgroups apart from age and sex. Non-health characteristics typically affecting life expectancy (such as ethnicity, socio-economic status or occupation) do not impact the 'ideal' life expectancy. People may lose healthy life years through illness or premature death. The DALY metric measures the gap between actual health and optimal health.

At the population level, DALYs are calculated as the adjusted number of years lived with disability (YLDs) and the number of years of life lost due to premature mortality (YLLs) or

$$DALY = YLD + YLL,$$

$YLD = Number\ of\ events \times duration \times disability\ weight$

$YLL = Number\ of\ deaths \times remaining\ life\ expectancy\ at\ the\ age\ of\ death,$

where the disability weight reflects the severity of illness and ranges from 0 (perfect health) to 1 (comparable to death). An illustration on how to calculate DALYs is provided in Box 21.17.

Box 21.17 Calculating DALYs

Let us revisit the example given in Box 21.14. This time consider calculating the number of DALYs lost by a woman in a period of 20 years, in which 10 years are lived in perfect health, then cervical cancer was diagnosed and treated for a period of 1 year (assigned disability weight: 0.383) while the remaining 9 years are lived with cured cervical cancer (assigned disability weights: 0.05). For this event history, the DALYs are:

$$10 \times 0 + 1 \times 0.383 + 9 \times 0.05 = 0.833\ DALYs,$$

corresponding to a loss of 0.833 years lived in full health.

Disability weights are typically based on the preferences of medical experts or the general population who rate the relative undesirability of hypothetical outcomes. The GBD project regularly publishes updated disability weights for many different diseases and conditions. If weights are unavailable from the published literature, they can be elicited using preference elicitation techniques. Alternatively, proxy health outcomes for which weights exist can be assigned, preferably through consultation with medical experts.

When mortality related to the health outcomes of interest is extremely rare, YLDs are a good approximation of DALYs. Box 21.18 provides an example where YLDs were used to quantify the disease burden due to different adverse events following immunisation.

Box 21.18 Years lived with disability for adverse events following immunisation

McDonald et al. (2018) explained in detail how to calculate years lived with disability (YLD) for adverse events following immunisation (AEFI). This involves determining the relative or absolute risks and background event incidence rates, selecting disability weights and durations and computing the YLD measure. They illustrated the proposed methodology for three recognised adverse reactions following three childhood vaccination types: idiopathic thrombocytopenic purpura (ITP); anaphylaxis and febrile convulsions after vaccination with diphtheria, tetanus, acellular or whole-cell pertussis (DTaP, DTwP); measles, mumps, rubella (MMR); or meningococcal C (MenC) vaccine. The results are in Table 21.11.

Table 21.11 Estimated AEFI-associated YLDs per 1,000,000 persons (with 95% UI), following vaccination with MMR, DTP and MenC (age group 13 months–4 years)

	Vaccination attributable incidence rate per 100,000 py (95% UI)	Disability weight	Disability duration	YLD per 1,000,000 vaccinated persons (95% UI)
DTaP-ITP	1.26 (0.32–3.16)	0.159	5 weeks	0.19 (0.049–0.48)
MMR-ITP	0.53 (0.51–0.55)	0.159	5 weeks	0.081 (0.078–0.084)
DTaP/wP- Anaphylaxis	0.10 (0.01–0.33)	0.552	1 day	0.002 (0.000–0.005)

(continued)

Table 21.11 Cont.

	Vaccination attributable incidence rate per 100,000 py (95% UI)	Disability weight	Disability duration	YLD per 1,000,000 vaccinated persons (95% UI)
MMR-Anaphylaxis	0.15 (0.08–0.29)	0.552	1 day	0.002 (0.001–0.004)
MenC-Anaphylaxis	0.14 (0.12–0.17)	0.552	1 day	0.002 (0.002–0.003)
MMR-Febrile convulsions	58.3 (32.3–103)	0.263	1 day	0.42 (0.23–0.74)

py: person-years.

For example, for ITP following DTaP vaccine, YLD = 1.26 × 0.159 × 5/52 = 0.019 per 100,000, or 0.19 per million vaccinated persons. For febrile convulsions following MMR, YLD = 58.3 × 0.263 × 1/365 = 0.042 per 100,000 or 0.42 per million.

DALYs may be used in much the same was as QALYs to evaluate the benefit–risk balance. Box 21.19 illustrates this for measles and rubella vaccination.

Box 21.19 DALYs for measles and rubella vaccination

Based on an extensive literature review, Thompson and Odahowski (2016) quantified the health impact of measles and rubella containing vaccines for different World Bank income levels. They characterised DALYs for measles and rubella infections and vaccine-related adverse health outcomes assuming optimal treatment in high-income countries and minimal treatment in low-income countries.

The authors found significantly more severe health consequences for measles or rubella disease than for vaccine use. For illustration, Table 21.12 shows the results for high-income and low-income countries, for measles in children.

The values in Table 21.12 are based on those at age 4 from (Thompson & Odahowski, 2016). The benefit–risk ratio contrasts the DALYs lost through disease per infection, to the DALYs lost through vaccination, per course (two doses). For measles, this approximates the benefit–risk ratio for direct effects of a vaccination programme achieving 100% coverage, compared to absence of a vaccination programme (since most children would acquire measles infections in the absence of a vaccination programme).

Table 21.12 DALYs estimation following measles vaccination, and following measles infection in childhood

Setting	Low income	High income
Vaccination (per 1,000 two-dose courses)	0.02	0.02
Disease (per 1,000 infections)	1,080	110
Benefit–risk ratio	54,000	5,500

Although benefit–risk assessments of vaccination programmes should ideally be done routinely, their use is still in its infancy. Such assessments ensure that all elements of the benefit–risk balance have been considered and rendered explicit, thereby improving transparency and communication in decision-making on vaccination programmes and policies.

Summary

- Assessing the benefit–risk balance of vaccination programmes is important to inform public health decision-making, although it is usually done informally.
- Benefit–risk methodologies aim to provide transparency to benefit–risk assessment by structuring the approach and making a clear distinction between evidence (prevented disease burden, induced risks) and value judgements (utility values, disability weights).
- Every benefit–risk assessment should start with clearly framing the benefit–risk question. To this end, descriptive benefit–risk frameworks can be used. They are developed to ensure that all elements important to the benefit–risk assessment have been considered and are rendered explicit.
- The benefit–risk ratio, numbers needed to vaccinate and to harm and the benefit–risk difference are commonly used benefit–risk measures.
- When several benefit and risk outcomes of varying severity are to be combined into an integrated benefit–risk measure, population health metrics are commonly used. These include QALYs and DALYs.

References

Abbas, K., Procter, S. R., van Zandvoort, K., Clark, A., Funk, S., Mengistu, T., … Lshtm Cmmid Covid-Working Group. (2020). Routine childhood immunisation during the COVID-19 pandemic in Africa: A benefit–risk analysis of health benefits versus excess risk of SARS-CoV-2 infection. *Lancet Glob Health*, 8, e1264–e1272.

Arlegui, H., Bollaerts, K., Salvo, F., Bauchau, V., Nachbaur, G., Begaud, B., & Praet, N. (2020). Benefit-risk assessment of vaccines. Part I: A systematic review to identify and describe studies about quantitative benefit-risk models applied to vaccines. *Drug Safety*, *43*, 1089–1104.

Arlegui, H., Nachbaur, G., Praet, N., & Begaud, B. (2020). Quantitative benefit–risk models used for rotavirus vaccination: A systematic review. *Open Forum Infectious Diseases*, *7*, ofaa087.

Bernard, D. M., Cooper Robbins, S. C., McCaffery, K. J., Scott, C. M., & Skinner, S. R. (2011). The domino effect: Adolescent girls' response to human papillomavirus vaccination. *Medical Journal of Australia*, *194*, 297–300.

Cho, B. H., Clark, T. A., Messonnier, N. E., Ortega-Sanchez, I. R., Weintraub, E., & Messonnier, M. L. (2010). MCV vaccination in the presence of vaccine-associated Guillain-Barré acute syndrome risk: A decision analysis approach. *Vaccine*, *28*, 817–822.

Escolano, S., Mueller, J. E., & Tubert-Bitter, P. (2020). Accounting for indirect protection in the benefit–risk ratio estimation of rotavirus vaccination in children under the age of 5 years, France, 2018. *Eurosurveillance*, *25*(33). https://doi.org/10.2807/1560-7917.ES.2020.25.33.1900538.

European Centre for Disease Prevention and Control (ECDC). (2020). Guidance on HPV vaccination in EU countries: Focus on boys, people living with HIV and 9-valent HPV vaccine. Retrieved from www.ecdc.europa.eu/en/publications-data/guidance-hpv-vaccination-eu-focus-boys-people-living-hiv-9vHPV-vaccine.

Gee, J., Naleway, A., Shui, I., Baggs, J., Yin, R., Li, R., … Weintraub, E. S. (2011). Monitoring the safety of quadrivalent human papillomavirus vaccine: Findings from the Vaccine Safety Datalink. *Vaccine*, *29*, 8279–8284.

Giuliano, A. R., Palefsky, J. M., Goldstone, S., Moreira, E. D. Jr., Penny, M. E., Aranda, C., … Guris, D. (2011). Efficacy of quadrivalent HPV vaccine against HPV Infection and disease in males. *New England Journal of Medicine*, *364*, 401–411.

Goldstone, S. E., Jessen, H., Palefsky, J. M., Giuliano, A. R., Moreira, E. D. Jr., Vardas, E., … Garner, E. (2013). Quadrivalent HPV vaccine efficacy against disease related to vaccine and non-vaccine HPV types in males. *Vaccine*, *31*, 3849–3855.

Hammond, J., Keeney, R., & Raiffa, H. (1999). *Smart choices: A practical guide to making better decisions.* Boston, MA: Harvard University Press.

Ikeda, S., Ueda, Y., Yagi, A., Matsuzaki, S., Kobayashi, E., Kimura, T., … Kudoh, K. (2019). HPV vaccination in Japan: What is happening in Japan? *Expert Review of Vaccines*, *18*, 323–325.

Jefferson, T., & Traversa, G. (2002). Hepatitis B vaccination: Risk-benefit profile and the role of systematic reviews in the assessment of causality of adverse events following immunisation. *Journal of Medical Virology*, *67*, 451–453.

Kelly, H., Carcione, D., Dowse, G., & Effler, P. (2010). Quantifying benefits and risks of vaccinating Australian children aged six months to four years with trivalent inactivated seasonal influenza vaccine in 2010. *Eurosurveillance*, *15*.

Kitano, T. (2020). Stopping the HPV vaccine crisis in Japan: Quantifying the benefits and risks of HPV vaccination in quality-adjusted life-years for appropriate decision-making. *Journal of Infection and Chemotherapy*, *26*, 225–230.

Ledent, E., Lieftucht, A., Buyse, H., Sugiyama, K., McKenna, M., & K. Holl. (2016). Post-marketing benefit-risk assessment of rotavirus vaccination in Japan: A simulation and modelling analysis. *Drug Safety*, *39*, 219–230.

McDonald, S. A., Nijsten, D., Bollaerts, K., Bauwens, J., Praet, N., van der Sande, M., ... Hahné, S. (2018). Methodology for computing the burden of disease of adverse events following immunization. *Pharmacoepidemiology and Drug Safety, 27,* 724–730.

Murray, C. J., Lopez, A. D., & Jamison, D. T. (1994). The global burden of disease in 1990: Summary results, sensitivity analysis and future directions. *Bulletin of the World Health Organization, 72,* 495–509.

Patel, M. M., Clark, A. D., Sanderson, C. F., Tate, J., & Parashar, U. D. (2012). Removing the age restrictions for rotavirus vaccination: A benefit–risk modelling analysis. *PLoS Med, 9,* e1001330.

Patel, M. M., Lopez-Collada, V. R., Bulhoes, M. M., De Oliveira, L. H., Bautista Marquez, A., Flannery, B., ... Parashar, U. D. (2011). Intussusception risk and health benefits of rotavirus vaccination in Mexico and Brazil. *New England Journal of Medicine, 364,* 2283–2292.

Sassi, F. (2006). Calculating QALYs, comparing QALY and DALY calculations. *Health Policy Plan, 21,* 402–408.

Simms, K. T., Hanley, S. J. B., Smith, M. A., Keane, A., & Canfell, K. (2020). Impact of HPV vaccine hesitancy on cervical cancer in Japan: A modelling study. *Lancet Public Health, 5,* e223–e234.

Thompson, K. M., & Odahowski, C. L. (2016). The costs and valuation of health impacts of measles and rubella risk management policies. *Risk Analysis, 36,* 1357–1382.

Torrance, G. W., Furlong, W., & Feeny, D. (2002). Health utility estimation. *Expert Review of Pharmacoeconomics and Outcomes Research, 2,* 99–108.

Index

Note: Where a topic is the main focus of a chapter or section, the corresponding index entry is referenced as nff: this denotes the first page (n) of the chapter or section and the pages immediately following it.

absolute risk 236, 368–370
active adverse events following immunisation (AEFI) surveillance 352ff; analysis of 358–360
active immunisation 7
active surveillance 234
acute flaccid paralysis (AFP) surveillance 147–8
adjusted vaccine effectiveness 202, 255, 291, 296, 305, 328
adjuvant 7–9, 12–13, 28, 345
adverse events following immunisation 12, 122, 140, 339ff; analysis of 356ff; in benefit-risk evaluation 407ff; causes of 339ff; estimation of 383ff; methodological principles 364ff; surveillance of 347ff; types of 340, 348
AEFI *see* adverse events following immunisation
affinity 21, 23, 27
age-specific vaccine effectiveness 309ff, 315, 318–320, 324–328, 330
aims of vaccination programmes 34, 38ff
all-or-nothing model 318, 320–323, 325–326, 328, 330
aluminium salts 9
analytical epidemiological studies 206, 215, 361
anaphylaxis 343, 354, 431–432
anthropological perspective 103, 109, 126
antibodies 6–7, 12, 19, 20ff; assays for 29–31, 135, 166; determinants of 28; in humoral response 20ff; interpretation of 163; isotypes 22; maternal 22, 42, 46, 64, 203; maturation of 21, 23, 27; and mucosal immunity 25; priming and boosting of 27, 81, 85; and protection 26–27, 163, 323–324; surveys 154ff; and vaccination 160, 210, 232, 343
antigens 7ff; and antibody tests 29, 134; and immunity 19–21, 23–24, 27–28; and potency 10–12
antimicrobial resistance 93–95
assay 10, 23, 29–30, 154–155, 161–167, 169, 206
assumptions: in impact assessment 175, 188; modelling 67, 169, 239–241, 262; in phylogenetic analysis 150, 210; sensitivity to 73, 252, 314, 328, 333; statistical 239, 392, 397–398
attitudes to vaccination 97ff, 103, 107–108, 339
attributable fraction 367–370
attributable risk 367–370
autism: and MMR 101–103, 108–109, 344, 366–367, 373, 385–386, 395; and thiomersal 103–104
average age at infection: in epidemic models 65–66; impact of vaccination on 86ff, 339
avidity 23; assays to determine 29, 31

B cell response 21–24
B lymphocyte 20
Bacille Calmette-Guérin vaccine (BCG) 8, 22, 313, 341, 356
basic reproduction number *see* reproduction number

before-and-after comparison 172, 174, 178ff
benefit-risk: assessment 51, 407ff; difference 422–423; frameworks 411ff; measures of 417ff; need for 408ff; ratio 417; table 412, 415, 416
bias 83; and adverse events 351–352, 359, 361, 373, 374ff; in assessing waning 326–327, 331; direction of 397; due to misclassification 248ff; in impact assessment 184, 189; information 122, 216, 245, 374, 390; in outbreak investigation 210, 215; selection 122, 165, 216, 252, 374, 390; in serological surveys 157, 164–165; in surveillance 131, 138, 140–142, 147; in vaccine coverage 122; in vaccine effectiveness 226–227, 245–246, 248ff, 253ff, 291–292, 298; *see also* confounding
bias-indicator study 256ff
biomarker 121, 154
booster response 27
boosting 27–28, 43, 81, 84–85
BRAT framework 411
Broome method 297, 299ff; *see also* indirect method
burden of disease 38, 99; and benefit-risk 407, 426, 430; and impact 75ff, 91, 172ff, 174–175; in outbreak investigation 200–201, 204–205; in setting programme aims 41–42; and vaccine effectiveness 236

carriage 58, 78, 90, 141, 145; and herd immunity 26; and outbreak investigation 214; and vaccine effectiveness 229, 231–233, 237–238, 300
case ascertainment 179, 245, 393
case-centred analysis 391
case-cohort 249, 296ff, 302, 313, 390
case-control study 215, 248, 255, 257, 409–410; for vaccine effectiveness 289ff; for vaccine safety 365, 368, 377, 383, 387ff; *see also* Broome method; case-crossover; screening method; test-negative design
case-coverage 296, 390–391
case-crossover 383, 400ff
case definition: in outbreak investigation 206, 208, 210; in surveillance 133–135, 148; and vaccine effectiveness 229, 232, 246ff, 250–252, 280–281, 286, 291, 294; validity of 133–134, 250–251
case finding 209–210, 251
catchment 136, 145, 360, 369
catch-up 43–44, 78, 83, 145, 157, 159–160, 162, 185–186, 203, 205, 305, 418
causal association 94, 358, 391, 410, 428

causality assessment 353, 357–358, 361, 408, 427
causes of outbreaks of vaccine-preventable diseases 196ff
CD4+ T cell 24
CD8+ T cells 24
cell-mediated immunity 19–20, 22, 24ff, 324; assays for 30
cellular immunity *see* cell-mediated immunity
certification of eradication 37, 40, 148, 150
chloropleth map 143
cholera vaccine 8, 78, 236–237, 295–296
citizen science 140
clinical trial 1, 5, 13–14, 47, 51, 103, 228, 246, 345, 347–348, 414, 425
cluster sampling 119, 165, 179
coding systems 140
cohort study 214–215, 295; compared to case-control 289; for vaccine effectiveness 93, 264ff, 320; for vaccine safety 370, 383ff, 389
coincidental adverse event 340, 348
cold chain 11, 148, 201, 204, 227, 253
combination vaccine 47, 101
communication 52, 108ff, 126–127, 216, 345, 411, 416, 433
compulsory vaccination 52, 98
concomitant vaccination 372, 397
conditional Poisson regression 392
confidence interval: calculation of 167, 290, 292, 349, 368; as measure of uncertainty 225
confounding 215, 359, 361, 364, 370; control of and adjustment for 268–269, 275, 279, 283–284, 286, 297, 370; in electronic databases 381, 387; factors 180, 293, 378, 386, 389; illustration of 254; by indication or healthy vaccinee effect 246, 256, 376–378; and matching 390; in self-controlled case series 393, 395–6; in studies of vaccine effectiveness 226, 253ff; in studies of vaccine safety 374ff; time-invariant 377; unmeasured 391
congenital rubella syndrome (CRS) 87, 93, 156–157, 199
conjugate 8, 13, 22, 58; and carriage 237; Hib vaccine 178, 231, 305; meningococcal vaccine 159, 428; pneumococcal vaccine 90, 145, 299
contact rate 56, 176; age-dependence of 160; changes in 180; effective 58, 62, 69, 71; and heterogeneity 68–69, 205; homogeneous 67; and indirect effects 76
contact survey 69
contact tracing 209

containment 37–40
contemporaneous comparison 176ff; control 172, 180; population 174
contraindication 42, 398–399
control infection 180–182, 186
control period 395–396, 399
control selection 294
controversy 98, 100, 102, 293, 409–410
convenience sample 164
co-primary case 279, 280–282, 285
correlate of protection 163ff, 323–324; see also antibodies
counterfactual 142, 172, 174, 183–185
COVID-19 35, 41, 379, 418
cowpox 6–7
critical immunisation threshold 55, 79, 80–81, 124, 170; estimation of 64ff; and heterogeneity 68–69; and reproduction numbers 60ff
critical vaccination coverage 241; see also critical vaccination threshold
critical vaccination threshold 40, 64, 80–81
CRM197 8
cross-protection 20, 90, 300
cross-reactivity 20–21
cumulative incidence 252, 258–260, 262; mathematical formulas 322, 328; ratio 270–271; and vaccine effectiveness 270–272; and waning 315–318, 320, 324, 329
Cutter incident 343–344
cytokine tests 30

danger-associated molecular patterns (DAMPs) 19
data linkage 101, 125, 349, 353–354, 393
data sources 132, 136, 141, 379; linked 353
data triangulation 132, 137
delay: in diagnosis 207–208, 215, 372–373; in protection 30, 278; in reporting 138, 143, 206, 359; in vaccination 229, 376–377, 397
delayed impact 81ff
Demographic and Health Survey (DHS) 118
descriptive epidemiology 204, 211, 214–215
differentiating infected from vaccinated animals (DIVA) vaccines 30
diphtheria tetanus acellular pertussis (DTaP) vaccine 8, 278, 384–385, 431–432
diphtheria tetanus pertussis (DTP) vaccine 76, 100, 116, 178, 330, 365–366, 354, 372, 374, 376–377, 384
direct effect 76, 172ff, 182, 187, 223, 419, 425, 432
disability-adjusted life years (DALYs) 426, 430
discordant pairs 292
disease modification 235

disproportionality analysis 358
dose effect 371, 389
dropout 125

Ebola vaccine 15, 229–230
ecology 89ff, 131, 144, 339
effect modification 269, 275
effectiveness see vaccine effectiveness
efficacy see vaccine efficacy
electronic health records 139–140
electronic registers and databases 379ff
elimination: and case definitions 134; definition of 39; and herd immunity 77ff; impacts of 87–88; modelling of 64; monitoring of 189ff; setbacks 106; surveillance for 147ff, 190–191; and vaccination strategies 41, 44–45; verification of 40
endemic transmission 40, 58, 63, 67, 77, 149
environmental surveillance 38
epidemic 35, 93, 100, 138, 226, 230, 234, 257, 281, 303, 312, 330, 357; cycles 55ff, 64, 142, 175, 180, 183; and outbreaks 195ff; period 86ff, 204; potential 60ff, 63, 147, 160; threshold 63, 147, 203–204
epidemic cycle see epidemic
equilibrium 64–65, 67
equity 34, 38, 41, 125
eradication: certification of 40; definition of 39; modelling of 64, 79; of polio 37–38, 43, 102–103, 148, 158, 215; of smallpox 1, 36–37, 46, 48; and surveillance 147ff, 150–151; and vaccination strategies 35, 41, 105
ethics: improprieties relating to 101; issues of 164, 228; perspective on 39, 408; requirement for 345
EuroMOMO 137–138
European Medicines Agency (EMA) 16, 50, 350, 391, 411
event-dependent vaccinations 397ff
excess mortality 137, 178
Expanded Programme on Immunization (EPI) 38, 48, 229, 418; coverage survey 121
extrapolation 183–184

failure to vaccinate 83, 196ff, 210–213
FAIR principles 143–144
follow-up 32, 44–45, 151, 229, 249, 260, 262, 264, 267, 273ff, 278–279, 281, 320–321, 348, 384–386, 420–421
Food and Drug Administration (FDA) 16, 50, 103, 349, 411
force of infection 56, 71, 170, 258; see also hazard
functional assay 29

generalised herd effects 91
generalised linear model 267, 272, 275, 282, 290, 305, 385
geometric mean titre (GMT) 167–168
Global Advisory Committee on Vaccine Safety (GACVS) 345
Global Alliance for Vaccination and Immunisation (GAVI) 48–49
Global Burden of Disease (GBD) 430
government 34, 48, 50, 98, 103, 122, 201, 350, 357, 410, 428
GrippeNet 140
group testing 167
Guillain-Barré syndrome (GBS) 148, 344, 354, 378, 398, 428–429

Haemophilus influenzae type b (Hib) vaccine 78–79, 116, 142, 231, 305, 354
harvesting effect 367
hazard 5, 258; ratio 277, 295–297, 313, 367, 370, 387; *see also* force of infection; incidence density
health inequalities 1, 75, 91
health-seeking behaviour 297
healthy vaccinee bias *see* confounding
hepatitis B vaccine 8, 24, 30, 41, 116, 228–229, 354, 387, 389–390, 401, 409–410
herd immunity 26, 39–40, 42, 55ff, 124, 143, 145, 231–232, 238, 321; and benefit-risk 425; and elimination 77ff; and impact 173, 182; loss of 106; principles of 55ff, 60; threshold 65; *see also* indirect effect
heterogeneity: of contacts 55, 61, 68ff, 170; individual 72; statistical 269, 285–286; of vaccine uptake 81, 125, 172
heterologous protection 92
high-titre measles vaccines 12
historical baseline 358
history of vaccines 6ff
homogeneous mixing 55, 64ff, 68
household contact studies 264, 278ff
human papillomavirus (HPV) vaccine 8, 25, 47, 79–80, 107, 162, 180–182, 188–189, 344, 410, 413–416, 427–428
humoral immune response 19–20
hypothesis 6, 101, 324, 365–366, 373; generation 142, 359–361, 367; null 214, 329; testing 237, 329, 360–361, 367, 386–387, 389

immune thrombocytopenia 354
immunisation: activities and campaigns 38, 43, 81, 117, 158, 197, 201; advice and policy on 48–49, 127; childhood 90, 255; definition of 6–7; level 86; modelling of 56; passive 22; programmes 46, 90, 125, 156, 357, 408, 410, 418; protection acquired by 30; schedule 159; *see also* adverse events following immunisation; critical immunisation threshold
immunisation anxiety-related reaction 340, 344
immunisation coverage 6, 116ff, 150, 165; *see also* vaccine coverage
immunisation error-related reaction 340, 344
immunisation information system 122
immunity 1, 5–8, 13, 18, 45, 163, 197; acquired 7; adaptive 19; cell-mediated 24ff, 324; cells associated with 9, 20, 30; correlates of 163ff; immune memory 7, 19, 26, 27, 341; immune response 7–9, 11, 14, 18, 28ff, 163, 223, 278, 323, 341; immune suppression 93; immune system 7–9, 12, 18ff, 42, 94, 101, 277; innate 19; mechanisms of 23, 25, 94; mucosal 13, 25ff, 43, 150, 163, 233; persistence of 26ff, 28ff; systemic 25ff; waning 143, 203–204, 211, 309ff; *see also* antibodies; antigens; herd immunity
immunogenicity 5, 8, 10ff, 14; assessment of 29; determinants of 28; and vaccination schedules 46–47
immunoglobulin 20, 22, 324; IgA 22, 25, 43, 161; IgD 22; IgE 22; IgG 22, 25, 31, 155; IgM 22, 23, 31, 208
immunological maturation 46; *see also* antibodies
immunological memory 27; *see also* immunity
immunosenescence 28
impact 1–2, 5, 39, 49–50, 55, 71–72, 75ff; on age at infection and inter-epidemic period 86ff; assessment of 172ff; on burden of disease 75ff; delayed 81ff; ecological 89ff; of herd immunity 77ff; and indirect effects 173–174; measures of 175, 424; on public health 91ff; surveillance to determine 131–132, 142, 145
imports: cases 39–40, 80, 147, 149, 176, 189; infections 40, 79; and surveillance for elimination 190–191
inactivated polio vaccine (IPV) 37–38, 161, 342
incidence density 258; *see also* hazard
incidence rate 78, 136, 175, 260, 277, 310–312, 324, 332, 351, 431–432; average 259–261, 273, 321; instantaneous 258–259; ratio 175, 273–276, 367, 392; *see also* cumulative incidence; hazard
indication bias 246, 256, 376–378, 391; *see also* confounding

indirect effect 57–8, 76, 80, 145, 172ff, 176, 182, 185–187, 224, 412, 417–418, 420, 422–426; *see also* herd immunity
indirect method: for elicitation of utilities 427; for vaccine effectiveness 297, 299ff
indirect protection 26, 41, 57, 97; *see also* herd immunity
infectious contact 55ff; *see also* contact rate
infectious disease models 70ff
infectious period 58–59, 61–62, 71, 88, 237–238, 266, 279–280
infectiousness 102; estimation of vaccine effect on 279, 281ff; immune response and 18, 25ff; transmission and 39, 44, 56, 58, 60, 239ff; vaccine effectiveness against 64, 77, 223–224, 237ff
influenza surveillance 138, 140; *see also* EuroMOMO
influenza vaccine 13, 41–42, 73, 93–94, 125, 139, 177, 226, 232, 236, 246, 256, 291, 297–299, 303, 350, 354–356, 360, 377–379, 391–392, 397–399, 401, 421–422
inoculation 6–7
instantaneous incidence rate 258–259
inter-epidemic period 86ff, 88–89, 204, 330
interaction 2, 5; social 68, 128, 160; statistical 269, 276, 278, 284–286
international collaborative networks 50
interrupted time series 172, 183ff; controlled 185
isotype switching 23

Jenner, E. 6
Jesty, B. 6
joint estimation 282–283
joint reporting form 125

killed vaccine 6–10, 35, 78, 161, 236, 341

laboratory accident 151
laboratory confirmation 134, 140, 148, 246, 250–251
laboratory surveillance 135–136, 147
latent period 39, 88, 279, 280; latency of VZV 85
leaky model 318; *see also* partial protection model
licensure 13ff, 47, 224, 345, 347–348, 353; post- 347–349, 353, 368, 370; pre- 51, 347–348, 355, 364, 407
life expectancy: in modelling 65–67; in health metrics 426, 430
live attenuated vaccine 8–10, 13, 27, 29, 37, 51, 93, 106, 161, 177, 341–342, 409
local reaction 12, 340, 343

logistic regression 290–292, 295, 299–300, 305, 390; conditional 292, 295, 387–389
low- and middle-income country (LMIC) 48, 92, 117–118, 127, 154, 198, 207, 345, 409, 423–424
lymphocytes 19–20, 26

major histocompatibility complex (MHC) 24
mapping: geographical 143; preferences 427
market authorisation 16, 50
marketing authorization holder (MAH) 50
mass vaccination programme 41, 49, 75, 131, 172–173, 196, 344
matching 254, 292–294, 297, 377, 388–389, 391; *see also* case-control study
maternal antibodies *see* antibodies
maternal vaccination 22, 42, 46
mathematical model 47, 70ff, 72, 160, 170, 241, 417–418, 420
maturation of antibodies *see* antibodies
measles and rubella (MR) vaccine 160–161
measles mumps rubella (MMR) vaccine 25, 83, 372; and aseptic meningitis 351; and febrile convulsions 354–355, 365–366, 369–370; and ITP 393–394; and measles 192, 357; and mumps 203, 217, 269–270, 313
measurement 100, 163; bias 138; error 372
measures of impact *see* impact
measures of risk 367ff
memory response 27
meningococcal vaccine 163, 212, 274, 428
meta-analysis 80, 164, 409
microbiome 26, 28, 91
military 35
misclassification: bias due to 210, 246, 248ff; of cases 286, 373; of cause of death 137; differential and non-differential 250; of vaccination status 122, 210, 286
missed opportunities for vaccination 125, 207
mixture model 168–169
modifications to vaccination programmes 32, 51, 410, 417
molecular clock 150, 210
molecular surveillance 149
monitoring 2, 5, 12, 18, 34–35, 38, 49, 195; of attitudes to vaccination 97ff, 115ff, 126; of coverage 115ff; of elimination 189ff; of immunity 158; of impact 52, 84, 94, 172ff; methods for 116ff; of new vaccines 355; of programmatic errors 227–228; purpose of 49; of safety 341, 345, 347ff, 352–353; sequential 360, 395; of vaccine effectiveness 223ff, 303; of vaccine failure 30–31; of vaccine-preventable disease 132ff, 137, 144ff, 150

mopping-up campaign 44–45
mRNA vaccine 9, 11
mucosal vaccines 12–13, 25
multi-dose vaccine 249, 301, 370ff, 372, 399
multiple indicator cluster survey (MICS) 117–118

national immunisation days 43
National Immunization Technical Advisory Group (NITAG) 48
national regulatory authority (NRA) 15–16
national vaccination programme 15, 35, 43, 47, 209, 340, 345
natural experiment 175
negative control 180, 185, 256, 396
nested case-control study 295, 387, 389–391
net health benefit 422, 428–429
non-acute events 373
non-governmental organisation (NGO) 48
non-specific effects 19, 94
notifiable disease 132–133
nowcasting 138, 143
number needed to harm 420
number needed to vaccinate 420

observation period 372–373, 393–399
odds ratio 270, 291, 293, 296–299, 367–368, 388–390, 392, 409–410; definition 289; expressions for 290, 292; and rare disease assumption 290, 295; screening 301–303
off-target impacts 92ff
opposition to vaccination 98–99, 201
oral fluid 135, 148, 165
oral polio vaccine (OPV) 9, 25, 37–8, 43, 102–103, 342–343, 375, 388–389
order of magnitude 351, 370
outbreak investigation 2, 31, 34, 50–51, 125, 134, 147, 195ff, 267, 302; aims of 204ff; caused by failure to vaccinate 196ff; caused by susceptible groups 203ff; caused by vaccine failure 201ff; report of 216; steps in 205ff
outbreak surveillance 190
overdispersion 269, 277

partial protection model 318, 320, 323–326, 328–333
passive immunisation 7, 22
passive surveillance 349ff; versus active 356, 358
pathogen adaptation 89ff, 94, 131
pathogen-associated molecular patterns (PAMPs) 19
pathogen surveillance 132, 136, 144ff
peripheral blood mononuclear cell (PBMC) 20

persistence of immunity 26ff
person-time 260, 273–376, 310–312, 320, 326–328, 333, 384, 386; at risk 260, 273, 311, 320
pharmacovigilance 50, 345, 349, 358
phylogenetic analyses 150, 210
plasma cells 20–21, 23–24, 26
point-of-care-tests (POCTs) 136
Poisson: assumption 277; conditional 392; error 275; model 186, 275–277, 385–386; quasi- 277; regression 183, 276, 384
polysaccharide 7–8, 29; vaccine 214, 233
pool of susceptibles 60, 69, 81ff, 160–161, 203
pooled sera 167
population health metrics 408, 426ff
porcine circovirus 10
positive predictive value 133–135, 148, 250–251
post-honeymoon outbreak 82–83, 203–204, 339
potency 5, 10ff, 12, 28, 204, 347
power: statistical 214, 239, 257, 293, 348, 379, 395
pre-qualification 15–16
preservative 9–10, 103, 345, 354
preventive fraction 224; see also vaccine effectiveness
primary case: in outbreaks 60; in household contact studies 253, 266, 279–283, 285–286
primary response 27
prior case or infection 246, 248, 252, 258, 285, 310–314, 325–259, 330–331, 333
ProACT-URL framework 411–413
profile likelihood 267, 274
programmatic approach 34
programmatic error 227–228
progression of disease 26–27, 224; vaccine protection against 224ff, 269; see also severe disease; vaccine effectiveness
project Tycho 144, 184
propensity score 254, 377
propensity to vaccinate 255
proportional hazards model 277–278, 296–297, 318, 384, 387
proportional reporting ratio 358, 360
protection 231ff; against disease 246; against infection 27, 64, 163ff, 231ff, 235, 238, 247, 282, 323; against progression 231ff; see also protective effectiveness; vaccine effectiveness
protective antibody threshold 322–3
protective effectiveness 106, 224ff, 232–233, 237–241, 248, 279, 282–284, 310
protein D 8
protocol 15, 50, 151, 227, 245, 358
pseudolikelihood 399

public engagement 110
pulse vaccination 43

quality-adjusted life years (QALYs) 426–429, 432

random sample 78, 119, 296, 301
rare adverse events 345, 366, 379
rare disease assumption 290, 295–296, 302; *see also* odds ratio
rash/fever surveillance 147
rate of infection 258, 260, 310, 315; *see also* risks and rates
rate-based vaccine effectiveness 261, 263, 270–273, 296, 314; *see also* risks and rates
reactogenicity 11–12
recall bias 390
record linkage 123, 165, 376
recurrent events 364, 374, 384
reference period 367
regression discontinuity design 186ff
regression model 183, 189, 254, 292, 313, 391
regulatory authority 15–16, 217, 355; medicines 50
relative incidence 367, 392, 394–400; *see also* incidence rate ratio
relative risk: for adverse events 359–360, 368; for benefit-risk 408, 423, 424; estimation of 225, 265–267, 270, 272, 280; and impact 189; and vaccine effectiveness 224ff, 234, 238, 257, 260, 310
reporting bias 351
reporting delays 138, 143, 359
reproduction number 55, 60ff, 64ff, 80: basic 61–63, 71, 170, 425; effect of heterogeneity on 68; effective 60–64, 160, 190–191; estimation of 64ff; and vaccine impact 224, 240–241
residual sera 164–165
residuals 10
reverse cold chain 148
ring vaccination 37, 45–46, 229
risk-based vaccine effectiveness 265–266, 271–273, 279, 281, 293, 295, 297, 315–317, 321–322
risk-benefit ratio 422, 426–428
risk difference 236, 368
risk of infection 39, 41, 58, 69, 91, 224, 231, 238, 250, 252, 258, 259–260, 279, 319, 325, 327; *see also* risks and rates
risk period 364, 365ff; and attributable fraction 368; choice of 365; indefinite 366, 390, 395; overlapping 372; pre-exposure 397
risk set 277, 295, 391–392

risks and rates 224, 257ff, 264, 314ff
robustness 122, 214, 228, 252–253, 214, 328, 379, 397, 417
rotavirus vaccine 10, 13, 230, 255, 399; withdrawal of 348, 368, 375, 408
routes of administration 5, 12ff
routine vaccination 35, 43–44, 157, 178–179, 182, 186, 197–198, 301, 417–418

safety *see* vaccine safety
safety profile 348, 350
sampling fraction 165
SARS-CoV-2 69, 110, 138, 140, 418
SCCS *see* self-controlled case series (SCCS)
scientific evidence 97, 101–102; communication of 108ff
screening method 205, 249, 289, 301ff, 311–312, 326–331, 390
screening odds ratio *see* odds ratio
screening study 302ff
SCRI *see* self-controlled risk interval (SCRI)
seasonality: confounding by 175, 180, 359–360, 376, 379, 384–385, 393–399; of contacts 60; of incidence 44, 92, 136, 138, 183; of vaccination 44, 375
secondary attack rate 238, 279–281, 285, 329
secondary case 190, 266, 279–282, 285
secretory IgA 25
selection bias *see* bias
selective vaccination programme 41–42, 75, 80, 140, 377
self-controlled case series (SCCS) 93, 392ff; for event-dependent vaccinations 397ff
self-controlled methods 358, 377
self-controlled risk interval (SCRI) 395
sensitivity: of case definition 133–134, 142, 233, 250; hyper- 343; of laboratory methods 165–166, 236, 247, 298; of surveillance systems 46, 132, 135–136, 147–148, 150, 199; to temperature 11; in understanding 103; and vaccine effectiveness 250–251
sensitivity analysis 73, 252, 300, 303, 314, 328, 331–333, 372, 390, 417
sentinel surveillance 136, 138–139, 145, 147, 297
sequential methods 355, 359–361, 395–6
seroepidemiology 29, 157, 164–166; *see also* serological surveillance
serogroup replacement 143
serological surveillance 84, 141, 147, 154ff, 178
serological survey: and parameter estimation 65, 70; and serological surveillance 69, 87, 154ff; *see also* serological surveillance
seroprevalence 154ff, 158, 164–166, 168–169,

332; seronegative 155–157, 162–163, 168–169; seropositive 154–155, 158, 162–163, 167–169
serotype replacement 26, 89ff, 94, 145, 301
serum 19, 22–23, 25–27, 29, 134, 154–155, 159, 162–165
severe disease 26, 31, 41–42, 146, 214, 390; vaccine protection against 231ff; *see also* progression of disease; vaccine effectiveness
severe event 356
sewage surveillance 147–148, 150, 342
SIA *see* supplementary immunisation activity (SIA)
side effect 9, 13, 46, 100, 106, 340–343, 347–348, 350–351, 353, 428
signal: in surveillance 350–351, 355, 356ff, 358–361, 412
SIR model *see* susceptible infected recovered (SIR) model
smallpox vaccine 6, 7, 13, 20, 36, 350
social media 126–129, 140, 356
specificity: antigen 21; of case definition 132–134, 142, 184, 233; of laboratory methods 166, 247, 298; of surveillance systems 147–148; and vaccine effectiveness 233, 250–251
spontaneous reporting 349–350
stabilisers 9–10
stability: political 199; vaccine 5, 10ff
standard error: formulas for the 265, 271, 274, 290, 292, 301
standardisation: in laboratory surveillance 136; of potency 10; of register data 122; of serological assays 166–167
stepped wedge design 177, 228–229, 231
strain replacement 300
Strategic Advisory Group of Experts (SAGE) 48
subclinical: infection 135, 157, 231, 233, 252, 328; infectious phase 39
subnational immunisation days 43
subunit vaccine 10
summary of product characteristics (SmPC) 7, 11
supplementary immunisation activity (SIA) 43–44, 117–118, 122, 197, 201–202
surveillance: of adverse events 347ff; for elimination or eradication 147ff; environmental 38; laboratory 135–136, 147; molecular 149; of mortality 137–138; of outbreaks 190–191; passive 349ff; pathogen 144ff; rash and fever 147; serological 154ff; sewage 147–148, 150, 342; syndromic 140; of vaccine effectiveness 303; of vaccine-preventable diseases 131ff; of vaccine safety 347ff

surveillance pyramid 141, 147
susceptibility gap 46, 157
susceptible infected recovered (SIR) model 71–72
syndromic surveillance 140
systematic review 107, 230, 256, 379, 409
systemic immunity 25ff
systemic reaction 12, 100, 345
systems serology 23, 30

T cells: cytotoxic 20–25; helper 20, 24; responses 21, 24; stimulation test 30
targeted vaccination programme 41, 75; *see also* selective vaccination programme
T-dependent B cell response 21–24
test-negative design 297ff
time series 89, 137, 142–143, 203, 213; *see also* interrupted time series
time since vaccination 32, 85, 202–203, 223, 305, 365–366, 387; and waning of vaccine effectiveness 309ff
time-varying: confounder 377; covariates 378, 399; exposure 277–278, 384; hazard ratio 277
timeliness: of surveillance 46, 122, 147; of vaccination 125
timing of events 370ff
T-independent B cell response 21
toxoid 7–8, 21, 278
training and test sets 185
transmission dynamics 2, 42, 55ff
transmission probability 56
transmission route 55
transudation 25

underreporting 141, 351
UNICEF 15, 48–49, 119, 125
United Nations (UN) 15, 48
universal vaccination 42–43, 64, 69, 84, 93, 101, 195–196

vaccination history 210, 245, 248
vaccination schedules 46ff
vaccine action 318ff, 322ff, 324–326, 330–333
vaccine associated enhanced disease 31, 343
vaccine coverage 1, 5, 40, 48–49, 176–177; assessment methods for 116ff; and case-coverage method 390–391; definition of 116; and impact 75–78, 80–84, 88, 172, 174–175, 179, 185, 187, 189, 192, 240–241; and infection dynamics 60ff, 64ff, 69, 72–73, 204; interpretation of 124ff; monitoring of 115ff, 147; and outbreaks due to failure to vaccinate 196ff; in screening method 301ff; and serological surveys

158, 162; statistics on 125ff; and vaccine hesitancy 104ff, 108; *see also* vaccine uptake
vaccine coverage target 40, 124–125
vaccine design 7
vaccine effectiveness 2, 5, 26, 32, 49, 63–64, 69, 73, 78–80, 223ff; age-specific 309ff; contrast with vaccine efficacy 227ff; and critical vaccination coverage 80–81; definitions of 223ff; estimation from case-control studies 289ff; estimation from cohort studies 264ff; estimation from household contact studies 278ff; estimation from screening studies 301ff; heterogeneity of 91; for infection, disease or disease progression 231ff; for infectiousness 237ff; methodological principles 245ff; in outbreaks 83, 93, 213, 215; pragmatic 227; protective 224ff; syndromic 235–237; for transmission 239ff; and vaccine uptake 107, 115, 205, 211; waning of 81, 85–86, 90, 164, 309ff; *see also* protective effectiveness; rate-based vaccine effectiveness; risk-based vaccine effectiveness
vaccine effectiveness profile 248
vaccine effectiveness surveillance 303
vaccine efficacy 5, 246, 416, 425; contrast with vaccine effectiveness 227ff
vaccine failure 18, 30ff, 201ff; primary 31, 83, 201–202, 211; secondary 31–32, 201–202, 210–211, 303; test for 31
vaccine hesitancy 97–8, 104ff, 110
vaccine injury compensation schemes 101
vaccine manufacturers 16
vaccine marketing authorisation holders 50
vaccine platforms 8
vaccine policy 48, 131–132, 141; role of outbreak investigation in shaping 195–196, 205, 211, 213–214, 216
Vaccine Position Papers 48
vaccine probe 236
vaccine product-related reaction 340; *see also* side-effect
vaccine quality defect-related reactions 340, 343
vaccine registers 117, 119, 122, 125, 210
vaccine safety 1, 5, 34, 106, 339ff; benefit-risk of 407ff; evaluation of 339ff, 383ff; definition of 10; methodological principles for 364ff; monitoring of 49–51, 347ff; in programme aims 39; surveillance of 347ff; and vaccine confidence 76, 99–100, 102–103, 106–107, 109, 126, 197; and vaccine coverage 115; and vaccine design 7–8; and vaccine trials 14; *see also* adverse events following immunisation
vaccine scares 99ff, 101, 104, 107, 110
vaccine trials 13ff, 29, 164, 227, 229–230, 353
vaccine uptake 69, 81, 87, 91, 104, 115ff, 188–189, 213, 249; and vaccine coverage 116ff
vaccinia virus 6–7
validity: of assays 166; of case definition 133; of choice of control populations 174, 178; of coverage estimates 118, 121; of extrapolation 184; of model assumptions 239, 277; of new diagnostic methods 213; of pathogen surveillance 146; of point of care tests 136; of study design 256–257; of vaccination status 121
value tree 414–415
variability: between studies 379; in confidence 106; sampling 262; statistical 269, 277; in vaccine effectiveness 226, 230
varicella vaccine 320–321, 355, 395–396
varicella zoster vaccine 22, 163
variola virus 6
variolation 6, 35
verbal autopsy 137
verification of elimination 40, 106
vertical vaccination programme 34
viral vector vaccine 9

waning vaccine effectiveness *see* vaccine effectiveness
waning vaccine immunity *see* immunity
WHO/UNICEF Estimates of National Immunization Coverage (WUENIC) 125–126
whole genome sequencing 191
World Health Organization (WHO) 12, 18, 36–37, 90, 102, 134, 158, 191, 340, 357, 409; certification and verification of disease control 40; and global vaccine safety 345

years of life lost 430
years lived with disability 430–431

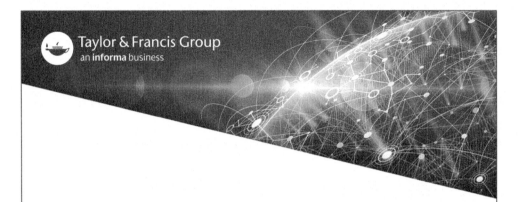

Taylor & Francis eBooks

www.taylorfrancis.com

A single destination for eBooks from Taylor & Francis with increased functionality and an improved user experience to meet the needs of our customers.

90,000+ eBooks of award-winning academic content in Humanities, Social Science, Science, Technology, Engineering, and Medical written by a global network of editors and authors.

TAYLOR & FRANCIS EBOOKS OFFERS:

- A streamlined experience for our library customers
- A single point of discovery for all of our eBook content
- Improved search and discovery of content at both book and chapter level

REQUEST A FREE TRIAL
support@taylorfrancis.com

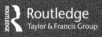 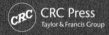